Postpartum Psychiatric Illness

Postpartum Psychiatric Illness

A Picture Puzzle

Edited by James Alexander Hamilton
and Patricia Neel Harberger

UNIVERSITY OF PENNSYLVANIA PRESS   Philadelphia

Library of Congress Cataloging-in-Publication Data
Postpartum psychiatric illness : a picture puzzle / edited by James Alexander Hamilton
and Patricia Neel Harberger.
   p.   cm.
   Includes bibliographical references and index.
   ISBN 0-8122-3137-6 (cloth). — ISBN 0-8122-1385-8 (paper)
   1. Postpartum psychiatric disorders.   I. Hamilton, James Alexander, 1907–   .
II. Harberger, Patricia Neel.
   [DNLM: 1. Mental Disorders.   2. Puerperal Disorders.   3. Puerperium—
psychology.   WQ 500 P858]
RG850.P67   1992
618.7'6—dc20
DNLM/DLC
for Library of Congress   91-30386
                                                                                  CIP

Contents

Illustrations

Tables

Preface

For psychiatric illness after childbirth, most of the twentieth century was a time of inactivity and denial. If textbooks of psychiatry or obstetrics mentioned postpartum illness at all, the topic was dismissed quickly with a pronouncement that these conditions were examples of the same varieties of mental disorder as those that occurred without relationship to childbirth. Pregnancy, delivery, or the responsibilities of child care were regarded as stresses that activated latent tendencies toward mental illness. Even the word "postpartum" and its synonyms were regarded as archaic, when used to qualify a psychiatric diagnosis.

The prevailing view stood in contrast to a strong nineteenth-century position that held that postpartum psychiatric disorders were unique in many ways. Scores of scholarly papers explored the unique features. Many believed that the study of these features would yield clues to the etiology and treatment of postpartum disorders.

In 1980, the pendulum began to move back toward the nineteenth-century interest when Ian Brockington, then at Manchester, England, called an international conference on postpartum disorders. Worldwide interest in these matters was kindled, and a substantial amount of new information was disclosed. Out of this conference came the Marcé Society, an international scientific organization to advance knowledge about postpartum illness. Scientific interest was mobilized.

During most of the twentieth century, postpartum illness was an affliction about which people did not talk. It was a condition without an identity. Many women who experienced postpartum disorders believed themselves stigmatized by a degrading disease. Then, as information began to emerge, support groups were created to provide information, guidance, and encouragement for the suffering women and their families. One support group led to another; the movement spread widely. Prominent coordinating organizations are Depression after Delivery, Postpartum Support International, and Post and Antenatal Depression Association (PANDA), in Australia. Some support groups arose from the initiative of women who had recovered from postpartum illness, while others were lead by health professionals.

Popular interest and the need for women to be informed were well served by Carol Dix's 1985 book, *The New Mother Syndrome* (Doubleday). The positive reception of this book is attested by the fact that it has gone through several editions and its scope has been extended by translations.

Early in the 1980s the media began to sense that new information, new attitudes, and new treatment possibilities were developing in the field of postpartum illness. Both scientific meetings and support group activities were covered with increasing interest and sophistication. Scientific papers and the media began to converge on a few central themes: mild postpartum symptoms, if not more severe disorders, are of fairly frequent occurrence; there may be much more to postpartum illness than a vagary of the mind; these conditions are not reflections of mental incompetence or character weakness; most patients recover completely; appropriate treatment and support hastens recovery; and responsibility must be borne by family members, health care professionals, and a variety of societal institutions, not the new mother alone.

Rare but devastating consequences of severe postpartum illness are suicide and infanticide. The media began to cover infanticide cases and the law enforcement actions that followed them. One of these tragedies took place in York, Pennsylvania. This well-informed and civic-minded community was shocked by the event and equally shocked by the lack of information that met questions of why and how this event could have happened. In 1987, the York Task Force Studying Postpartum Stress and Depression was organized and set about a systematic investigation. York Hospital took an important role in the task force. A support group was initiated. Then York Hospital and the Infant Mental Health Coalition of York organized a joint medical and public conference which was held at the hospital in April 1988. The interest displayed at the conference encouraged the hospital to stimulate the creation of a book on postpartum illness. World leaders in many aspects of the problem were asked to write chapters, and they did so with unanimity.

This book is an outgrowth of that conference and represents the work of thirty-one authors who have made major contributions to research, treatment, and thinking in this field. The authors are from different specialty fields and different continents. At this stage of interest revival, and rapid accumulation of information, it is to be expected that different opinions and interpretations will be found. The editorial policy encouraged the expression of individual thinking. As new information is put with the old, and when new research is brought forth and evaluated, wide areas of agreement have become apparent.

The mystery that has shrouded the phenomenon of psychiatric illness after childbirth is disappearing. In its place is emerging a picture of an illness that can be fairly well defined and for which effective methods of prevention and treatment are available today. Clues exist that point toward treatment possibilities which could reduce significantly the duration and severity of postpartum psychiatric illness.

Acknowledgments

The editors are indebted to many who made this book a labor of love: to our beloved families: James Harberger; Quincy, Lincoln, and Seneca Harberger; and Marjorie Hamilton who encouraged us and made many sacrifices so that we might remain committed and complete this valuable project; to the authors who have been generous with their time and tolerant of our demands; to the York Task Force Studying Postpartum Stress and Depression; to Patricia Smith, our editor at the University of Pennsylvania Press who has been consistently supportive; to Maryann Zaremska, the medical librarian at Saint Francis Memorial Hospital in San Francisco, to Barbara Bevan, its former director, and Beth Evitts, its current director; to Shirley Cooper, Virginia Grove, Gail Diehl, and Diane Robinson of the York Hospital Hoover Library for their enthusiastic assistance; to Glenn Cannon, Alex Burger, Rod Pabst, and Gloria Heard of the Media Services Department of York Hospital for their critical assistance with our art work; to Erma Dettinger in the York Hospital mailroom who guided our perpetual flow of correspondence from the East Coast to the West Coast and vice versa; to Betty Altland who typed, beautifully, the chapters over and over; and to the York Hospital Auxiliary, an 1,800-member group without which the hospital would be poorer in many ways. The auxiliary made an unprecedented grant to our book production project, for which we are most grateful. There are many impediments to completing a project of this magnitude. One of the persons most responsible for helping to overcome these impediments and gain early and continued support was Dr. David R. Fink, Jr., Director of Education—Department of Medical Affairs, York Hospital. We gratefully acknowledge Dr. Fink's unhesitating encouragement and his role in providing a critical stimulus to insure continued progress on the book.

Introduction

The 1980s have witnessed an explosion of knowledge regarding post-partum illness, and a parallel expansion of interest on the part of both the public and many individuals in the health professions. When this book was proposed in 1988, the editors examined questions that were asked by many thoughtful and interested people. These questions appeared to fall into four categories, which became the four parts of the book. Part I examines many unique qualities of postpartum illness and describes the main syndromes that appear. Part II presents the best of current treatment methods. Part III examines in detail evidence implicating organic changes during the puerperium in the etiology of postpartum illness. Part IV looks at problems that exist because post-partum psychiatric illness has been virtually overlooked by modern science. The question of what should be done to catch up is asked, and some of the answers are suggested.

Parts I and III present evidence from a variety of sources suggesting that postpartum psychiatric syndromes implicate a *range* of patho-physiology which is fairly extensive and extended in time. Looked at as individual variables, a very complex phenomenon is suggested.

These data can be viewed as a dynamic mechanism that induces many changes in the reproductive and endocrine systems during the puerperium. With this approach, many clinical details, organic trends, and irregularities begin to take on the outline of a model, or a picture puzzle as it is being assembled.

One does not put a picture puzzle together in an instant. Similarly, the details of postpartum illness and its physiology cannot be coalesced readily into a short description. This book tries to indicate the pre-sumptive outline of the picture, present as many details as possible, and then fit these details into the overall picture. The picture is looked at from different perspectives and thus involves some purposeful repe-tition.

Finally, in Chapter 25, when the picture is fairly advanced, its plausibility is questioned. The nearly complete picture is used to set up critical tests of its validity. If the tests validate the picture, effective treatments could be available in the near future. If the tests disprove the picture, pursuit of other inquiries is encouraged.

Each of the four parts has its own introduction. The introduction to Part IV suggests the diversity of problems that arise when an area of knowledge falls behind. Humanitarian problems exist along with the scientific ones. All of these problems can be solved. Their solution has been hastened by the acknowledgment of postpartum illness.

Part I
The Qualities
of Postpartum
Psychiatric Illness

The art of clinical description was highly developed in the nineteenth century. Disorders were described in great detail, and their courses were traced from inception to recovery, or death. When many cases of postpartum illness were studied, it became apparent to leading nineteenth-century physicians that these cases exhibit a remarkably wide range of symptoms and signs and that one pattern of symptoms often gives way to another. The changeability of these cases is a striking quality. Two broad categories of illness were distinguished: an agitated, highly changeable psychosis with an onset usually during the first two weeks after delivery and a depression that began insidiously three or more weeks after delivery, worsened slowly, reached a plateau, and then improved or stabilized at a level of mild or moderate depression. Some cases began with the agitated psychosis but developed into a condition indistinguishable from the second type of depression.

The early writers noted many qualities, such as confusion, hallucinations, and a timing and progression, all of which they associated with known organic disorders. They suspected a relationship with changes in the generative organs.

Chapter 1 describes the patterns of postpartum illness as seen by the nineteenth-century observers. Chapter 2 examines old and new information which suggests that the observed patterns of postpartum illness have many qualities which are unique and distinguish postpartum illness from schizophrenia or other so-called functional disorders. These unique qualities support the earlier inferences that postpartum syndromes reflect *organic pathology*. Chapter 3 recognizes the confusion that has followed imprecise and misleading terminology. An informal nomenclature is proposed to facilitate communication. The logic that has guided the development of this nomenclature could be applicable to an eventual modernization of the official terminology.

Chapter 4 attempts to convey the depth of feelings, the intensity of sensations, the terror, and the shame of many postpartum patients by quoting their actual words. The authors, Patricia Harberger, Nancy Berchtold, and Jane Honikman, have heard these words and many more like them in support groups and telephone contacts as new mothers call "warm lines" to cry for help. The unique themes and feelings so characteristic of these disorders emerge in stark clarity.

Chapter 1
Patterns of Postpartum Illness

James Alexander Hamilton

The searchlight of investigative enthusiasm almost completely avoided psychiatric illness after childbearing for the first 80 years of this century. Many careful and insightful observations of the nineteenth century were misquoted or forgotten. Twentieth-century discoveries relevant to postpartum illness were disregarded. The result of this aberration may have been the needless suffering of tens of thousands of very sick women, the partial disability of millions of others, and the immeasurable disruption of and hardship to their families.

New attitudes about and rethinking of postpartum problems began in 1980 when Ian Brockington, then at the University of Manchester, England, called a conference on postpartum psychiatric illness. Suddenly, scores of independent investigators and practitioners throughout the world learned of each other's work and thinking. They founded the Marcé Society, an international organization to advance knowledge and improve the treatment of postpartum patients (Brockington and Kumar 1982).

Much has been learned since 1980. Information is scattered and incomplete, and little is known with absolute certainty. Nevertheless, when information from many sources is fitted together, as a picture puzzle is fitted together, a fascinating image emerges, which has very favorable implications for prevention and definitive treatment of postpartum illnesses.

The puzzle analogy as a model for constructive thinking in this area of neglected opportunities was provided by Professor Ralph Paffenbarger of Stanford University and Harvard. In a masterful application of epidemiological and statistical analysis, he put it this way: The clues to postpartum illness "are arranged in a tantalizing fashion, much like the pieces of a picture puzzle partly fitted together. The question remains whether all of the pieces will match, or indeed whether they are all on hand" (Paffenbarger 1961).

Since Paffenbarger's statement in 1961, many more pieces of the puzzle have become available, and it is time to bring the picture up-to-date. As this is done, opportunities for research and clinical applications become apparent immediately.

The first important pieces of the puzzle were generated by very able nineteenth-century physicians as they observed patients, tried to understand what they saw, and attempted to devise remedies. The observations of these physicians were carefully made and meticulously recorded. Their observations provide valuable information about the various manifestations of postpartum illness, the patterns in which symptoms are arranged, and the way in which individual cases evolve with the passage of time and the transitions of female physiology. The detailed nineteenth-century clinical descriptions are particularly valuable because psychoactive medications, widely used for these illnesses today, tend to blur distinctive features that were previously seen and recorded.

Although reports of mental illness related to childbearing date back to antiquity, the first systematic study of the phenomenon was reported by Jean Etienne Dominique Esquirol and summarized in a forty-three-page review of ninety cases in his two-volume textbook, *Des maladies mentales* (Esquirol 1838). Esquirol divided his cases into three groups: those occurring *during* pregnancy, those occurring *soon after* childbearing, and those developing *several weeks or longer* after delivery. His pregnancy cases had a high incidence of earlier psychiatric illness, and the patients were seen as resembling cases unrelated to childbearing. Among cases that developed within a few days after delivery he noticed a high incidence of delirium. Esquirol's concept of delirium was close to that of today: an acute deviation in thinking and behavior characterized by disturbances of perception and consciousness, disorganization, hallucinations, confusion, transitory delusions, and marked changeability. Esquirol was very familiar with delirium, having seen it in association with high fever. Noting all degrees of disability and great variability in recovery time, he suggested that the incidence of postpartum illness might be much higher in the general population than was indicated by hospital statistics. He believed that many suffered silently at home.

A New York physician, James MacDonald (1847), reported on his study of sixty-eight postpartum cases and was able to sharpen the distinction between the categories noted by Esquirol. The group of early onset after delivery seemed to develop rapidly after a few hours or days of restlessness, irritability, insomnia, feelings of exhaustion, and confusion. The severe phase was manifested by extreme agitation, bizarre behavior, hallucinations, transitory delusions, mania, occasional violence, and usually great changeability. The group of later onset, those beginning three or more weeks after delivery, began insidiously and deteriorated gradually. Their mood was characteristically depressive.

Over half of MacDonald's cases recovered. However, some became chronic, including members of both groups. The chronic cases resembled dementia, and after the elapse of many months there was little or nothing to distinguish members of the first group from members of the second.

Bethlem Hospital, near London, was a center for the care of postpartum patients during the nineteenth century as it is today under R. Kumar. J. Webster (1848) reported on 131 cases, comprising 13 percent of a sample of female admissions to Bethlem. He criticized the common practice of bleeding postpartum patients and advocated sedation with opium and Indian hemp.

The French tradition of concern regarding these problems, initiated by J.E.D. Esquirol, was continued by Louis Victor Marcé. After completion of his training at the medical school at Nantes, Marcé took a position at the hospital at Ivry-sur-Seine, which had been founded by Esquirol and had a tradition in the treatment of postpartum cases. Marcé became affiliated with the University of Paris and quickly immersed himself in the study and treatment of postpartum cases. Reviewing seventy-eight cases of his own plus hundreds of cases from other studies and other hospitals, he published his *Traité de la folie des femmes encientes* (Marcé 1858). Four years later he published a textbook of general psychiatry, *Traité pratique des maladies mentales* (Marcé 1862). He died in 1864 at the age of 36.

Marcé divided a sample of 310 cases into three groups. Of these, 9 percent began *during pregnancy* (*folie des femmes encientes*), 58 percent began during the *first six weeks* after delivery (*folie des nouvelles accouchées*), and 33 percent began *after six weeks* (*folie des nourrices*). He took note of the common observation that pregnant women were said to experience an exaggeration of eccentricities during pregnancy, develop cravings for special foods, complain of annoying physical symptoms and sometimes experience excessive fatigability. Nevertheless, when he reviewed the symptoms and behavior of his twenty-seven cases originating during pregnancy, he could find no important features that distinguished the psychoses of pregnancy from the psychoses unrelated to childbearing (Marcé 1858).

This was not the case with the other two groups, the 180 cases that developed during the puerperal period and the 103 cases that developed later. Each of these two groups was seen to have its own unique qualities, and both postpartum groups were quite distinct from other forms of mental illness, said Marcé.

Marcé's descriptions of the two postpartum groups of early and late onset are important for several reasons:

1. The unique qualities he noted in each group include many characteristics that separate them from run-of-the-mill functional psychoses.
2. These unique qualities afford clues to specific organic mechanisms that may be prominent in each group.
3. Marcé's excellent case histories and the syntheses of case histories into descriptions of illness patterns are of great value today. The findings and tools of modern medicine can now be applied to these disease patterns to adduce probable disease mechanisms and promising therapeutic and preventive strategies.
4. Marcé is quoted again and again in the twentieth century as an authority for the position that postpartum psychiatric illnesses were identical to functional illnesses such as dementia praecox (schizophrenia) and manic-depressive psychosis (bipolar disorder). His position was precisely the opposite. It strains credulity to accept that any person who had read either of Marcé's books could quote him as authority for the position that postpartum psychiatric illnesses were not distinct clinical entities.

Marcé noted that the agitated syndrome of early onset, the *folie des nouvelles accouchées,* with onset usually between Day 3 and 10, often began with insomnia, confusion, and agitation. This moved into episodes of delirium with bizarre behavior, hallucinations, distortions of thinking, changing delusions, and loss or distortion of memory for acute episodes. Violence and exhaustion were frequent. Wild mania could be followed by severe melancholia. Marcé commented that one predisposing factor to this early syndrome was hemorrhage at delivery.

Marcé's depressed syndrome of late onset, the *folie des nourrices,* was said to develop slowly, with the first symptoms usually after three weeks, sometimes much later. The first symptoms were often headache and excessive fatigability. Depression usually followed. Patients were said to have "poor nutrition," indigestion, and often anemia. Marcé said that these patients had "poor circulation," but from his text it is not clear whether this meant cold extremities or peripheral edema. The predominant characteristic of these patients was said to be "profound exhaustion." Eventually, many patients developed severe melancholia. Others began to level off and to recover after a few months. As Marcé reviewed carefully taken histories, it appeared to him that the physical complaints preceded the "intellectual disorders" (meaning, psychiatric symptoms) in these cases of late onset.

Marcé also noted that some patients began with symptoms of early agitated psychosis but then evolved into the late depression. Other patients alternated between agitated psychosis and depression.

In Marcé's time, the art of descriptive psychiatry was well advanced. His textbook, the *Traité pratique des maladies mentales*, reveals an awareness of the symptoms and the behavior of a wide range of psychiatric patients (Marcé 1862). It was quite apparent to Marcé that many kinds of physical illness were associated with characteristic psychiatric symptoms and signs and that these were quite different from the symptoms and signs found in cases without physical illness. Later, the first group became known as the symptoms and signs of organic disease. Prominent among these indicators of organic illness were confusion, delirium, hallucinations, temporary disturbances of memory, errors in recognition, and lapses in logical thinking. It did not escape Marcé's attention that many of the symptoms and signs of both early and late postpartum syndromes pointed toward an organic etiology.

In the twentieth century, the adjectives "organic" and "functional" have come to have fairly definite meanings in psychiatry. An organic psychosis or symptom has a definite physical cause, a toxin, an injury, a metabolic abnormality, or some obvious deterioration of brain tissue, such as Alzheimer's disease. Organic psychoses contrast with functional mental disorders, such as schizophrenia, and the mood disorders, mania and depression. The latter are regarded as chronic dysfunction of complex mind-body interactions. Recent developments suggest that mood disorders may involve deficits, excesses, or imbalances of neurotransmitters; this is a suggestion of organic etiology on a different level. Nevertheless, the label "functional" for schizophrenia and mood disorders is an acceptable colloquial designation. "Organic symptoms and signs" suggest an inflammatory, toxic, or metabolic interference that involves central nervous system neurons. Although the collective term "organic symptoms and signs" was not in use in Marcé's time, his observation of the predominance of confusion and delirium led him toward the conclusion that postpartum psychiatric illness had a distinct physical etiology.

When Marcé reviewed his cases of late onset, it was apparent that he had indications of physical illness beyond the psychiatric signs and symptoms usually referred to as organic. Exhaustion was one such complaint regarding a physical condition, unless one chose to ascribe it to the imagination. Marcé's first inclination was to ascribe it to physical depletion caused by lactation, but then he noted that most women nursed their infants without suffering exhaustion. Indigestion, poor nutrition, weakness, constipation, and anemia had the appearance of a physical illness. The depression of mood in cases of late onset could be a purely psychological phenomenon, yet it seemed to be *preceded* by physical complaints and physical exhaustion.

When Marcé looked at the total picture of postpartum illness, he saw other phenomena that directed him toward organic interpretations. He saw that some patients began with the early agitated psychosis and then moved gradually into the late depressive syndrome. Their illness did not evolve in the reverse direction. Marcé saw a few patients deteriorate gradually into a state of dementia, a condition he regarded as similar to senile dementia, and this he knew was often associated with physical changes in the brain. He sensed a parallel course between the psychiatric illnesses and the involution of the organs of generation as they returned toward the prepregnancy state. The consistent differences between early and late syndromes was one reason for his belief. Another was the common occurrence that a patient would seem to recover and then experience a relapse before the first menstrual period. In his 1862 textbook, Marcé quotes a report of M. Baillarger, read to the Société de Médecine, stating that, of forty-four cases of *folie puerpérale*, eleven became ill *précisément au moment* of the return of the menses (Marcé 1862, page 146). Marcé's discussion of postpartum illness is treated in the chapter *Des causes de la folie*, the section *Causes physiques*, the subsection *Causes physiologiques*.

Marcé was convinced that postpartum psychiatric illnesses were physical illnesses.

That which gives puerperal psychosis its special quality is the coexistence with it of a functional and organic modification of the uterus and related organs. . . . The coexistence of this organic state raises an interesting question of pathologic physiology: one immediately asks if there exist connections between the uterine conditions and the disorders of the mind, and if these disorders do not develop in consequence of modifications of the genital apparatus; in a word, if the psychosis is sympathetic.*

Marcé went one step farther: he proposed that the connection he had observed be called "morbid sympathy." Since Marcé's books were writ-

*Ce que donne à la folie puerpérale son caractère spéciale, c'est la coexistence d'une modification organique et fonctionelle de l'utérus et de ses annexes. . . . La coexistence de cet état organique soulève tout d'abord une intéressante question de physiologie pathologique: on se demande involontairement s'il existe des connexions entre l'état utérin et les désordres de l'intelligence, si ces dernières ne se sont développés que consécutivement aux modifications subies par l'appareil génital; en un mot, si la folie est sympathique" (Marcé 1858, pages 7–8). The Appendix has a selection of pages reproduced from Marcé's books.

ten prior to the discovery of the endocrine system, a mechanism whereby widely separated parts of the body could communicate by chemical messengers had not been proposed. Hence, the state of knowledge in 1858 did not permit Marcé to spell out the relationship which he sensed by his clinical intuition.

Marcé's 1858 book was the principal authority on postpartum illness for the rest of the century, although important information was added by others. In Germany, C. Fürstner (1875) reported in detail about the confusion, anxiety, and delirium of the early syndrome of postpartum illness. He was particularly interested in the fact that, while delirium was accompanied by fever in other medical diseases, most postpartum patients were afebrile. Another important German researcher was L. H. Ripping (1877), who reported on the remarkable variety and changeability of the symptoms of postpartum patients. He cited several instances in which mania and transitory hallucinations evolved into a set of fixed delusions. He pointed out that postpartum patients often seemed to have symptoms of two or more diseases or syndromes at the same time. Among his patients suffering from severe depression, he noted a peculiar "dreamy condition," which was not present in the usual case of depression.

In England, George Savage (1875) studied and reported on postpartum patients at Bethlem Hospital, stating, "We cannot classify them with any degree of precision into mania, melancholia and dementia. We shall note typical cases of each of these variables, but I must premise by saying it is common for one to pass through all these common forms."

During the last two decades of the century, bits of information regarding the endocrine system began to emerge. One condition that attracted early attention was myxedema, an illness now known to be the result of marked deficit of thyroxine. It is characterized by swelling of tissues throughout the body. When a swollen extremity is cut with a knife, a thick mucinous substance oozes out. In many cases, swelling of the thyroid gland is visible. Early microscopists looked at preparations of these swollen glands and found the tissues to be abnormal. Patients with myxedema are slow-moving, slow-thinking, and often depressed.

In 1883, the Clinical Society of London decided to find out about myxedema and appointed a committee to investigate it. Five years later the committee reported on 109 cases which had been studied very carefully (Ord 1888). Of the cases studied by the Committee, ninety-nine were females, most of them depressed.

It is worthy of note that a large proportion of the female patients were married, and that nearly all had borne children. In a significant proportion, the child-bearing had been excessive, and in some cases there appears to be little doubt that the early symptoms of the disease date from childbirth, though curiously enough, in other instances there is a history of temporary diminution of the myxoedematous condition during pregnancy. . . . One case has certainly presented a remarkable variation of myxoedema in connection with pregnancy. The patient, after presenting the full physiognomy of myxoedema, became pregnant, whereupon the swelling passed away, to return after the birth of the child. This succession of phenomena occurred three times in seven years. . . . Insanity occurs in nearly half of the cases and takes the form of acute or chronic mania, melancholia, or dementia, with a marked predominance of suspicion and self-accusation. In about one-third of the cases, wakefulness is recorded, and sleep is often disturbed by horrible dreams and sensations. Among physical complaints was a high instance of occipital headache. The body temperature was subnormal, although occasionally it rose to normal or a degree or two higher. Patients got along very poorly in cold weather (Ord 1888).

In 1888 it was suspected that myxedema was caused by a lack of the "substance" of the thyroid gland. However, efforts to prepare an extract of the substance failed at first because the molecule of thyroxine was destroyed easily by heat and by many solvents. Soon after 1888 it was discovered that a preparation suitable for oral administration could be prepared by vacuum drying of animal thyroid glands. Administered to myxedema cases, the thyroid preparation produced very favorable results. Medical enthusiasm was great, and thyroid was tried on many illnesses, including psychiatric illnesses. Results were negative or questionable in cases not clearly related to thyroid deficit.

Ord and his 1883–88 committee demonstrated great insight by stressing these observations: (1) a 10-to-1 predominance of women patients with a thyroid disorder, (2) a high incidence of psychiatric symptoms associated with thyroid deficit, and (3) the fact that most of the victims became ill after childbearing. The implications of these observations for psychiatry remained fallow for a century, but they were revived in the excellent review, "Behavioral Aspects of Thyroid Disease in Women," by Victor I. Reus (1989).

Desiccated thyroid was used with great success in one case of postpartum depression, reported in the medical literature and then forgotten. On December 24, 1906, a German physician, K. Stössner, was called to a farm in the Rhineland to see a child with the measles (Stössner 1910). The child's mother he found to be "completely hopeless." After the delivery of her last child, she had noted an "inability to be happy," difficulty in thinking, and a feeling of stiffness in her face. Her memory and hearing became poor. Movement and speech were slowed, and she noted a loss of tone in her speech. Emotional responsiveness was decreased. She had amenorrhoea, loss of hair, and swelling of her legs and feet.

Stössner noted the physical signs that suggested myxedema and then began to administer thyroid. The patient was somewhat better within a month and was quite normal by March 12, 1907, both with respect to physical signs and the depression. The thyroid was discontinued, and she suffered a relapse. When the thyroid was resumed, she recovered and remained well. Although Stössner reported his case in a prestigious medical journal, his discovery received no attention.

The Picture Puzzle Partly Fitted Together

Psychiatric illness after childbearing was observed thoughtfully and described in detail by many nineteenth-century physicians. Led by J.E.D. Esquirol and L. V. Marcé, there was consensus that two distinct patterns of symptoms could be seen: an agitated psychosis, which usually began a few days after delivery, and a depressive reaction, which usually began three or more weeks after delivery. In some patients, the first pattern was followed by the second, and cases with qualities of both syndromes were not unusual. Common to both patterns were pervasive symptoms such as confusion, a tendency for the course of illness to change and to follow changes in the organs of reproduction, and a plethora of associated physical signs and symptoms late in the course of illness. These observations led Marcé and others to suspect a critical physiological connection between postpartum psychiatric illnesses and the reproductive system.

Knowledge regarding the endocrine system began to emerge toward the end of the nineteenth century, and many physicians believed that it would be relevant to the understanding and treatment of many diseases. Early studies of myxedema, or adult hypothyroidism, indicated that this disease had associations with childbearing and psychiatric manifestations similar to those observed in postpartum psychiatric illness (Ord 1888). With these meticulous observations and discerning inferences, quite a few pieces of the picture puzzle of postpartum psychiatric illness were on hand. Then the course of psychiatric history turned abruptly to a different direction, and the picture puzzle received scant attention for most of the twentieth century.

References

Brockington, I. F., and Kumar, R. (Eds.) (1982). *Motherhood and Mental Illness*. London: Academic Press.

Esquirol, J.E.D. (1838). *Des maladies mentales considérées sous les rapports medical, hygiénique et médico-légal*, Vol. 1. Paris: J. B. Baillière.

Fürstner, C. (1875). Ueber Schwangerschafts- und Puerperalpsychosen. *Arch. Psychiatr.*, 5:505–43.

MacDonald, J. (1847). Puerperal insanity. *Am. J. Insanity*, 4:113–63.

Marcé, L. V. (1858). *Traité de la folie des femmes enceintes, des nouvelles accouchées et des nourrices.* Paris: J. B. Baillière et Fils.

———. (1862). *Traité pratique des maladies mentales.* Paris: J. B. Baillière et Fils.

Ord, W. M. (1888). Report of a committee of the Clinical Society of London, nominated December 14, 1883 to investigate the subject of myxoedema. *Trans. Clin. Soc. London (Suppl.)*, 21:1–215.

Paffenbarger, R. S., Jr. (1961). The picture puzzle of the postpartum psychoses. *J. Chron. Dis.*, 13:161–73.

Reus, V. I. (1989). Behavioral aspects of thyroid disease in women. In B. L. Parry (Ed.), *Women's Disorders.* Vol. 12:1 of *Psychiatr. Clin. North Am.*, March, 1989.

Ripping, L. H. (1877). *Die Geistesstörungen der Schwangeren, Wochnerinnen und Säugenden.* Stuttgart.

Savage, G. H. (1875). Observations on the insanity of pregnancy and childbirth. *Guy's Hospital Reports*, 20:83–117.

Stössner, K. (1910). Ein Fall von Myxödem im Anschluss an Gravidität. *München Med. Wochenschr.* 57:2531–33.

Webster, J. (1848). Remarks on the statistics, pathology and treatment of puerperal insanity. *Lancet* 2:611–12.

Chapter 2
The Issue of Unique Qualities

James Alexander Hamilton

A doctrine, well-established throughout the world and quite strong in the United States, maintains that psychiatric illnesses after childbearing have little or no relationship to the physiological events of the reproductive process. It is held that the stresses of pregnancy, delivery, and child care uncover latent psychiatric illnesses, such as schizophrenia and the affective disorders.

The contrary position maintains that postpartum psychiatric illnesses are primarily a reflection of physiological changes, particularly endocrine changes, which occur during the first few weeks after childbearing. While all of these changes may not be known, this position holds that enough is known to regard postpartum disorders as a set of organic syndromes and to encourage the vigorous use of the vast amount of information which supports this position. In this second viewpoint, psychological factors and stresses are not ignored; indeed, they may be enormous, but they are considered secondary to the organic factors.

As indicated in Chapter 1, many nineteenth-century physicians made observations and compiled detailed records of psychiatric illness after childbirth. Many of them noticed the frequent occurrence of symptoms usually associated with known organic illnesses of the nervous system, such as confusion and delirium. They noticed an apparent correlation of the known physical changes during the puerperium, with the appearance of psychiatric symptoms. These observations led many physicians to suspect a close connection between the physical changes and the psychiatric disorders. Then, just as twentieth-century technology began to provide tools for exploring the suspected connection, the belief of most psychiatrists shifted to the doctrine that the connection was of little significance, perhaps nonexistent.

These contrasting views represent a clear-cut dichotomy in medical opinion that is reflected in the treatment of patients. It is, therefore, appropriate to review the development of each position.

The doctrine that postpartum physiological changes have a minimal or negligible relationship to postpartum psychiatric illness will be examined first. In the early years of the twentieth century, giant steps were taken to relate medical and surgical diseases to their causes. Discoveries in pathology and bacteriology led to the development of rational preventive and treatment measures in medicine and surgery. Many diseases were given new names that reflected their etiology.

In psychiatry, efforts were made to seek out the causes of the major psychiatric illnesses and to develop a consistent nomenclature. The search for the causes of most types of mental illness proved futile. Without etiology as a basis for the classification and naming of psychiatric disorders, the next best alternative seemed to be the identification of psychiatric disorders on the basis of behavior patterns or clusters of symptoms. This seemed to work fairly well, and three broad categories were visualized: dementia praecox (later called schizophrenia) was seen to be a disorder in thinking. Manic and depressive syndromes were seen to be disorders in emotional (or affective) reactions. Toxic-exhaustive psychoses (later called organic psychoses) were seen to be illnesses in which toxic, metabolic, neoplastic, degenerative, or traumatic agents interfered with the function of central nervous system neurons. For each of the three principal categories, typical patterns of signs and symptoms were designated. Some overlapping was observed, but most psychiatrists were comfortable with the tripartite division of mental illness.

Most of the varieties of mental illness could be fitted into the new system of classification. There was one outstanding exception: psychiatric illness after childbearing resisted classification into one or the other of the main categories. After beginning with confusion and delirium, signs of organic psychoses, these patients could become delusional, a criterion of the schizophrenic category, or they could experience mood changes characteristic of depression or mania. Worse than that, the patients could change rapidly from one pattern to another, or exhibit criteria of two or even all three of the categories at the same time. This was not only frustrating, but the eager classifiers sensed that the pleomorphism of postpartum illness was a threat to their new system. Some of the leaders suggested that these undisciplined patients be tagged according to the symptom pattern which was most prominent at the time of diagnosis. Concurrently, it was suggested that the term "postpartum" and all of its synonyms be expunged from the official lexicon of psychiatry.

One of the most influential of America's psychiatrists was Edward A.

Strecker, coauthor with Franklin G. Ebaugh, of the most popular clinical psychiatric textbook of the first half-century (Strecker and Ebaugh 1940). An often quoted paper by the two began with the statement, "Old names die hard" (Strecker and Ebaugh 1926). They went on to say, "All others (in addition to ourselves) who have studied this problem are unanimous in the belief that there is no psychosis which may be designated as 'puerperal.'" The paper cited nine references from 1894 to 1915, all of which provided tabulations of cases divided into the three chosen categories. No contrary papers were cited. Their own work was to pick fifty case histories of postpartum illness from the records of three hospitals and to find that they could be arranged in three groups, dementia praecox, manic-depressive psychosis, and toxic-exhaustive psychosis (psychosis with an identified organic cause). When symptoms were tabulated, there was an annoying pervasiveness of confusion and delirium in the dementia praecox and the manic-depressive categories. This intrusion of organic signs and symptoms into the other two categories was explained away by this statement, "It would seem reasonable to put forward the hypothesis that labor . . . does exert a modifying influence on the psychotic reaction."

David A. Boyd, Jr., was very prominent in the organizational activities of American psychiatry at midcentury. In 1952 he wrote a long review, "Mental Disorders Associated with Childbearing," for the *American Journal of Obstetrics and Gynecology* (Boyd 1942):

In 1847, James MacDonald reported a series of cases of "puerperal insanity" and maintained that a special form of insanity could be distinguished. . . . Marcé, in 1858, was the first to challenge the traditional views and maintained that there was nothing specific about puerperal mental disorders and that these did not differ from psychoses occurring in nonpuerperal women of the same age. Unfortunately, his contributions were disregarded for fifty years and physicians continued to believe that a specific type of "puerperal insanity" existed.

Boyd went on to cite eighteen papers between 1875 and 1899 which accepted the position that postpartum illness was a separate entity, and which dealt with a range of observed unique qualities. Boyd deemed the studies worthless, "inasmuch as no such nosological entity exists."

Boyd's alleged quotation of Marcé, presenting a position exactly the opposite of that which Marcé held, is worthy of note from the standpoint of scholastic standards. (Marcé's position is outlined in Chapter 1, and excerpts are given in the Appendix). When an authority or a research paper is cited, the least a reader can expect is that the author has seen the document and has tried to read, understand, and convey it accurately. Both before and after Boyd there are dozens of references to Marcé which misquote him, as Boyd misquotes him. The possibility that all of these authors read and misunderstood Marcé seems improbable.

The incidents of faulty quotation of Marcé might be dismissed as unimportant were it not for the catastrophic effects that followed. Marcé was *the* nineteenth-century authority on postpartum illness, and his alleged denial of the uniqueness of postpartum syndromes constituted a powerful support for the doctrine that psychiatric illnesses after childbirth have little or no relationship to the physiological events of the puerperium. The words "postpartum" and "puerperal" became archaic words in psychiatry. The vast majority of psychiatrists followed suit and denied the uniqueness of these conditions. The ample nineteenth-century literature fell to a trickle.

The final success of Strecker and his followers was achieved in 1952 with the first edition of the official U.S. nomenclature, the *Diagnostic and Statistical Manual of Mental Disorders* (*DSM*). The word "postpartum" and its synonyms were expunged from the official diagnostic terminology. (E. A. Strecker was a member of the Nomenclature Committee that formulated the manual.) The policy of avoiding postpartum diagnoses continues in the third revised edition, *DSM-III-R* (American Psychiatric Association 1987).

The doctrine which holds that psychiatric illness after childbearing is not significantly different from psychiatric illness unrelated to childbearing is expressed unequivocally in the official nomenclature handbook, the *DSM-III*, with the statement, "There is no compelling evidence that postpartum psychosis is a distinct entity," (American Psychiatric Association, 1980, page 373).

The contrary position is that there *is* compelling evidence that postpartum psychiatric illness is a distinct entity, or group of entities. Support for this contrary position consists of a great many pieces of evidence from many sources. Much of this book is devoted to presenting the evidence. In this chapter, a broad outline of information is sketched out, as major configurations of a picture puzzle are assembled. Smaller, but important pieces are filled in later.

The conclusion of this chapter will be that many unique qualities of postpartum illness reflect deficits and imbalances in the endocrine system, as this system moves rapidly from the hyperactivity of pregnancy down to, and sometimes beyond, the levels of the nonpregnant state. Superimposed upon, but secondary to, the organic factors are stresses that are unique to the responsibilities and the anxieties of new motherhood.

The outline presented in this chapter suggests that several endocrine glands and their hormones play specific roles in the development of postpartum illness, and these roles are coordinated with the sequence of endocrine events that follows childbirth. Consideration of the progression of postpartum psychiatric symptoms indicate that this progression follows the march of endocrine readjustment.

The Thyroid

An association between thyroid deficit, childbearing, and a high incidence of psychiatric illness was indicated clearly in the report of the Clinical Society's committee to investigate myxoedema (Ord, 1888). The focus of interest was on the physical illness, and there is no evidence that the psychiatric findings were ever put to work. Stössner reported in 1910 on the use of desiccated thyroid on a single case of depression and myxedema after childbearing (Stössner 1910).

Kilpatrick and Tiebout (1926) studied seventy-six patients and found twelve who became chronic. Among these patients, physical debility was prominent. The authors suggested that their findings indicated that an unknown physical process was operative in postpartum illness. The New York physician G. M. Davidson had studied German endocrine research, and his speculations led him to try ovarian and pituitary extracts, to which he added one grain of thyroid extract daily if patients were depressed or apathetic. He reported "favorable results in some cases," but his mixing of hormones and the inadequate presentation of data do not permit definite evaluation of his results (Davidson 1936). A. A. Baker found thyroid extract effective for postpartum women with three different kinds of complaint: depression of mood with loss of energy, diminished sexual responsiveness, and insufficient lactation (Baker 1967).

Almost without exception, those who reported on the use of desiccated thyroid attributed their discovery to accident, not astute medical inference. This was the case with the author of this chapter, whose introduction to this field was through a patient referred in 1949 because of failed treatment. Three weeks after delivery she had had the first symptoms of depression. After two months of office treatment by a psychiatrist, she had gone to the Mayo Clinic in Rochester, Minnesota, where a diagnosis of postpartum depression had been made. She was referred to a psychiatric facility where a course of electroconvulsive treatments (ECT) was given. The response to ECT was good, but when she returned to San Francisco, she became depressed within one week. She was then referred to me, and with medical help we undertook a thorough medical and psychiatric assessment. Laboratory studies revealed a thyroid deficit. She was treated with 1 grain per day of desiccated thyroid and in six weeks she was well. She had no recurrence of depression.

From 1949 to 1956 the author treated thirty patients who were hospitalized with major postpartum depression. Thyroid studies ranged from midnormal to low, with one marked elevation. Thyroid was given to twenty-nine patients, beginning at ½ grain and working up to 1 to 2 grains in gradual increments. The results with twenty-seven patients were excellent. Two had short relapses, returned to the hospital, and then recovered. Except for a few patients whose thyroid measurements were quite low, the use of desiccated thyroid was empirical. Although thyroid appeared to be remarkably effective in these twenty-nine patients, a rationale was absent, and this created serious doubts about the treatment.

In 1956 triiodothyronine became available, and this active analogue of thyroxine was seen as an opportunity to observe an accelerated thyroxine-like action. Four patients were tried on triiodothyronine after a small initial dose of desiccated thyroid. Striking improvement was seen within three days. A study group of fourteen psychiatrists and obstetricians, with representation from two medical schools, was formed to work with the new thyroxine analogue. Ten more patients were treated successfully and had quite rapid recoveries with the combination of triiodothyronine and desiccated thyroid (Ballachey et al. 1958).

Aspiring to achieve a degree of experimental control, the study group set up a double-blind study with daily divided doses compared with daily divided placebos. Some hospitalized patients were included in the study for a few days, and striking differences between days were noted. When the code was broken, it was apparent that the bad days were placebo days. The double-blind experiment was then begun with six outpatients with late postpartum depression of moderate severity. Frequent telephone reports were encouraged, and it was soon learned that the on-and-off quality of mood had a disturbing effect on patients. Two patients appeared to become suicidal, were hospitalized and recovered eventually with desiccated thyroid therapy. Further double-blind experiments were discontinued.

Review of the limited amount of data available suggested that while the effect of triiodothyronine might be dramatic, it was preferable to take more time and seek more stable effects with thyroxine or desiccated thyroid. This decision was reinforced when early reports suggested that triiodothyronine might have a greater depressing effect on the activity of the thyroid gland than thyroxine.

After the triiodothyronine experiment, thyroxine or desiccated thyroid was used with several hundred patients, preceded by one or a series of serum thyroid studies. There was never an indication for desiccated thyroid before the third week postpartum, since thyroxine remains in the high range for two to three weeks. A series of thyroid studies, repeated pulse determinations, and observations of body and peripheral temperatures is important in deciding the initiation and amount of thyroid medication. While high serum thyroxine levels were a contraindication for thyroid medication, midnormal and low-normal values did not exclude the administration of this hormone. Early postpartum psychosis was treated during my active practice with moderate amounts of a phenothiazine, plus a variety of sedatives and tranquilizers sometimes in large doses, but adjusted constantly to fit the immediate condition of the patient. Antidepressants were not used.

More recently, the work of the Tokyo thyroidologist N. Amino and others (1978) have added an important new concept to the assessment of postpartum thyroid function. The new information relates to pregnancy and postpartum changes with this hormone and is reviewed in the context of information developed many years ago by T. S. Danowski and colleagues (1953).

At delivery, the serum thyroxine of almost all women tends to be higher than the average for nonpregnant women, often 1½ times that average as determined by protein-bound iodine. From the date of delivery, thyroxine tends to drop. On the average, the falling curve passes through the nonpregnant level at about three weeks postpartum. The fall usually continues beyond this and then levels off at a value somewhat below the nonpregnant average, which holds steady for about a year. Danowski's paper graphed the postpregnancy fall for many patients, and all of them demonstrated a downward trend.

Amino has found an exception to the smooth drop in thyroxine that is attributable to an autoimmune reaction. Serum thyroxine may rise briefly soon after delivery, the patients may become agitated, and this is associated with an autoimmune reaction of the thyroid gland. Thyroid enlargement may occur. This stage is often followed by a stage of hypothyroidism, which is a reaction associated with antithyroid microsomal antibodies in the serum. Treatment for the hyperthyroid phase is conservative, and antithyroid drugs should not be employed. For the second hypothyroid stage, thyroxine may be appropriate. In most cases the thyroid gland returns to its normal functional level in about a year.

Mild to moderate hypothyroidism was advocated as an important factor in the etiology of postpartum depression in 1962 (Hamilton 1962). This advocacy met resistance from a popular belief that hypothyroidism was an all-or-nothing phenomenon. This view was weakened a decade later by D. C. Evered and associates (1973) at Newcastle-upon-Tyne, who distinguished three levels of primary hypothyroidism. The intermediate group, with only an elevated thyroid-stimulating hormone (TSH) as a laboratory index, had symptoms such as excessive tiredness, dry skin, constipation, and hair loss.

A final step in the definition of "mild postpartum hypothyroidism" was taken by C. C. Hayslip and coworkers (1988) at Walter Reed Army Medical Center. Blood was drawn from 1,034 consecutive obstetrical patients on the second day postpartum. Seventy-two, or 7 percent, were found seropositive to antimicrosomal antibodies. Of these, thirty-five were given an intensive thyroid work-up at three to six months postpartum. They were then separated into two groups: seventeen who were determined to be hypothyroid and eighteen who were eu-thyroid. Psychological evaluation was then done by questionnaire and by a trained interviewer who had not been apprised of the laboratory results. The hypothyroid group was significantly higher in a diagnosis of depression (9 to 0). Symptoms in which the hypothyroid group was significantly high were impairment of concentration, impairment of memory, and carelessness, i.e., frequently making mistakes. Other symptoms in which the hypothyroid group scored high were resting fatigue, inability to complete work, cold intolerance, nervousness, and nightmares. These symptoms, together with those already noted by Evered, are remarkably similar to those of postpartum depression.

With the discovery of a serum thyroxine fall-off from a fairly common puerperal immune reaction, it is apparent that two independent mechanisms may act to lower serum thyroxine and produce depressive symptoms after childbearing. One, immune thyroiditis, is primary. The other is secondary to a sluggish postpartum pituitary, a mechanism described later in this chapter. These are not necessarily either-or mechanisms; they could be additive. A practical conclusion from the discovery of the postpartum autoimmune mechanism for inducing postpartum hypothyroidism is that greater consideration should be given to the thyroid in all instances of late depression after childbearing. Another implication is that assessment of the postpartum thyroid state is a difficult task which is not accomplished by a single test at a single moment in time.

The Adrenal Cortex

Cortisol is a hormone of the adrenal cortex essential to many life processes. When cortisol is lacking many kinds of illness may develop, including acute psychotic reactions. The drug cortisone, an analogue of cortisol, became available in 1949. Its remarkable efficacy for treatment of many illnesses was soon recognized, and cortisone was used extensively, often in very large doses. Unfortunately, many toxic reactions developed. When cortisone was discontinued, psychotic reactions from adrenal insufficiency occurred frequently.

The internist Ione Railton saw many cases of psychosis associated with adrenal insufficiency and cortisone withdrawal when she was a resident at the University of California, San Francisco (UCSF) in the 1950s. For the most part, these psychoses were treated by medical services, since the essential element of treatment was to provide just enough of a cortisol analogue to hold the psychosis in check. After Doctor Railton's residency, she received a fellowship to work on the psychiatric service, saw a few cases of early postpartum illness, and immediately noticed a striking resemblance to the psychoses induced by cortisone withdrawal. Patients exhibited confusion, hallucinations, and a remarkable tendency for symptoms to change, exacerbate, and go into temporary remission. Aided by the endocrinologist Peter Forsham, she worked out a program to test the apparent similarity to the cortisone-withdrawal psychoses. Small doses of prednisolone, an analogue of cortisol, were given to the postpartum cases. Railton's study included sixteen test cases and a control group of sixteen patients who were fairly comparable to the experimental group. The prednisolone, 10 mg two times per day for two to three weeks, appeared to be a very effective regimen that decreased the severity of symptoms and shortened the illness duration substantially (Railton 1961).

There was no response to this paper. Railton returned to medicine and became associate clinical professor of medicine at UCSF. In 1984 she reported to the Marcé Society on ten additional cases treated successfully with prednisolone (Railton 1984). She died in 1986, leaving what I believe may be the most important single contribution to the treatment of postpartum psychosis of this century. Her experimental work was done almost thirty years ago. Because the use of any cortisol analogue involves an element of risk and a requirement of medical judgment, I believe that her findings should be verified and that the limits of drug use should be spelled out. Railton's discovery does fit snugly into the overall picture puzzle of postpartum illness as the next section on the pituitary gland shows.

The Pituitary Gland

The Swiss psychiatrist V. S. Bürgi addressed the problem of physical signs and symptoms in postpartum psychiatric patients who failed to recover and had been ill for a long period of time (Bürgi 1954). He recalled that Marcé had studied patients of this kind and had noted the following: weakness, pallor, anemia, gastrointestinal disorders, excessive sweating, menstrual absence or irregularity, and "poor circulation." From his own observations, Bürgi added these signs and symptoms: headache, tiredness, insomnia, excessive sleepiness, dizziness, increase in blood pressure, hair loss, skin changes, especially dryness of the skin, peripheral edema, constipation, marked changes in appetite that were reflected in body weight (either marked loss or gain), and a decrease in sexual responsiveness.

Pondering on the variety and characteristics of the observed signs and symptoms, Bürgi concluded that, together and separately, they were similar to the signs and symptoms apparent in patients who have disease of the diencephalon. (The diencephalon consists of organs derived from the posterior part of the embryonic forebrain and includes the thalamus, the hypothalamus, and part of the pituitary gland. In most definitions, the entire pituitary is included. Although it is a gland, it is adjacent to the hypothalamus and functions closely with the hypothalamus in several vital functions.)

Since the listed signs and symptoms occur in chronic cases of postpartum illness, Bürgi noted, can we not infer an affliction of the diencephalon in postpartum illness? He indicated this position succinctly in the title of his paper: "Puerperalpsychose oder Diencephalosis puerperalis?" (puerperal psychosis or disease of the diencephalon after childbearing?).

The pituitary is a small mass of glandular tissue that lies directly under the brain and just posterior to the point at which the optic nerves cross and enter the brain. The pituitary rests in a bony cavity, roughly the size of that part of the thumb under the nail, the sella turcica. The pituitary is divided into two parts. The following discussion focuses on the larger part, or anterior pituitary.

The anterior pituitary secretes more than a dozen hormones that stimulate and control the activity of many glands and processes throughout the body. Among pituitary hormones are those that stimulate the thyroid, the adrenal cortex, the organs of generation and lactation, the growth of muscles and bone, and the pigmentation of the skin. Of principal interest here is the thyroid stimulating hormone (TSH) and adrenocorticotropic hormone (ACTH).

The bony cavity in which the pituitary gland lies, the sella turcica, is open at its upper end where the pituitary is contiguous with the hypothalamus, a small mass of brain tissue. Veins that drain the hypothalamus exit directly into a network of veins which surround and permeate the anterior pituitary gland. Neurons in the hypothalamus synthesize and excrete tiny amounts of chemicals. These are picked up by capillaries in the hypothalamus and carried by small veins to the vein network in the pituitary. These chemicals from the hypothalamus are called "releasing hormones" and cause the pituitary to secrete specified hormones. Thus, thyroid-releasing hormone (TRH) signals the pituitary to discharge thyroid-stimulating hormone (TSH), which in turn activates thyroxine production by the thyroid gland.

The hypothalamus itself is a very remarkable part of the brain. With a total mass equivalent to about one teaspoonful, it is a center and relay station for many autonomic and automatic activities of the body. Among these are the bodily reactions to stress, fear, and anger and the preparation of the body to engage in intense physical activity, the fight-or-flight response. One part is a cellular mechanism that senses a deficit in cortisol, signals the pituitary through their common vein network to produce ACTH, and *this* hormone is carried by the bloodstream to the adrenal glands. The "detector" in the hypothalamus is a specialized kind of neuron that reacts to low cortisol. In reacting, it secretes the releasing hormone that stimulates the pituitary to secrete ACTH.

The hypothalamus is served by many incoming nerve pathways, such as those from the cerebral cortex, which carry messages that danger is perceived. The hypothalamus has outgoing nerve pathways that go through the autonomic nervous system to mobilize the body for vigorous physical activity, actions such as accelerating the activity of the circulatory system. These are messages carried by nerve pathways of the sympathetic nervous system.

As noted earlier, both the hypothalamus and the pituitary are frequently included as part of the diencephalon, the general area which Bürgi pointed toward in his examination of patients who had had postpartum psychiatric reactions and had failed to recover.

During the last trimester of pregnancy the pituitary gland has a marked increase in blood supply. The secretory cells of the pituitary exhibit evidence of increasing activity. The target organs, especially the adrenal glands and the thyroid increase their activity, and this is reflected in serum hormone levels that range 50 percent higher than those during the nonpregnant state. The fall toward and often beyond the averages in the nonpregnant state for serum cortisol and thyroxine is paralleled by a postpartum fall in ACTH and TSH (Tulchinsky 1980).

In 1909 the German pathologists J. Erdheim and E. Stumme published exquisite drawings of the microscopic appearance of circulatory and cellular changes in the pituitary during normal pregnancy and the puerperium (Erdheim and Stumme 1909). During the third trimester, the increase in size as well as in the number of capillaries, secretory cells, and secretory granules is very apparent. It is a striking contrast to the shrunken, pale pituitary a week after delivery, with greatly diminished cells and granules.

Morris Simmonds (1914) described a case of widespread endocrine deterioration and psychiatric symptoms that was associated with traumatic destruction of the pituitary gland. This condition, which was eventually given the name of Simmonds' disease, was reviewed extensively by Roberto Escamilla and H. S. Lisser (1962). Beginning in 1937, Professor Sheehan began to report on a condition he described as "Simmonds' disease due to postpartum necrosis of the anterior pituitary." Sheehan and many others pursued the investigation of this postpartum phenomenon for almost a half-century, and this work culminated in a remarkable book, *Post-Partum Hypopituitarism* (Sheehan and Davis 1982). Destruction of the pituitary following childbirth is known widely as Sheehan's syndrome.

The endocrinologist Roberto Escamilla was a member of the study group mentioned earlier in this chapter, and he participated in many speculative discussions regarding the etiology of postpartum psychiatric illness. He urged the study group to consider the hormonal events likely to have preceded what appeared to be a postpartum drop in thyroxine production, and he was probably responsible for an inquiry addressed in 1961 by the author to Professor Sheehan regarding the psychiatric symptoms in Sheehan's syndrome (Escamilla 1956–66). The inquiry described many of the symptoms of postpartum psychiatric illness and asked if Professor Sheehan had seen such symptoms in his cases.

Sheehan (1961) replied that his cases exhibited two varieties of symptoms:

a) The patient has a permanent apathy and indolence similar to that of a myxoedema. b) She is liable to have attacks of insanity which are often very short and transient and appear to be due to biochemical disturbances. Both these psychological conditions are cured by treatment. There is no doubt at all about the organic nature of the psychological disturbances . . . the electro-encephalographic abnormalities are really very specific.

In discussing the similarities between the psychiatric symptoms of postpartum psychiatric illness and the symptoms of postpartum hypopituitarism, Professor Sheehan suggested that they might be of similar origin, with the principal difference being that "they were seen by different eyes, those of the psychiatrist and those of the endocrinologist." Additional information implicating the pituitary gland in postpartum psychiatric illness appeared in the 1980s, and the correspondence with Professor Sheehan was resumed in 1987. Unfortunately, he suffered a fractured hip in 1987 and died in 1988. Chapter 15 of this book by Collin Davis and Mohammed Abou-Saleh, Liverpool associates of Professor Sheehan, provides extensive information regarding the psychiatric symptoms and the pathophysiology of Sheehan's syndrome.

At this point it is appropriate to note or recall several bits of information that are congruent with the hypothesis of related involvement of the thyroid and the adrenal glands, through the pituitary, in postpartum psychiatric illness:

1. The two reports of Ione Railton (1961 and 1984), indicating a therapeutic effect of prednisolone, a cortisol analogue, on early postpartum symptoms, support the hypothesis of Professor Sheehan. While experimental controls were not optimal, some weight should be attached to Railton's reputation as an unusually able observer.

2. The book by Sheehan and Davis (1982) reports details of successful treatment of postpartum hypopituitarism with a combination of thyroxine and cortisone acetate. Rapid alleviation of the psychiatric symptoms of this disorder is a notable feature of the hormonal treatment.

3. If Sheehan's syndrome, with permanent damage to the majority of pituitary cells is on a continuum with the psychiatric disorders, where the pituitary insufficiency is temporary, one might expect that there would be intermediate cases between the two. Such cases are now being found. The author has seen one, confirmed by pituitary imaging. Another case, with two well-documented episodes of postpartum psychosis, has multiple physical stigmata of Sheehan's syndrome. She has not had an adequate medical work-up because she is in jail for infanticide. Chapter 14 has a case from Japan. S. Khanna (1988) has reported a case from India.

4. While cortisol and thyroxine deficits provide the most obvious signs and symptoms of pituitary insufficiency, it might be expected that other functions or organs controlled by the pituitary might sometimes provide an indication of pituitary insufficiency. The author examined a recovered case of postpartum depression and found her to have changed from a person who tanned deeply to one who was unable to develop skin pigmentation. Susan Hickman explored this phenomenon informally with former postpartum psychiatric patients in a support group and found that it was not uncommon (personal communication 1988).

None of the above bits of information can be considered to be positive proof that a limited and usually temporary degree of pituitary insufficiency is a critical factor in the development of postpartum psychiatric symptoms. However, these and other information add credibility to a picture of hormonal pathophysiology that could have great explanatory and therapeutic utility.

The experience in Professor Sheehan's clinic indicates that when pituitary destruction is documented, thyroxine alone is only partly helpful, treatment with a cortisol analogue is only partly helpful, but that treatment with a combination of thyroxine and cortisone is very effective, even with massive destruction of the pituitary (Sheehan and Davis 1982, pages 304–7).

Hormones of the Placenta

During the last trimester of pregnancy, serum estrogen and progesterone rise to levels many times the maximum values ever registered during the nonpregnant state. Almost all of these substances are derived from the placenta, since ovarian production is arrested at this time. With the loss of the placenta, the principal secretion site is lost. The serum levels of these hormones plunge to near zero within 24 to 48 hours.

Prevention of a postpartum psychiatric reaction becomes a very serious consideration in cases where a prior postpartum episode has occurred. The risk of a recurrence is unacceptably high. Chapter 17 presents details of preventive measures, including the administration of estrogen or progesterone immediately after delivery and continuing it in decreasing doses for two to four weeks. The result is to cushion the fall of estrogen or progesterone from 24 to 48 hours to a smooth slow fall of many days or weeks.

The details and the limitations of this form of prophylaxis are not discussed here. It is pertinent to note that in the case of estrogen prophylaxis, the method with which the author has had extensive experience, the likelihood of a recurrence is markedly reduced, even with patients who are at very high risk.

If the administration of estrogen at delivery, for example, acts to prevent a postpartum psychiatric reaction, it is a simple logical step to predicate that the sudden postpartum fall of this substance may be the first step in the sequence of events that may provoke symptoms of a serious psychiatric disorder in susceptible individuals. The estrogen fall after the loss of the placenta is probably not the immediate cause of psychiatric symptoms, since these do not emerge for at least three days, sometimes much longer. Rather, it would appear that other processes must intervene, probably physiological processes, before the stimulus to psychiatric symptoms develops. The other time-consuming processes are provided in the hypothesis that models a temporary post-partum pituitary insufficiency. This may initiate an early onset of a cortisol deficit. Later on, the pituitary insufficiency may initiate a thyroxine deficit. Or the pituitary insufficiency may initiate an early cortisol deficit and a later thyroxine deficit. The earlier appearance of symptoms ascribed to cortisol deficit are accounted for by its relatively short half-life in the serum. The storage of thyroxine in the body and the serum is greater, and it is released much more slowly, smoothly.

Summary

This chapter has addressed two conflicting positions regarding psychiatric illness after childbirth. The first position, and probably the one most followed in the United States, equates the various patterns of postpartum illness with the variety of psychiatric syndromes or disorders that occur without reference to or involvement in the physiological processes of childbirth, syndromes that occur in males as well as females. The succinct statement of this position is in the *DSM-III*, the authoritative handbook of the American Psychiatric Association (1980) is, "There is no compelling evidence that postpartum psychosis is a distinct entity."

A second position holds that much information supports the contrary view, "There *is* compelling evidence that postpartum psychosis (as well as major postpartum depression) is a distinct entity."

As this second position is advanced in this chapter, a considerable number of physiological mechanisms, mostly endocrine, have been implicated. These mechanisms are not involved in the vast array of psychiatric conditions unrelated to childbearing. (There are very marginal or rare conditions in which hormonal factors are critical in nonpuerperal mental illness, for example, psychoses secondary to neoplasm or infection of the pituitary or adrenals and myxedema unrelated to pregnancy. However, the exceptions highlight the rarity of a critical hormonal factor outside postpartum psychiatric illness.

This chapter followed two parallel and related courses. One was a collection and presentation of information from sources widely separated in time, distance, and research orientation. Part of this information related to observations wherein the development of postpartum illness revealed unique abnormalities pathognomonic of endocrine pathology, mostly deficiencies. Another part of the information related to observations wherein the administration of one or another hormonal substance appeared to influence the course of postpartum illness. Hormones of the placenta, pituitary, thyroid, and adrenals each appear to have some role in postpartum illness. These hormonal factors and the reported responses are unique to postpartum illness. It follows from this information alone that postpartum disorders are unique.

As the involvement of one hormone after another in postpartum illness is implicated, another unique quality of postpartum illness is revealed: the hormonal factors appear to fit together in a pattern of relationships that extend in time from the high serum levels of the third trimester through readjustment and reequilibration toward the nonpregnant state. This process can take a year or more, and sometimes patients can reach a hormonal equilibrium that is less than optimal and produces only milder symptoms.

A simplified picture that is emerging has these contours: the high levels of many serum hormones appear to be maintained by the high levels of placenta-produced hormones, certainly estrogen. The fall of estrogen initiated by delivery sets in motion a chain of responses that eventually diminishes the trophic hormones of the anterior pituitary. Their reduction is reflected in diminished secretion by the glands that are targets of pituitary trophic hormones, notably cortisol and thyroxine, both of which are essential to proper function of cells. Substantial but not incontrovertible evidence points toward relative or absolute deficits in these substances as critical to the emergence of symptoms of postpartum psychiatric illness.

Thus, in addition to the many indications of hormonal influences in postpartum illness, there is emerging a time-related pattern of the integrated activity of hormones, in postpartum illness as well as in health. This picture of probable integrated action is a second consideration in assessment of the uniqueness of postpartum illness.

The foregoing is submitted in support of the position that there is compelling evidence that postpartum psychiatric illness is a distinct entity. Many details and applications require exploration. This book presents many details and many paths for exploration.

References

American Psychiatric Association (1952, 1980, 1987). *Diagnostic and Statistical Manual of Mental Disorders, DSM, DSM-III, DSM-III-R.* Washington, D.C.: American Psychiatric Association.

Amino, N., Miyai, K., et al. (1976). Transient hypothyroidism after delivery in autoimmune thyroiditis. *J. Clin. Endo. and Metab.,* 42:296–301. Also: Amino, N. 1984. Communication to the Marcé Society. Also see: Leading Article (editorial) 1978. Thyroid disease and pregnancy. *Br. Med. J.* 6143:977–78.

Baker, A. A. (1967). *Psychiatric Disorders in Obstetrics.* Oxford: Blackwell.

Ballachey, E. L., Campbell, D. G., Claffey, B., Escamilla, R., Footer, A. W., Hamilton, J. A., Harter, J. M., Litteral, A. B., Lyons, H. M., Overstreet, E. W., Poliac, P. P., Schaupp, Jr., L. L., Smith, G., and Voris, A. T. (1958).

Response of postpartum psychiatric symptoms to 1-triiodothyronine. *J. Clin. and Exper. Psychopath.*, 19:170.
Billig, O., and Bradley, J. D. (1946). Combined shock and corpus luteum hormone therapy. *Am. J. Psychiatr.* 102:783–87.
Boyd, Jr., D. A. (1942). Mental disorders associated with childbearing. *Am. J. Obstet. and Gynecol.*, 43:148–65, 335–48.
Bürgi, V. S. (1954). Puerperalpsychose oder Diencephalosis puerperalis? *Schweiz. Med. Wochenschr.* 84:1222–25.
Christian, E. P. (1889). What is puerperal mania and what constitutes puerperal insanity? *Ann. Gynaecol.* 2:449–57.
Dalton, K. (1980, 1988). *Depression after Childbirth: How to Recognize and Treat Postnatal Illness.* London: Oxford University Press, 1988. Progesterone prophylaxis used successfully in postnatal depression. *The Practitioner* 229:507–8, 1985.
Danowski, T. S., et al. (1953). Is pregnancy followed by relative hypothyroidism? *Am. J. Obstet. and Gynecol.* 65:77–80.
Davidson, G. M. (1936). Concerning schizophrenia and manic-depressive psychoses associated with childbirth. *Am. J. Psychiatr.* 92:1331–46.
Erdheim, J., and Stumme, E. (1909). Über die Schwangerschaftsveränderung der Hypophyse. *Beitr. Pathol. Anat. (Zeigler)* 46:1–132.
Escamilla, R. (1956–66). Personal communication with author.
Evans, J. J., Sin, I. L., et al. (1987). Estrogen-induced transcortin increase and progesterone and cortisol interactions. *Ann. Clin. Lab. Sci.* 17:101–5.
Evered, D., Ormiston, B. J., et al. (1973). Grades of hypothyroidism. *Br. Med. J.* 1:657–62.
Gull, W. W. (1874). On a cretinoid state supervening in adult life in women. *Trans. Clin. Soc. London* 7:18–85.
Hamilton, J. A. (1962). *Postpartum Psychiatric Problems.* St. Louis: C. V. Mosby.
———. (1967). Puerperal psychoses. In J. J. Sciarra (Ed.): *Gynecology and Obstetrics.* Hagerstown, MD: Harper and Row.
Hayslip, C. C., Fein, H. G., et al. (1988). The value of serum antimicrosomal antibody testing in screening for symptomatic postpartum thyroid dysfunction. *Am. J. Obstet. and Gynecol.* 159(1):203–9.
Hickman, S. (1988). Personal Communication.
Karnosh, L. J., and Hope, J. M. (1937). Puerperal psychoses and their sequelae. *Am. J. Psychiatr.* 94:537–50.
Khanna, S. A., Ammini, S., Saxena, D., et al. (1988). Hypopituitarism presenting as delirium. *Int. J. Psychiatr. Med.* 18:89–92.
Kilpatrick, E., and Tiebout, H. M. (1926). A study of psychoses occurring in relationship to childbirth. *Am. J. Psychiatr.* 6:145–59.
Lisser, H. S., and Escamilla, R. F. (1962). *Atlas of Clinical Endocrinology.* 2d. ed. St. Louis: Mosby.
Marcé, L. V. (1858). *Traité de la folie des femmes enceintes, des nouvelles accouchées et des nourrices.* Paris: J. B. Baillière et Fils.
———. *Traité pratique des maladies mentales.* Paris: J. B. Baillière et Fils.
Meyer, A. (1925). The evolution of the dementia praecox concept. In E. C. Winters (Ed.), *The Collected Papers of Adolf Meyer,* Vol. 2. Baltimore: Johns Hopkins University Press.
Ord, W. M. (1888). Report of a committee of the Clinical Society of London to investigate the subject of myxœdema. *Trans. Clin. Soc. London (Suppl.)*, 21:1–215.

Page, E. (1959). Personal communication. Also: Dodek, S. M. (1961). Personal communication.

Railton, I. E. (1961, 1984). The use of corticoids in postpartum depression. *J. Am. Med. Women's Assoc.* 16:450–52, 1961. The use of prednisolone for postpartum psychiatric problems. Report to the Marcé Society, 1984.

Sheehan, H. L. (1961, 1987). Personal communications.

Sheehan, H. L., and Davis, J. C. (1982). *Post-Partum Hypopituitarism.* Springfield, IL: C. C. Thomas.

Simmonds, M. (1914). Über hypophysischevund mit todlichem Aufgang. *Deutsche med. Wehnschr.* 40:322–23.

Stössner, K. (1910). Ein Fall von Myxödem im Anschluss an Gravidität. *München Med. Wochenschr.* 57:2531–33.

Strecker, E. A., and Ebaugh, F. G. (1926, 1940). Psychoses occurring during the puerperium. *Arch. Neurol. and Psychiatr.* 15:239–52.

Tulchinsky, D. (1980). The postpartum period. In D. Tulchinsky and K. J. Ryan (Eds.), *Maternal-Fetal Endocrinology.* Philadelphia: W. B. Saunders.

Chapter 3
The Problem of Terminology

James Alexander Hamilton, Patricia Neel
Harberger, and Barbara L. Parry

The medical records of patients hospitalized for psychiatric illness after childbearing often reveal a striking lack of uniformity in the terms used for the description and the diagnosis of these patients. From one page to the next, the same patient may appear to be suffering from a half-dozen or more maladies. Among the officially approved diagnoses are schizophreniform disorder, schizoaffective disorder, atypical psychosis, bipolar disorder—manic, bipolar disorder—depressed, major depressive disorder, organic mood disorder, and organic mental disorder not otherwise specified. When current professional jargon intrudes upon official terminology, the following designations appear on medical charts: puerperal psychosis, postpartum psychosis, and postpartum depression (PPD). Terms with wide acceptance in the general language appear occasionally: postpartum blues, maternity blues, postnatal depression, and even the abbreviation PPD. With all of these words running freely through hospital charts, the casual observer might suspect that the nomenclature of psychiatric illness after childbearing is in a state of chaos.

Problems exist, but they are not insoluble. This chapter proposes some solutions for the communication problem. Other rational solutions are possible. The authors of chapters in this book are not confined to the terms developed in this chapter, but in some instances their chosen terminology may be tied to the proposed solutions by footnotes.

Historical events have contributed to the present situation, and it is appropriate to review some of them. The art of medical communication goes back over 300 years. In 1676 the great English physician Thomas Sydenham established principles of disease study and nomenclature by insisting, in his *Medical Observations,* that the correct delineation of a disease required study of its cause, if known, its onset, its course (with the progression of symptoms), treatments which have been found effective, and the termination of the disease (Sydenham 1763). Naming by pathophysiological causes was preferred, but with a cause undetermined, it was urged that names be used which would facilitate identification of diseases. Sydenham's concept of longitudinal analysis was applied to postpartum psychiatric illnesses by J.E.D. Esquirol (1838), L. V. Marcé (1858) and many other early investigators. The leading twentieth-century exponent of longitudinal analysis of postpartum illness is Bernhard Pauliekhoff of Münster (Pauliekhoff 1964). Professor Pauliekhoff is the author of Chapter 18 of this book.

The variegated nomenclature of current official terminology is the result of an effort to name and classify postpartum illnesses according to their presenting symptoms, a snapshot approach usually made on the basis of the symptoms first seen, as contrasted with names that represent longitudinal analysis. One of the unique qualities of postpartum illness is the multiplicity of symptoms and symptom constellations that manifest themselves and the tendency of these presentations to change. The diversity of official terms reflects this quality. The encroachment of professional jargon in terms such as "puerperal psychosis" represents an effort of professionals to communicate meaningfully with each other and with patients. The further encroachment of popular usage, such as "postpartum depression," represents an effort on the part of the public and the media to find a general term.

Many reasons can be adduced to explain the 1952 decision to ordain a nomenclature based on predominant presenting symptoms (American Psychiatric Association 1952). One reason was that psychiatrists early in this century were anxious to develop some kind of an official classification system for mental illnesses. Unlike the situation in general medicine, where causes or pathophysiology were accessible keys to classification, it was not possible to determine specific causes of most mental illnesses. The symptom-pattern solution was conceived as a substitute. Schizophrenia had patterns of thinking aberrations; mania and depression had patterns of mood aberrations; organic psychoses had confusion, delirium, hallucinations, and transitory delusions. Patients with psychiatric illnesses after childbearing could have any or all of these constellations of symptoms, or they could jump from one pattern to another.

Postpartum patients were a threat to the system of classification, or so it appeared. A simple solution was to expunge the term "postpartum" and its synonyms from the official lexicon and require that these patients be classified in an orderly manner according to predominant symptoms at the time of examination. The result of this decision is a disaster for communication. Even in professional meetings, the term "depression" is sometimes used to designate a major psychiatric illness that requires psychiatric hospitalization, sometimes to designate the malaise that troubles one woman in ten after childbearing.

Effective communication between health professionals, adequate treatment of patients, and productive research depend on the availability of a realistic and accurate nomenclature. The fourth edition of the *Diagnostic and Statistical Manual of Mental Disorders* is due in 1993 or 1994. Whether an adequate or acceptable system of nomenclature can be adopted in time for this edition is not certain. A task force charged with editing *DSM-IV* must be satisfied. It is quite possible that no significant change in the official nomenclature of postpartum illness will be in operation before the twenty-first century.

The need for a meaningful vocabulary for communication is urgent. This chapter presents a suggested terminology that reflects current knowledge of the disorders and syndromes that occur after childbearing. The terminology rests partly on categories that were distinguished during the nineteenth century and partly on professional jargon. It is also appropriate for use with patients, relatives of patients, and the public as well as in courts of law.

A basic feature of this terminology is that it ties the diagnosis of patients into the postpartum state and thereby establishes a distinction between postpartum patients and those who are victims of chronic "functional" mental illness. This alerts physicians to the facts that they are dealing with acute illnesses which have a characteristic onset, course, and termination; that the illnesses have an excellent prognosis; and that they have unique hazards and unique therapeutic opportunities.

The Major Disorders

Postpartum Psychotic Depression

This is very close to the *folie des nouvelles accouchées* of Esquirol (1838) and Marcé (1858).

The onset of *postpartum psychotic depression* occurs usually between the third and the fifteenth day after delivery. It begins with confusion, anxiety, and insomnia and often moves quickly to delirium. Hallucinations and transitory delusions are frequent. This clinical picture may give way to periods of deep depression. The disorder is remarkable for its mercurial changeability, and lucid intervals may give a false impression of recovery.

Some cases of *postpartum psychotic depression* recover completely after a few days or weeks. Others exhibit a gradual diminution of their symptoms and evolve into a state where the predominant mood is mild to moderate depression, usually with some confusion. However, these patients occasionally exhibit an exacerbation of psychotic thinking and behavior that has the florid agitation, hallucinations, and delusions of the disorder early in the puerperium. These exacerbations may occur many weeks or months after delivery.

Two other terms are used in the professional jargon for *postpartum psychotic depression*: "postpartum psychosis" and "puerperal psychosis." Both are acceptable, and their meanings are understood by knowledgeable professionals, but both have limitations. Postpartum psychosis leaves out the important depressive component that is a prominent feature of the disorders. Puerperal psychosis has the limitation of using an adjective that implies a period which continues for only about six weeks after delivery. This can cause problems if a legal or health insurance issue arises when the patient is several months after delivery.

Neither the term "postpartum psychosis" nor "puerperal psychosis" is totally misleading, as are some names that are attached to this disorder. The suggested alternative, *postpartum psychotic depression*, equally unofficial, is recommended because it is more accurate and less subject to misinterpretation.

Major Postpartum Depression

This disorder is a slowly increasing depression of mood that begins after the third week postpartum. The mood changes are often associated with markedly diminished energy and multiple physical symptoms and signs. The patient often believes that she is a failure at motherhood, and this may be associated with a grave suicidal risk.

When Marcé's case histories of "folie des nourrices" are examined, some fall into this category. Others, with depression mixed with psychotic thinking or behavior, would fit the "postpartum psychotic depression" category. The criterion we propose as critical to distinguish the two groups is the presence or absence of definite psychotic thinking at any stage of the illness. The obsession of failure, which may come close to a delusion in some cases of postpartum depression, is not regarded as fulfilling the criterion of psychosis.

The severity of major postpartum depression may be assessed as mild, moderate, or severe. The severe category includes mainly those patients who should be cared for in a hospital with psychiatric controls. Lesser categories of severity are used for patients who are deemed appropriate for outpatient care.

The depressed patients seen and hospitalized by Esquirol and Marcé as well as those treated by present-day psychiatrists are products of a selective process whereby the patient or somebody else, perhaps a physician, reacts to symptoms, complaints, or behavior, and this leads to psychiatric referral. In other words, somebody has feared that the patient is sick. The total number of depression referrals who are hospitalized is less than one in one thousand births, since this figure includes psychoses as well as depressions. There is no good estimate of the number of mild and moderate major postpartum depressions who are treated as outpatients. However, it seems unlikely that they would exceed one in one hundred births, well over ten times the incidence of the severe cases.

In recent years, the designation "postpartum depression" has been applied to another population: those members of a cross-section obstetrical population who make certain affirmative answers to questions on a questionnaire or formal interview. Those designated as depressed comprise 10 percent or more of most obstetrical populations which have been studied. These individuals with "test-derived" postpartum depressions are therefore at least one order of magnitude more numerous than the clinically derived cases of postpartum depression (O'Hara and Zekoski 1988).

Are the foregoing samples comparable? Are the test-selected cases on a continuum with the clinically derived depressions? Are conclusions derived from the study of test-selected depressions applicable to clinically derived depressions? The evidence that might provide answers to these questions is not in. This is an important reason for having a special designation for patients who come to health professionals for help.

The second development that pertains to the naming of clinically derived cases of depression after childbearing is the recent widespread interest in postpartum illness. With this interest and subsequent media coverage, the term "postpartum depression" has been applied to all varieties of symptoms and illnesses, from severe psychosis to transitory fluctuations of mood. If the identity of clinically derived or medically defined illness is to be preserved, the term major postpartum depression, or a meaningful equivalent, is desirable.

Differential Diagnosis

Important differences distinguish *postpartum psychotic depression* from major postpartum depression. The first is the time of onset, and this difference was made the basis for Marcé's different names. *Postpartum psychotic depression* usually begins acutely, within the first fortnight, while major postpartum depression begins insidiously after two or three weeks. The outstanding feature of the former is its aberrations of consciousness, its psychotic episodes. Also, the psychosis is remarkably mercurial and unpredictable. The major postpartum depression is more consistent and steady. Psychotic thinking is absent. Physical complaints are prominent. Confusion is prominent in both disorders, but more striking with the psychotic episodes.

There are mixtures of these two disorders. Cases may begin as psychoses and evolve to conditions in which the clinical picture is a major depression. The occurrence of mixtures makes for disagreement regarding the relative incidence of the two disorders.

Do these mixtures negate the need for separating them as two disorders? An important argument for separation is that the psychosis, once identified, carries with it the otherwise poorly predictable hazard of injury to the infant as well as to the new mother. There is a real suicide hazard with major depression, but it is a hazard more easily identified. Once *postpartum psychotic depression* has been identified, it is prudent to hold this diagnosis throughout the course of the illness.

Still another reason for separating the disorders in nomenclatures is that their onsets and courses suggest different etiologies. It is necessary to think about etiologies if specific pharmacotherapy is ever to be entertained as a goal.

Maternity Blues

This is a term for the tearful, anxious, sleepless, exhausted episodes occurring in 30 to 80 percent of all new mothers, usually three to ten days after childbearing. It lasts from a few hours to a few days. Because of its high incidence, it is regarded by many as a normal event of the puerperium.

A remarkable feature of maternity blues is the fact that its timing of onset and its early symptoms are very much like those of *postpartum psychotic depression.* Many cases of the latter disorder are first dismissed as maternity blues. Continued worsening of symptoms after one or two days is a signal that the serious disorder is a possibility. Jan Campbell describes maternity blues in Chapter 7 and reviews its tantalizing clues regarding physiological mechanisms. She advances the position that this syndrome may be a fortuitous model for testing hypotheses regarding the mechanisms of *postpartum psychotic depression.*

Postpartum Panic Disorder

Discrete periods of severe anxiety during the puerperium are usually described as symptoms associated with affective or psychotic disorders.

Sometimes this panic syndrom appears in isolation, without either psychotic or affective syndromes. At other times patients recall that the first indications of their illness were panic attacks without any known stimulus. Patients have reported their own inferences that later disturbances of mood or thinking were "caused by" apprehensiveness or preoccupation incidental to their efforts to find an explanation for the panic attacks.

The syndrome of panic attacks after childbearing has been described by Metz and coworkers (1988) who suggest that therapeutic goals may be best achieved by regarding this condition as a separate entity—postpartum panic disorder.

Definitions

A few terms, used frequently in this book, will be defined. The definitions are congruent with those of most medical dictionaries and the *DSM-III*.

A "symptom" is a complaint or phenomenon that arises from a particular condition and serves as an indicator of that condition. A "sign" is an objective indication of a disease process. The word "symptom" is often used to cover both symptoms and signs. A "syndrome" is a pattern of symptoms and/or signs that often go together and constitute a recognizable condition. The term "syndrome" is less specific than "disorder" or "disease." A disorder or a disease may have more than one syndrome. The term "disease" implies a knowledge of cause and/or pathophysiological process. The term "disorder" is used frequently to designate psychiatric conditions whose etiology is not yet determined. This book adheres to the practice of using "disorder" for the two major postpartum conditions, *postpartum psychotic depression* and *major postpartum depression*.

This chapter notes a tradition in general medicine to identify disorders by etiology or by the longitudinal course of illness, a practice which follows the seventeenth-century suggestion of Thomas Sydenham. The current official names for psychiatric illness after childbirth follow neither etiology nor the course of illness. It is suggested in this chapter that both clinicians and patients have been confused by the official terminology. Physicians with wide experience in treatment of these conditions report that the provision of childbirth-related names for these disorders has a strong, positive therapeutic effect on patients; confusion regarding nomenclature has an adverse effect (see Chapters 6, 8, and 9). In Chapters 21 and 22 it is suggested that the present terminology may confuse the criminal justice community, often with sacrifices of the rights and interests of ill women. Chapter 23 indicates how the official terminology may deprive many patients of insurance coverage to which they are entitled by their insurance policies and the law. Part III, "The Organic Matrix," provides information that pertains to etiology. Chapters 18 and 19 present longitudinal descriptions of the two major disorders. The disorder names suggested in the present chapter were developed after a consideration of all these matters.

References

American Psychiatric Association (1952, 1980, 1987). *Diagnostic and Statistical Manual of Mental Disorders, DSM, DSM-III, DSM-III-R.* Washington, DC: American Psychiatric Association.

Esquirol, J.E.D. (1838). *Des maladies mentales considérées sous les rapports medical, hygiénique et médico-légal,* Vol. 1. Paris: J. B. Baillière et Fils.

Marcé, L. V. (1858). *Traité de la folie des femmes enceintes, des nouvelles accouchées et des nourrices.* Paris: J. B. Baillière et Fils.

Metz, A., Sichel, D. A., et al. (1988). Postpartum panic disorder. *J. Clin. Psychiatr.* 49:278–79.

O'Hara, M. W., and Zekoski, E. M. (1988). Postpartum depression: A comprehensive review. In R. Kumar and I. F. Brockington (Eds.), *Motherhood and Mental Illness.* London: Butterworth.

Pauleikhoff, N. (1964). *Seelische Störungen in der Schwangerschaft und nach der Geburt.* Stuttgart: Ferdinand Enke.

Sydenham, T. (1763). *The Entire Works of Dr. Thomas Sydenham—Newly Made English from the Originals,* 5th ed. John Swan, Translator. London: R. Case. (Stanford Historical Collection).

Chapter 4
Cries for Help

Patricia Neel Harberger, Nancy Gleason
Berchtold, and Jane Israel Honikman

Introduction

Before the prevention or treatment of postpartum psychiatric illness is
possible, first must come the realization that, in fact, women and their
loved ones cry out for help. Unfortunately, such pleas often go un-
noticed until significant damage has occurred. In an arena immobilized by the stigma of mental illness, the normal communication
process breaks down.

Not infrequently, the health community fails to hear women's cries
for help. Interactions between caregiver and care-receiver become
distorted because of misinformation and denial by both parties, and
there is a failure to regard critical messages. Questions asked, responses given, and decisions made by uninformed persons can reinforce the woman's silence, perpetuate her isolation, and facilitate
deterioration in her condition (Gondolf 1988).

The authors of this chapter suggest that such damaging interactions
can be avoided, that women's messages can be heard and appropriate
steps taken to promote healthy postpartum development for the family. For those who are concerned there exists an exciting challenge. One
must anticipate that families may be experiencing difficulty and view
their method of communication as a *unique language*.

Cries for help are usually transmitted "in code." The new mother,
who is supposed to be enjoying her baby, has no explanation for what is
happening to her. She fears the worst and is ashamed. Confused and
frightened, she may seek help *through* her baby (Margison 1982, Trout
1985, 1987, Ziporyn 1984, page 2067). It is the obligation of those in a
position to hear the cries to "decode" them, to appraise correctly what
is happening, and to take appropriate action. Unnecessary heartache

TABLE 4.1. Prenatal suggestions.

1. Encourage realistic expectations.
2. Assess risk status.
3. Provide for adequate support (instrumental and emotional).
4. Consider prophylaxis for high-risk women.
5. Maintain open communication.

and sometimes tragedy can be avoided by learning the *language* illustrated in this chapter, by providing an atmosphere that promotes trust and acceptance, and by asking a few open-ended questions. Family members, friends, physicians, nurses, social workers, and members of the clergy can make important contributions to creating a healthy, supportive environment for the new mother and her child.

Having worked with women and their families over a period of several years, the authors have been in a position to hear the cries, to be advocates for and to educate couples, and to influence community efforts that promote mental health in the postpartum period. They have established support groups and "warm lines," both at the local level and nationally, which provide immediate support for women who are experiencing emotional problems as well as their families.

A new mother may refer herself or become associated with a support group via referral from a physician, nurse, friend, or social service agency representative. Often she or a relative telephones a "warm line" whereby there is contact with an informed listener, an individual who is familiar with postpartum illness. Through the call, support and reassurance are given, an individual conference is arranged, information regarding a support group is shared or a referral is made to a professional who has been successful in treating postpartum disorders.

In this chapter, the experiences of new mothers are described in their own words. Common responses of family members as well as professionals are illustrated. The quotations are reports of firsthand communication and convey the vividness, urgency, and level of detail that go beyond ordinary clinical descriptions of illness. Recommendations are also made to aid in early recognition of postpartum emotional difficulties thereby allowing for early intervention before problems reach crisis proportion (Tables 4.1 and 4.2).

The Scope of the Problem

One component of the problem involves large numbers of women with a relatively mild illness which, when recognized, is easily treated. The second involves a relatively small number of women with a severe

TABLE 4.2. Seven simple postnatal suggestions.

1. Expect distress to occur.
2. Create a safe environment for expression.
3. Ask open-ended questions.
4. Listen for "coded messages."
5. Communicate hope.
6. Refer appropriately.
7. Provide close follow-up.

illness, also easily treated when recognized in time. Evidence suggests that the former may be a "little sister" of the latter (Hamilton 1989, Ziporyn 1984) (see also Chapters 3, 7, 14, 15, and 19). Both are affected by numerous biological, psychological, and social factors and can be viewed on a continuum (Figure 4.1). The duration and prognosis of both are dependent upon recognition of the cries for help. One of the major challenges in dealing with postpartum psychiatric illness has been early recognition. The aspiration of this chapter is to make that job easier.

Hearing the Cries

Motherhood is expected to come naturally. When the umbilical cord is cut and the baby passes into the new parents' eager arms, maternal aptitude is expected to flow like breast milk. In fact, just as there are physical and psychosocial barriers to free-flowing breast milk, so there are barriers to the ease of adjusting to parenthood.

During the early weeks and months after birth, the newborn infant is fussed over by family and scrutinized by health professionals. Unfortunately, the mother's condition is often overlooked. Predictably, she will be tired. The expectation is that she will be awakened throughout the night and early each morning. Typically, she has many responsibilities beyond the care of the new baby. Clearly, she needs help with the maintenance of the home and infant feedings, and critical to her ability to function, she needs good nutrition for herself. Adequate help and nutrition, however, may not come. In the United States, new mothers leave the hospital within the first 24 to 72 hours following birth and are not seen again by a health professional for six weeks. In our highly mobile society, young families have often moved away from their relatives and the network of traditional helpers is unavailable. The natural mechanism for protecting and monitoring the new mother's health is missing (Stern and Kruckman 1983, Paykel et al. 1980, O'Hara et al. 1983, Cutrona 1982, Boston Women's Health Book Collective 1984).

LESSER SEVERITY → GREATER SEVERITY

"Maternity Blues" ("Baby Blues")	Postnatal Depression (Mild–Moderate Postpartum Depression) (Postpartum Panic Disorder)*	Major Postpartum Depression (Severe Postpartum Depression)	Postpartum Psychosis (Puerperal Psychosis)	Postpartum Psychotic Depression (Pauliekhoff's Amentia)
Affects 50–85%	Affects 10–20%	(Affects 1 in 3 or 4 with a history of a previous episode)	Affects 0.1%–0.2%	
Minimal dysfunction	Moderate dysfunction		Maximal dysfunction	
Self-limiting				
Onset Day 3–10	Insidious development	Slow onset	Early onset (May be confused with "baby blues")	Combined qualities of both postpartum psychosis and major postpartum depression
	Numerous physical signs and symptoms	Numerous physical signs and symptoms		
	Often unrecognized	Rapid improvement may be followed by relapse	Vivid hallucinations and delusions	Episodes of hallucinations and delusions (often concealed) alternate with periods of apparent lucidity
	Deleterious effect on maternal-child relationship, marriage, and family life	Grave suicidal concerns	Mercurial changeability	
	Hangs on interminably			
Enlightened support of family and friends effective		Skilled professional intervention vital		
Help-seeking behavior discouraged by social pressure	Help-seeking behavior often discouraged and trivialized		Help-seeking behavior discouraged by stigma of mental illness and severe dysfunction	
Potential for violence low			Potential for violence high (suicide and infanticide)	
Excellent prognosis	Excellent prognosis with recognition and treatment	Excellent prognosis with recognition and treatment	Excellent prognosis with recognition and treatment	
Self-limiting				

*Postpartum panic disorder is atypical in that symptoms are primarily anxiety and fear rather than depression. Development may not be insidious, and the incidence is unknown.

Deterioration in a new mother's condition and her need for help cannot be detected if she is caring for her infant, alone. Thus, the mobility of our modern society is directly related to the recognition of postpartum emotional disorders.

Ours is an age where stoic independence is prized. Women struggling to fulfill perceived high expectations of their ability to handle motherhood with ease may be reluctant to seek help. In case upon case, however, women reveal that, early on, they sense that "something is wrong." A vague and nameless uneasiness is experienced as a prodrome to further difficulty. Interestingly, sleep disturbances in the absence of pain or a crying baby has been found to be a very common early warning. However, women experiencing postpartum distress often have great difficulty articulating their problem.

You feel this terrible uncertainty. Is this the way all new mothers feel? Since this is my first child, I'm not sure what is normal. I just don't feel like me. *Something is wrong.* It is so different from what I expected.
—Postpartum depression support group participant (1988)

The first signs of postpartum psychiatric illness may appear immediately after birth, or weeks or even months later. If left unrecognized and untreated, the woman's illness may continue for years. Postpartum emotional problems test the strength of marriages. They destroy lives, and women who might otherwise recover quickly may become chronically depressed (Holden et al. 1989, Timmerman 1987, Kruckman and Asmann-Finch 1986 page xv, Ziporyn 1984, page 2062).

Twenty-five years ago, I went through postpartum depression. That time of my life still haunts me. I never had any more children for fear it would happen again.
—Fifty-year-old physician (1987)

She was such a beautiful baby, as were her two brothers. But I was so depressed. Really, it has gone on for years. There was no one I felt could understand or help me. I could barely function after each baby was born. I had never had a problem before. My husband finally gave up, and divorced me after our third. I know Laura's problems exist because I was such a terrible mother when she was little!
—Mother of a 13-year-old, being treated for an eating disorder in a family therapy session (1988)

Ignoring the cries for help can result in tragedy, and not always in the form of headline-grabbing stories involving maternal suicide or infanticide. Less recognizable damage may occur that leaves lasting scars on the woman, her marriage, the baby, and other relationships (Cogill et al. 1986, Robson 1980, Brockington and Kumar 1982, Atkinson and Atkinson 1983, Margison 1982, Richman 1976, Bagedahl-

Strindlund 1987, O'Hara et al. 1989, Kumar et al. 1984, Weissman et al. 1984, Caplan et al. 1988, Murray 1988, Field 1984, Harvard Medical School Mental Health Letter 1989).

Getting help, especially having other women to talk with has saved my life, our marriage, and my sanity. My family just doesn't understand. Our doctor never asks how I am doing.
> —Postpartum depression support group participant (1986)

This thing that's happening to me is destroying our marriage. My husband keeps telling me to snap out of it . . . but I can't!
> —Warm Line telephone call (1988)

The myth of blissful parenthood is ingrained in our society. Anxiety and depression after the birth of a baby is unacceptable. Often, it seems the stigma of mental illness creates insurmountable barriers to recognition and treatment.

We can't talk about that in childbirth classes . . . it's so rare . . . it will scare everyone . . . they'll think they're going to get it. . . . Besides, couples don't want to hear about negative things.
> —Supervisor of prenatal classes in a teaching hospital (1987)

If early recognition is to occur, postpartum emotional health issues must be discussed in childbirth classes and during obstetrical office visits. Information on warning signs for a variety of birth-related problems such as abruptio placenta, postpartum hemorrhage, and sepsis has long been given to expectant mothers. Why not the spectrum of postpartum emotional responses? Childbirth educators and others have a responsibility to apprise expectant couples of these concerns. In addition, screening measures could be administered routinely during visits to the obstetrician, nurse-midwife, family physician, or pediatrician (Cox et al. 1987, Kumar et al. 1984).

I feel like everyone expects me to be happy. How can I tell them I'm not when I have such a good baby? I don't understand what's wrong with me.
> —Support group participant (1989)

Recognizing the Clues

Emotional reactions following childbirth range from the most mild form of "baby blues" to the more serious symptoms that include bizarre delusions, obsessions, and hallucinations (See Table 4.3).

Often women who are suffering conceal their thoughts and are determined not to tell anyone. Sneddon emphasizes caution regarding the so-called "smiling depression." (See Sneddon, Chapter 8.)

Traditionally, physical illness has been viewed as an acceptable rea-

TABLE 4.3. Symptoms suggestive of postpartum psychiatric illness.

Crying for no apparent reason which continues beyond one week.
Inability to sleep.
Loss of appetite or overeating.
Extreme anxiety regarding the baby's health or safety.
Feelings of inadequacy, numbness, helplessness, and profound inexplicable sadness.
Exaggerated mood swings.
Lack of feeling for the baby or others.
Inability to care for the baby.
Fear of being alone.
Confusion.
Inability to concentrate.
Feeling overwhelmed and unable to make decisions.
Inability to sit still, talking incessantly.
Physical complaints which suggest a panic attack.
Uncharacteristic silence and reclusiveness.
Experiencing bizarre thoughts or frightening dreams.

son for seeking help. Physical symptoms are worthy of special attention and follow-up and should not be taken lightly. They may suggest an organic basis for a woman's complaints. Although physical symptoms can be the woman's "ticket to enter the theater" the emotional upheaval being experienced by a new mother can easily be overlooked as conscientious health professionals proceed to investigate an array of physical complaints to the exclusion of her feelings. Sophisticated technological evaluations may miss what an informed and sensitive history-taker may decipher.

The intensity of physical signs and symptoms is particularly striking in cases of postpartum panic disorder described by Metz and coworkers (1988). (See Chapters 3, 9, and 17.)

What is wrong with me?! I feel like my whole body is in a panic. My heart is pounding out of my chest. I can't sit still. I have no appetite. My hair is falling out. I can't think straight. I feel confused. I start to change the baby, and then walk off before I even get his diaper on. I can't sleep. I can't make decisions. I have never experienced anything like this before. A year ago, I was a competent attorney!

—"Warm-line" telephone call (1985)

I felt like someone was walking on my chest. I couldn't breathe. I was sure I was going to have a heart attack. The implication was that it was all in my head— but it wasn't! It was real!

—Support group participant (1989)

Uncharacteristic silence or reclusiveness on the part of an ordinarily vivacious woman can be a relevant piece of the puzzle.

I didn't want anyone to know I was so strangely sad—after all—I had a beautiful little girl, a lovely home, and a successful husband. What did I have to be depressed about?! So I stayed to myself, at home. I didn't go anywhere for a couple of months, and I didn't want anyone to visit. I just tried to hide myself from the world and hoped it would get better . . . but it got worse.
—Lamaze class participant pregnant with second child (1982)

Excessive concern about the baby's health can be another clue.

After six years of infertility, I don't want to screw up but *I feel so nervous.* I keep calling the pediatrician about the baby, but *I guess I'm really worried about me.*
—Warm line telephone call (1989)

An infant's failure to thrive may result from emotional deprivation and can be a warning sign that the mother is experiencing postpartum distress. Her apparent detachment or lack of interest in her child should not be judged harshly but rather seen as an indication that she may be ill and unable to function. The unspoken message may be that she seriously doubts her ability as a mother. Although easily misinterpreted as "bad mom" behavior, judgmental remarks serve only to reinforce her poor self-image. It is imperative that a child who is not thriving be treated from a family systems perspective.

Something is going on with this mother I am seeing in the clinic. I can't put my finger on it. I have her coming in every week because the baby isn't gaining weight. *She never misses an appointment* but she looks so apathetic. She seems uncomfortable holding the baby, or making eye contact with me.
—Request for consultation by a family medicine resident in a teaching hospital (1987)

We're worried about this 20-year-old mother . . . she brought her four-week-old baby to us. She left in tears, saying she was afraid to take care of him and *wanted to leave him where he would be safe.*
—Director of a child abuse prevention center (1988)

What appears to be intentional neglect in the care of a baby may be an important behavioral clue.

Tell me where I can get help for my daughter-in-law. She refuses to care for the baby. She says she's afraid she will drop him or stick him with a diaper pin. My son flatly denies there is a problem. He thinks I am overreacting. I'm worried. I just know something is terribly wrong. Could it be PPD [postpartum depression]?*
—Telephone call from New York (1988)

---

*Postpartum depression is an umbrella term used by both the lay community and professionals to refer to a variety of postpartum disorders.—Eds.

How Mothers View Themselves and Are Perceived by Others

Whatever the severity of the postpartum woman's distress, her pain is compounded by the utter surprise that what she is experiencing is not what she expected.

We were so prepared for the birth but totally unprepared for what happened when we brought the baby home. Why don't they tell you about this in Lamaze classes? They talk about everything else! We felt betrayed.
—"Warm-line" telephone call (1986)

In addition, the birth of a baby can be regarded as a combination of several dramatic losses, such as the loss of a cherished ambition, the loss of independence, and the loss of a career (Cox 1988).

We wanted a baby for so long. After six years of infertility, how can I admit I'm not happy staying home with my daughter. I never dreamed I would feel this way. I'm afraid to tell my husband or my doctor.
—1988

Upon experiencing postpartum anxiety, women often see themselves as failures and their self-esteem plunges. Convinced they are not living up to the expectation of a madonna-like motherhood, they experience an extraordinary amount of guilt. They are embarrassed and ashamed. The masquerade of easy and uneventful early parenthood is a tremendous burden.

I remember it seemed like all the other mothers I knew were so capable. I couldn't let on . . . I don't want my daughters-in-law to suffer like I did. I am glad someone is finally putting an end to this conspiracy of silence.
—New grandmother and attorney (1988)

Mothers are supposed to love their babies! *I don't have any feelings* toward mine. *I just feel numb.* What's wrong with me?
—Support group participant (1986)

I felt like I was going crazy but there was no one I could tell. I was so afraid they would take my baby away. The whole thing was so unlike me. It was nothing like what I expected. God! If people only knew. Finally, my family doctor said "Carrie, you're having a real hard time, aren't you? Tell me what's going on." He saved my life!
—Graduate student (1985)

Dr. J. S. Price (1978) has written poignantly about how it *feels* to be depressed:

The patient is isolated. Because depression reduces affection for others, there are ideas of unworthiness. Others can't stand to see the suffering. Outward depression is socially unacceptable and there tends to be a great cover-up. This results in an inability to reveal the severity of the problem.

New mothers engage in the practice of denial. They may convince themselves that if only they try harder, everything will be all right. They may appear to be champions under duress, organized and efficient with endless amounts of energy. Skillful concealment disguises their deteriorating condition as they strive to perform like a "walk-on-water woman."

I fooled everyone—especially myself. I breast-fed, went back to work, exercised, and entertained until I collapsed.
—Lamaze class participant (1979)

Even when postpartum illnesses are relatively mild, women are confused about what is happening to them. Their inability to problem-solve and perform at their usual level sets them up for self-blame. At a time of heightened vulnerability they often feel isolated. Fear of disapproval by friends and family members, particularly husbands, prevents self-disclosure. An atmosphere of unconditional acceptance of the new mother's postpartum emotional experiences is imperative. Fear of rejection is a most formidable barrier to seeking help.

By the time my baby was three weeks old, I still had not had one night's sleep. I became a clinging vine with my husband. I cried when he left the house in the morning. *I was petrified of being alone.* Gradually, I could feel myself losing touch. I felt dizzy. When I tried to tell my husband, he said, "You're crazy, Susan!" My doctor said, "Calm down. Relax. You're making a big deal out of everything." My parents told me, "Susan, grow up. You're a mother now, with responsibilities!" I was so scared. No one seemed to understand.

Finally, I was hospitalized. It broke my heart. I was not allowed to see my baby or my three-year-old son. I embarrassed my family. They have never forgiven me. I vowed I'd never have another baby but now I'm pregnant again!
—Warm line telephone call (1979)

Antecedents of Violent Behavior

Postpartum psychiatric illness in its most severe form (postpartum psychotic depression) is characterized by mercurial fluctuations between periods of apparent lucidity and episodes of bizarre delusions and vivid hallucinations, which frequently have a religious theme. Some women experience frightening thoughts and disturbing dreams that may involve harming themselves or their baby. They may be afraid of touching knives or may have thoughts of drowning or dropping the baby.

Consider the shocking dilemma of a new mother who, having successfully completed her pregnancy, labor, and birth, suddenly hears voices advising her to "jump off a bridge" or "drown" her crying child to "put him out of his misery." Women have reported, through their tears, that they could see themselves throwing their tiny infant down the stairs. They relate being on the brink of following the commands of auditory hallucinations urging them to end both their life and that of their child.

> When my son was two weeks old, I parked the car in a parking garage. When I lifted him out of his safety seat to go shopping, I began having thoughts of throwing him over the edge. We were on the fifth level! I have never been able to tell anyone until now.
> —Educator, conference attendee (1987)

Such horrific thoughts are for many women unspeakable; consequently, they struggle to survive alone. Most have escaped violence against themselves or their baby. Some have not. A skilled listener can facilitate the expression of such abhorrent thoughts and the concomitant relief which is felt by the woman no longer alone with them.

Although postpartum psychosis is relatively rare (one or two per one thousand births), the potential for tragedy is obvious. The risk increases substantially, to one in three or four women with a history of a previous postpartum psychotic episode (Hamilton 1985, 1987, 1989, Brockington et al. 1982, Paffenbarger 1982). (See also Chapters 16 and 17.)

It is incumbent upon anyone who is in contact with a new mother to inquire about how she is feeling. If she is found to be in distress, further information can often be elicited by simply asking "How are you feeling? Are you having any frightening thoughts or dreams?"

> It is so awful, I just can't say it . . . when she finishes breast-feeding and I place my daughter against my shoulder to burp her, I find myself thinking about how my hand could so easily fit around her neck and strangle her. Sometimes when I look at a paper grocery bag, I can see myself putting her in and closing it. Oh God! why is this happening to me?
> —Telephone call from the mother of a three-week-old (1988)

> I could hear voices telling me that Billy was the devil, that I should drown him, and then my husband who was Jesus Christ, could raise him from the dead. I was psychotic but it made sense at the time.
> —Telephone call (1985)

It is well known that postpartum psychosis typically appears in the early days and weeks following birth. In its early stages, and to the uninformed eye, a psychosis may be indistinguishable from the infamous maternity blues (Hamilton 1989). (See also Chapters 3, 7, and 17.)

I began laughing and then crying while still in the hospital. The nurses told me it was just the baby blues. I never told anyone that I saw knives every time I closed my eyes. Is it any wonder I couldn't sleep? I could have been one of those mothers who kills their baby. I was lucky! I felt like my old self in about six months.

—Description of an incident that occurred in 1969

I called my obstetrician twice and tried to tell him about the voices but I just couldn't get the words out. . . . He kept saying "Mary, you have a beautiful, healthy son. You should be enjoying him. Get some sleep and stop worrying so much." If only he had known the truth. My husband, who was in the Navy, was away at sea. I was so frightened.

—Support group participant (1986)

The stress-filled weeks and months following the birth of a premature or ill baby is a predictable time of distress for both parents. Having a difficult baby or one with neonatal complications has been associated with the diagnosis of postpartum psychiatric illness (Hopkins et al. 1986). Early separation of mother and baby has been shown to place both at risk for attachment disorders (Klaus and Kennel 1976, Dix 1988, Brazelton et al. 1974, Robson and Kumar 1980). (See also Chapter 8.)

My son was born ten weeks early with lots of problems. They rushed him to the medical center in a helicopter. I was sent home the next day. The doctors and nurses seemed so at ease while I felt so clumsy. They thought I didn't love him when I said he shouldn't come home yet. No one will ever know how much I ached for him.

When he came home three months later, he was so small. I knew I wasn't capable of taking care of him and there was no one to help me. I was so depressed. I knew God was punishing me for using birth control pills. We are Catholic. I kept seeing knives with blood and hearing guns go off. I knew everyone would be better off without me. I couldn't think of anyone who would take care of Johnny . . . so I shot him and then shot myself.

—Panel participant (1988)

I couldn't eat. I couldn't sleep. I just paced the floor every night while everyone else was asleep. They never knew. When I asked my mother if she ever had a problem after any of us was born, she said, "Oh, heavens, no . . . I never had time for that." I just couldn't tell her how desperate I was. I was too ashamed.

—A woman imprisoned for infanticide (1986)

We should have known something was wrong. Her baby "almost drowned" in the bathtub the week before. She called 911 herself! We were so out of it! We could have asked her a few simple questions and avoided a tragedy. In retrospect, I know she was trying to tell us in the only way she could.

—Emergency room nurse (1987)

Husbands—Neglected and Blamed

It is most likely the husband or a close relative with whom the distressed mother attempts to discuss her dilemma. New fathers often react with confusion, shock, denial, and anger. They too have subscribed to the myth of blissful parenthood and are likely to be ill-prepared for the demands placed upon them.

As Thomas Gordon has pointed out, anger is a secondary feeling (see Kieschnick and Zener 1980). Primary feelings include confusion, frustration, fear, helplessness, and a sense of inadequacy (Figure 4.2). Fear and anger have been described as allied emotions resulting from stress and a feeling of being threatened, cheated, or duped. Both function as emergency emotions signaling impending danger. Without an understanding of their origin, false solutions to problems are frequently seized upon (Gaylin 1989, Freud 1949, Becker 1975) (see Figure 4.3).

The husband is the invisible victim of this illness. The first feeling I had was shock. This can't be happening to my wife. . . . I lost my friend. I lost my partner. I lost my life. . . . for a little bit. It wasn't easy to be the strong one. You lose your home life . . . the fantasy of what this is supposed to be like! I'd come

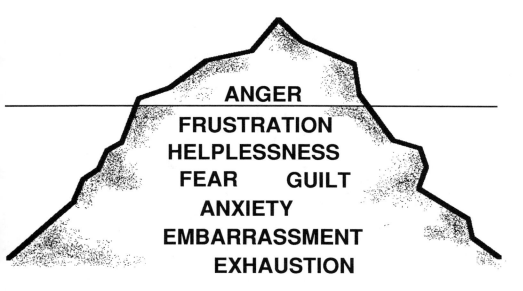

Figure 4.2. "Gordon's Iceberg." Adapted with permission from a concept developed by Thomas Gordon, Ph.D. (Kieschnick and Zener 1980).

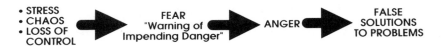

Figure 4.3. The pathway to false solutions.

home from work and I didn't want to deal with it . . . not every day. At work, I couldn't get her off my mind and that threatened my job. When there are financial pressures, this becomes a devastating reality. And then there was the anger . . . God! did I feel angry, but under the anger was a sense of *isolation*. No one wanted to talk about it! Plus I was *afraid* she would never get better.
    —Report from a husband and father at the second annual meeting of Postpartum Support, International, Princeton University Medical Center, Princeton, New Jersey, June 1988 (Smith 1988)

The cries for help from husbands often involve anger, as witnessed by numerous telephone calls to the authors over the years. Sometimes the first contact with a professional is an appointment for marital counseling. Being faced with what seems an insoluble problem can be emasculating. Unable to cope, husbands may spend more time away from home and involve themselves more deeply in their work. In the absence of needed information and support, an overburdened husband may threaten to or actually abandon his wife.

The husband's behavior provides critical clues to what is happening in the family. Studies have shown that the husband's understanding and support is critical to the woman's recovery from postpartum psychiatric illness (Atkinson and Atkinson 1983, O'Hara 1985, Timmerman 1987, Paykel et al. 1980, Pitt 1968, Cutrona 1982, Kumar et al. 1984). His concerns must be attended to if there is to be success in solving the picture puzzle of postpartum psychiatric illness.

It was a real shock when my wife was so unhappy after our son was born. If you had known her before—she was so full of life. At first, I told her to just snap out of it—but she couldn't. I didn't know what to do. No one seemed to want to talk about it—like we should just ignore it and it would go away. It affected my concentration at work. I couldn't leave home without her crying. Now I realize it wasn't her fault. Thank God she didn't kill herself.
                                                                                    —1987

Why don't they tell you about this in prepared childbirth classes? No one warned us! We thought we were prepared for anything. No one mentioned a word about postpartum depression.
    —Angry husband's remark during a support group meeting (1989)

I know I could and should have done more. We as a family did not want to accept mental illness in our lives. Because of this stigma, Sharon suppressed

her feelings after Garrett's birth. Had we ever imagined infanticide or suicide might result, something would have been done.
—Glenn Comitz, husband of a woman imprisoned for infanticide
(Comitz 1988, *Beyond the Blues* 1989)

Depression robbed her of the sense of a past and the hope of a future. . . . The first lesson Pat and I learned is that we waited too long to get help. . . . *Depression doesn't just happen to one person alone. It happens to the whole family.*
—John Timmerman, *A Season of Suffering* (1987)

Conclusion

Families and professionals unconsciously deny that there may be a problem. Each of us would like the postpartum period to play out uneventfully, like a beautiful fairy tale.

Recognition that there may be a problem requires that we take some action. In our busy fast-paced lives, this can be inconvenient. For too long we have been ignorant and lax regarding postpartum mental health issues. We have been impatient, judgmental, and even angry with new mothers. Often we have trivialized their cries for help. We have looked upon postpartum psychiatric illness as a problem that belongs to women alone. We have argued about diagnoses and, worse still, perpetuated the conspiracy of silence by using labels that are threatening and inappropriate. We have neglected research, so critical to the quality of care we render.

It is the belief of the authors that an investment of research, education, and support for young families will reap immeasurable rewards for the future.

Healthy mothers nurture healthy, productive future citizens.

Postpartum psychiatric illness crosses all socioeconomic lines and affects women of varying educational backgrounds. It may strike without warning. Families experiencing such difficulties do cry out for help. It is imperative that we listen and respond with knowledge, skill, and compassion.

Acknowledgments

The assistance of the following individuals in the preparation of this chapter is gratefully acknowledged: our loving families, especially My Dars; innumerable victims of postpartum illness, particularly Lisa, Chanda, Angela, Melinda and Sharon; members of the York Hospital Library Staff, Rob Pabst, Alex Burger; and of course, Betty Altland.

Resources

The Family Resource Coalition

The Family Resource Coalition of Chicago, Illinois, is a national organization working with preventive, community-based family resource and support programs which provides technical assistance to practitioners working with families. Readers are encouraged to contact the coalition at the following address for an up-to-date list of support groups or centers in specific locations:

> Family Resource Coalition
> 230 North Michigan Avenue #1625
> Chicago, IL 60601
> Telephone: (312) 726–4750

The Marcé Society

The Marcé Society was founded in 1980 and is an international society for the understanding, prevention, and treatment of mental illness related to childbearing. For information contact:

> Honorary Secretary
> The Marcé Society
> Queen Margaret College
> Clerwood Terrace
> Edinborough EH12-8TS
> United Kingdom
> Telephone: (031) 339–8111

Postpartum Support International

Postpartum Support International (PSI) was formed in 1987. Its goals include increasing awareness of postpartum mental health issues, maintaining international communication, advocating for women and their families, and promoting research. PSI also sponsors an annual conference. Membership is open to individuals and organizations worldwide who are interested in promoting healthy postpartum development. For further information contact:

> Postpartum Support International
> 927 North Kellogg Avenue
> Santa Barbara, California 93111
> Telephone: (805) 967–7636

Depression After Delivery

The Depression After Delivery (DAD) Support Network is a self-help mutual aid organization managed by women who have experienced postpartum disorders. Originally started as one small support group in 1985, it has become a growing network of support groups. DAD extends to every state and Canadian province through a telephone "warm line" and provides information packets and support to women, families, and professionals. For further information contact:

> Depression After Delivery
> Post Office Box 1282
> Morrisville, Pennsylvania 19067
> Telephone: (215) 295–3994

Pacific Postpartum Support Society

> Pacific Postpartum Support Society
> 1416 Commercial Drive
> Vancouver, British Columbia V5L-3X9
> Telephone: (604) 255–7999

The National Childbirth Trust

> The National Childbirth Trust
> Alexander House
> Oldham Terrace
> Acton, London W36NH
> Telephone: (01) 992–8637

The Association for Postnatal Illness

> The Association for Postnatal Illness
> 25 Jerdan Place
> Fulhan, London SW6-1BE
> Telephone: (01) 731–4867

Post- and Ante-Natal Depression Association

> PANDA
> 18 Elysee Court
> Strathmore, Victoria
> Australia 3041

References

Atkinson, S., and Atkinson, T. (1983). Through a husband's eyes. *Health Visitor.* 56:17.

Bagedahl-Strindlund, M. (1987). *Parapartum Mentally Ill Mothers and Their Children.* Stockholm.

Becker, E. (1975). In L. Levi (Ed.), *Emotions—Their Parameters and Measurement.* New York: Raven Press.

Beyond the Blues. March 1989. Lifetime Cable Network. Signature Series. Documentary.

Boston Women's Health Book Collective (1984). *The New Our Bodies, Ourselves.* Boston: Simon & Schuster.

Brazelton, T. B., Koslowski, B., and Main, M. (1974). The origins of reciprocity: The early mother-infant interaction. In M. Lewis and L. A. Rosenblum (Eds.), *The Effect of the Infant on the Caregiver.* New York: John Wiley and Sons.

Brockington, I. F., and Kumar, R. (Eds.) (1982). *Motherhood and Mental Illness.* London: Academic Press.

Brockington, I. F., Winokur, G., and Dean, C. (1982). Puerperal psychosis. In I. F. Brockington and R. Kumar (Eds.), *Motherhood and Mental Illness.* London: Academic Press.

Caplan, H. L., Cogill, S. R., Alexandra, H., Robson, K. M., and Kumar, R. (1988). The effect of maternal postnatal depression on the emotional development of the child. *Br. J. Psychiatr.*

Cogill, S. R., Caplan, H. L., Alexandra, H., Robson, K. M., and Kumar, R. (1986). Impact of maternal postnatal depression on cognitive development of young children. *Br. Med. J.,* 292:1165–67.

Comitz, G. (1988). Commutation Hearing for Sharon Comitz. Harrisburg, Pennsylvania. December, 1988.

———. (1987). Personal communication.

Cox, J. L. (1988). The life event of childbirth: Sociocultural aspects of postnatal depression. In R. Kumar and I. F. Brockington (Eds.), *Motherhood and Mental Illness,* Vol. 2.

Cox, J. L., Holden, J. M., and Sagovsky, R. (1987). Detection of postnatal depression: Development of the ten-item Edinburgh Postnatal Depression Scale. *Br. J. Psychiatr.,* 150:782–86.

Cutrona, C. (1982). Nonpsychotic postpartum depression: A review of recent research. *Clin. Psychol. Rev.,* 2:487–503.

Dix, C. (1988). *The New Mother Syndrome.* New York: Simon and Schuster.

Field, T. (1984). Early interactions between infants and their postpartum depressed mothers. *Infant Behavior and Development,* 7:517–22.

Freud, S. (1949). *Inhibitions, Symptoms and Anxiety.* London: Hogarth Press.

Gaylin, W. (1989). *The Rage Within.* New York: Simon and Schuster.

Gondolf, E. W. (1988). *Battered Women as Survivors: Alternatives to Treating Learned Helplessness.* Toronto: Lexington Books, D.C. Heath Publishing Company.

Hamilton, J. A. (1982). The identity of postpartum psychosis. In I. F. Brockington and R. Kumar (Eds.), *Motherhood and Mental Illness.* London: Academic Press.

———. (1985). Guidelines for therapeutic management of postpartum disorders. In D. Inwood (Ed.), *Postpartum Psychiatric Disorders.* Washington, D.C.: American Psychiatric Press.

———. (1987). Personal communication.

———. (1989). Postpartum psychiatric syndromes. *Psychiatr. Clin. North Am.,* 12(1):89–93.

Harvard Medical School Mental Health Letter (1989). Postpartum disorders—effect on the child, 5(11):3.

Holden, J., et al. (1989). Counselling in a general practice setting: Controlled study of health visitor intervention in treatment of postnatal depression. *Br. Med. J.* 298:223–26.

Hopkins, J., Campbell, S. B., and Marcus, M. (1986). The role of infant-related stressors in postpartum depression. *J. Abn. Psychol.,* 96:237–41.

Kieschnick, M., and Zener, A. E. (1980). *Dr. Thomas Gordon's Parent Effectiveness Instructor's Guide.* Solana Beach, CA: Effectiveness Training, Inc.

Klaus, M. H., and Kennel, J. H. (1976). Parent to infant attachment. In D. Hull (Ed.), *Recent Advances in Pediatrics.* London: Churchill Livingston.

Kruckman, L. D., and Asmann-Finch, C. (1986). *Postpartum Depression—A Research Guide and International Bibliography.* New York: Garland Publishing, page XV.

Kumar, R., Robson, K. M., and Smith, A.M.R. (1984). Development of a self-administered questionnaire to measure maternal adjustment and maternal attitudes during pregnancy and after delivery. *J. Psychosom. Res.* 28:43–51.

Margison, F. (1982). The pathology of the mother-child relationship. In I. F. Brockington and R. Kumar (Eds.), *Motherhood and Mental Illness.* London: Academic Press.

Metz, A., Sichel, D. A., and Goff, D. C. (1988). Postpartum panic disorder. *J. Clin. Psychiatr.,* 49:278–79.

Murray, L. (1988). Effects of postnatal depression on infant development: Direct studies of early mother-infant interactions. In R. Kumar and I. F. Brockington (Eds.), *Motherhood and Mental Illness,* Vol. 2. London: Academic Press.

O'Hara, M. W., et al. (1983). Postpartum depression: A role for social network and life stress variables. *J. Nerv. Ment. Dis.* 171(6):336–41.

O'Hara, M. W. (1985). Psychological factors in the development of postpartum depression. In D. G. Inwood (Ed.), *Recent Advances in Postpartum Psychiatric Disorders.* Washington, DC: American Psychiatric Press.

O'Hara, M. W., and Engeldinger, J. (1989). Postpartum mood disorders—detection and prevention. *The Female Patient,* 14:19–27.

O'Hara, M. W., Rehm, L. P., and Campbell, S. B. (1982). Predicting depressive symptomology: Cognitive-behavioral models and postpartum depression. *J. Abn. Psychol.,* 91(6):457–61.

Paffenbarger, R. S., Jr. (1982). Epidemiological aspects of mental illness associated with childbearing. In I. F. Brockington and R. Kumar (Eds.). *Motherhood and Mental Illness.* London: Academic Press.

Paykel, E. S., Emms, E., Fletcher, J., and Rassaby, E. S. (1980). Life events and social support in puerperal depression. *Br. J. Psychiatr.* 136:339–46.

Pitt, B.M.N. (1968). Atypical depression following childbirth. *Br. J. Psychiatr.,* 114:1325–35.

Price, J. S. (1978). Chronic depressive illness. In D. W. Goodwin and S. B. Guze (Eds.), *Psychiatric Diagnosis,* 4th ed. London: Oxford University Press, 1989.

Richman, N. (1976). Depression in mothers of preschool children. *J. Child Psychol. Psychiatr.* 17(1):75–78.

Robson, K. M., and Kumar, R. (1980). Delayed onset of maternal affection after childbirth. *Br. J. Psychiatr.* 13:347–53.

Smith, J. (1988, 1989). Personal communication.

———. (1988). Report from a husband and father. Second Annual Meeting of Postpartum Support, International. Princeton University Medical Center. Princeton, NJ, June 1988.

Stern, G., and Kruckman, L. (1983). Multi-disciplinary perspectives on postpartum depression: An anthropological critique. *Soc. Sci. Med.* 17(15):1027–41.

Timmerman, J. H. (1987). *A Season of Suffering: One Family's Journey Through Depression.* Portland: Multnomah Press.

Trout, M. D. (1987). Notes on postpartum depression: Seeking help through the baby. *The Marcé Society Summer Bulletin.*

————. (1985). Personal communication.

Weissman, M. M., Prusoff, B. A., Gamon, G. D., Merikangas, K. R., Leckman, J. F., and Kidd, K. K. (1984). Psychopathology in the children (ages 6–18) of depressed and normal parents. *J. Am. Acad. Child Psychiatr.* 23:8–84.

Ziporyn, T. (1984). Rip Van Winkle period ends for puerperal psychiatric problems. *J.A.M.A.* 251(16):2061–67.

Part II
Recognition, Treatment, and Support

In the United States, where medical surveillance of new mothers often lapses between discharge from the hospital and physical checkup several weeks later, the recognition of postpartum illness is left mainly to chance. Even severe cases of postpartum psychotic depression or major postpartum depression may continue for days or weeks, their symptoms concealed or dismissed as "baby blues," neuroticism, or character weakness. Elizabeth K. Herz, a distinguished physician and educator, addresses these problems in Chapter 5 and outlines broad objectives and methods for prevention and treatment. Others in Chapters 6, 8, and 9 discuss the best of current psychiatric and pharmacological resources and optimally adapt them to postpartum illness. The authors of these four chapters have outstanding records of successful treatment. They add *art* to modern medicine. As these chapters indicate, it is apparent that there are many areas of agreement. These areas merit serious attention since their neglect is sometimes associated with failed treatment or unduly protracted duration of illness. There are differences in some of the recommended treatment details, and this is to be expected where *art* plays a role in medical practice. The reader has an opportunity to synthesize several very successful approaches.

Maternity blues is an important topic, since incipient psychosis must be distinguished from this self-limiting phenomenon. In Chapter 7, Jan Campbell describes this distinction. Also, through her examination of biological aspects of maternity blues, she comes to the proposal that this condition could be a model for exploring biological aspects of postpartum psychosis.

Certain features of the health system in the United Kingdom, reviewed by Ian Brockington in Chapter 10, appear to facilitate the early recognition of psychiatric illness after childbirth. Many third-world and less technologically developed cultures have rituals for special treatment and support of new mothers. It has been observed that such rituals appear to be associated with a limited occurrence of postpartum symptoms. Laurence Kruckman reviews some of these rituals in Chapter 11, and suggests that families and support groups may provide similar protection in Western cultures.

Chapter 5
Prediction, Recognition, and Prevention

Elizabeth K. Herz

The emotional anguish of women with postpartum psychiatric illness can be described in the words of a new mother who experienced it herself:

> When our daughter was born it was the happiest moment of my life. Everything was so perfect. But then without any reason I became so sad. I lost my energy and I felt that it was all my fault that it was happening. Then I got these feelings of hurting myself and kept asking myself, "Why?" I felt stupid having these feelings and didn't want anyone to know because I thought I could fight it on my own. It was like there was something going on inside of me which I had no control over. I didn't want these feelings but they came up when least expected. Inside I would say, "You might as well give up, something is telling you to. There is no use in going on." These thoughts terrified me and I would shake my head and say, "What the hell are you saying! This isn't what I want." But I also felt that nothing would straighten me out and I would never feel like me again. And then I became panicky for fear I would harm my daughter. I know I won't do anything extreme, I haven't even attempted anything. But these thoughts are ruining me inside. I see terrible visions and can't seem to shake them off completely. I have been remaining silent because of being ashamed, guilty, and isolated. I don't feel I'm insane. I also had thought that they would take me away to a mental hospital if I admitted what I was feeling and I definitely don't want that. But I do need some help to recover. I can't seem to do it myself.

This short but eloquent description contains so many of the typical elements of postpartum depression: blissful happiness and then bewilderment about the unaccountable sadness, self-blame, lowered self-esteem, the feeling of losing control over thoughts and emotions, helplessness, hopelessness, and the overwhelming fear of doing harm to the child. Her guilt, shame, and fear of the consequences prevent disclosure of her torment. But this woman, at least, was finally able to reach out for help when she accidentally learned that she was far from being the only new mother to go through this experience (Pugh et al. 1963, Paffenbarger 1961, Weiner 1982).

In fact, postpartum mental disorder is possibly the most prevalent postpartum complication and can cause protracted morbidity. Particularly with the increased risk of suicide in depression, postpartum psychiatric illness constitutes a potentially fatal postpartum complication.

In addition to the risks for the woman, the impact on the infant must be considered. There exists a direct correlation between the severity of the maternal disorder and infant morbidity caused by problems ranging from difficulty in bonding and poor feeding, all the way to the battered child syndrome and infanticide. And of course, it causes severe strain in the marriage and other relationships.

In view of its prevalence and potential severity, it is surprising that more attention has not been devoted to this complex disorder. How can we understand this omission? One reason is that the disorder lies between obstetrics and psychiatry. Much controversy has taken place among different schools of thought which stressed either physiological or psychological causation (Dalton 1971 and 1980, Hamilton 1962, Sandler 1978). Increasing numbers of researchers in this field now believe that an either-or proposition is not the appropriate conceptualization and that we are dealing with many factors that work together in determining postpartum mental disorders. That is, psychological and social environmental factors interact dynamically with hereditary and biochemical ones in affecting maternal vulnerability to postpartum mental disorders (Kendell 1985, Butts 1969, Oakley and Chamberlain 1981, Cox 1983).

Differences of opinion persist between researchers about the relative importance attributed to these factors. But the main ongoing controversy centers on whether postpartum mental disorders present specific nosologic entities causally related to childbirth or functional psychiatric disorders coincidental to the puerperium (Inwood 1985, Brockington and Kumar 1982 and 1988). As long as postpartum mental disturbances are not classified as a special category, a definition cannot be conclusively formulated nor can the hypothetical concept of a spectrum disorder (from mild depression to psychosis) be entertained. The lack of definition stymies research and diminishes the usefulness of prior or ongoing studies for meaningful comparisons. For instance, the temporal proximity to childbirth is currently the only criterion to define postpartum depression. The length of the postpartum period assigned by different authors, however, varies from three weeks to one year. Disagreement also exists about incidence, symptoms, course, and severity of postpartum mental disorder.

Prediction

It is therefore not surprising that data on predictive factors for the development of PPD are inconsistent, and the evidence in research studies is often contradictory. In addition to the lack of uniform definition, the comparability of data is further compromised by the variety of methodologies used (e.g., prospective or retrospective, self-rating or interview) and the interdisciplinary differences in concepts. The overriding issue remains the confounding number of interacting variables that potentially influence maternal adjustment. Despite inconsistencies of data, however, some vulnerability factors emerge repeatedly and seem to carry more weight in their predictive value. The monumental review by O'Hara (1987) illuminates the confounding heterogeneity of the literature.

Potential risk factors can be divided into physiologic, demographic, psychological, interpersonal, or contributing variables.

Physiologic Variables

The generally presumed contributory role of physiologic changes on the development of postpartum illness is still without conclusive proof. Extensive studies evaluating gonadal hormones, prolactin, cortisol, thyroid hormones, tryptophan, and neurotransmitters have produced inconclusive results. One explanation may be that women vary in their sensitivity even to apparently normal blood levels of various biochemical substances. A higher incidence of postpartum illness has been reported for women with *dysmenorrhea* and premenstrual syndrome, however, suggesting some significance to the *endocrine profile,* but the data are not consistent.

The clinical observation that more previously *infertile women* develop postpartum illness than women after a successful pregnancy at first intent appears paradoxical. One hypothesis postulates a common endocrinologic cause, especially for idiopathic infertility. But infertility can also become "the identified problem" for all the unhappiness a woman may experience, thus preventing realistic acceptance of other problems. The impossible expectations of resolving all unhappiness through the birth of a baby will naturally result in disappointment. The realization of previously unacknowledged problems together with the disappointment of her unrealistic expectations can put a woman into a tailspin of depression.

One prospective study found more psychiatric symptoms in women given *oral contraceptives* shortly after childbirth compared to controls using other forms of contraception. It is interesting to note that some PMS-sufferers also feel worse on oral contraceptives. Subsequent research could not confirm these findings.

An association of *physical complications during pregnancy and delivery* with postpartum illness has not been consistently demonstrated. One study found a higher incidence of depression after caesarean section but this finding could not be replicated in other studies.

Consensus does exist regarding the significance of *hereditary factors* for psychiatric illness particularly for postpartum psychosis.

Thus far, no uncontested logitudinal cause-effect relationship between a physical factor and PPD has been established. It is generally acknowledged that an etiologic explanation of postpartum illness relying solely on physiologic changes is insufficient. Such a reductionistic approach would also not explain why relatively few women develop PPD despite the fact that all women undergo the biochemical changes of pregnancy and why postpartum illness can be experienced by adoptive mothers, too.

Demographic Variables

Both *primiparous women and grand multiparas* seem to be at higher risk for postpartum illness from evidence in the literature.

In some studies *very young and older women* appear to be more vulnerable to depression.

Long and very short intervals between pregnancies may be potential risk factors for postpartum illness.

Low socioeconomic status and the *single mother* have also been implicated in some studies but contradicted by others.

Overall, various demographic data show no consistent association with postpartum illness, except the high risk for primiparas.

Psychological Variables

A history of *previous psychiatric illness* is identified as a significant risk factor in the majority of studies, particularly when the depressive episode was postpartum or developed during the pregnancy. Many women, however, experience their first episode of affective disorder in the postpartum period; other women are affected exclusively in the puerperal phase.

In other words, the stress of pregnancy, delivery, and childrearing may precipitate depression in a previously healthy woman or prompt a recurrence in a woman with a preexisting affective disorder. One might wonder if more consistent findings could be reported if three distinct groups of women with depressive disorders were created: women with new-onset postpartum illness, women with previous history of affective disorder who develop postpartum illness, and women with reactive depression (e.g., depression associated with a stillbirth).

Subgrouping might shed light on the unresolved question of whether a distinct entity of postpartum psychiatric illness exists with different symptomatology from the recurrent or reactive depression. Distinguishing characteristics, especially in postpartum psychosis, have repeatedly been pointed out by leading researchers but may only apply for a specific subgroup and get lost in studies that lump all groups together.

Various personality types with a predisposition for postpartum illness have been postulated. Such examples are the overly anxious woman with external locus of control and the overcontrolling introvert. The most common personality trait is recurrent maladaptation to change in developmental tasks (Hayworth et al. 1980, Rosenwald 1972).

A predictor of high significance for postpartum psychiatric illness is continued ambivalence or negative attitude toward the maternal role. The phrase "maternal role conflict" was coined by Gordon and Gordon (1957) in addressing a problem of some high-achieving career women who consciously or unconsciously reject traditional female roles and/or experience these roles as threats to their identities. One dilemma for the working mother is the issue of if and when she wants to or has to return to her job. Not infrequently, she finds herself trapped by arrangements made before the delivery and realizes that her reaction to being a mother is opposite from what she had expected. This is true for the woman who plans to return to work, and when the time comes, she cannot bear to leave her child. This may be just as true for the woman who plans to stay home and then cannot cope with the loss of her professional identity and contact with the adult world.

Interpersonal Variables

Poor marital relationship is probably the most significant risk factor for postpartum illness. The adjustment to the parental role constitutes a developmental crisis or a turning point, and the necessary adaptations depend on the mutuality of both partners. Many conflicts can result from disappointed expectations regarding the participation of the partner in the child care and sharing of responsibilities. An unavailable husband and marital tension can undermine successful maternal adjustment.

The suggestion has been made to replace the term "postpartum depression" with "maternal" or even "parental depression." The term "postpartum depression" links the disturbance to pregnancy and delivery but may disregard the many stresses of motherhood. While the contribution of hormonal changes, psychodynamic processes, and birth is not discounted, more emphasis is placed on psychosocial stressors for corrective interventions (Chalmers and Chalmers 1986).

A significant association between a *poor relationship with her own mother* and postpartum illness has emerged in several studies (Uddenberg 1975, Kumar and Robson 1984). To become a mother herself, a woman quite naturally relies on her own mother as a role model. This can revive what was good in their own relationship, but the woman may be more likely to recall situations that she would not want her own child to undergo. If she rejects her mother as a role model, she may feel at a loss and very much alone in knowing how to cope.

The *absence of the extended family* deprives the woman of the traditional support of more experienced relatives and prevents prior apprenticeship in caring for infants. The lack of competence and proper guidance is a major source for anxiety and depression. *Isolation from family and friends* correlates significantly with postpartum illness.

The infant can also contribute to the development of postpartum emotional disorders especially if there is a poor match between the mother's and child's temperaments. Positive reinforcement to her caretaking may be lacking, particularly if the mother misreads the infant's cues. A flawed interaction can become the source for her frustrations, anger, guilt, and depression. Furthermore, an unplanned child can make it even more difficult for a woman to correctly respond to the demands and accept unwanted responsibilities.

Stressful life events such as separations by moving or losses of loved ones during pregnancy may predict depression (Paykel et al. 1980, O'Hara et al. 1982). Similarly, postpartum emotional disorders are also more prevalent in mothers with high-risk infants.

Despite the ambiguities some of the researched factors have potential predictive value—for example, lack of the husband's support and marital tension, preexisting psychiatric disorder and/or family history of psychopathology, a poor relationship with one's own mother, isolation from a support network, and ambivalence about the maternal role as well as stressful life events. Other potential predictors should also be kept in mind because the development of postpartum illness is probably contingent not only on the severity but also the number of interacting risk factors and the woman's individual perception of their gravity.

Contributing Variables

In addition to the potential predictors of depression among new mothers, one finds totally unrealistic expectations of motherhood that may contribute to the emotional distress. Such unrealistic expectations include a sense of intuitive mothering competence, sustained blissful happiness, a feeling of unremitting self-sacrificing love for the child, equal sharing of the infant care with the father, and the "Supermom" myth.

Some approaches in prenatal teaching contribute to false expectations regarding the woman's conduct during labor (Stewart 1985). When romanticized ideas inevitably clash with reality, many women ascribe the resulting difficulties to their own inadequacy. A negative self-perception regarding her childbirth experience can precipitate a depressive reaction. The lack of adequate preparation for parenthood and minimal prenatal exposure to the realities seem to be important contributors to the development of postpartum emotional disorders.

Recognition

An incipient mental disorder may often go undetected because the new mother generally does not volunteer her emotional distress out of shame, guilt, or fear. Furthermore, the focus of the six-week postpartum checkup is the medical aspects of her reproductive system. Sleep and eating disturbances, diminished energy, and mood fluctuations are such typical concomitants in the postnatal phase that a woman who voices such complaints usually is reassured without further investigation. But these complaints can also be cardinal symptoms of a major depressive disorder.

Other potential indicators can also be easily brushed aside as temporary occurrences in the maternal adjustment process: a decrease in social activities and contacts can mean that the mother enjoys spending time with the baby but could also indicate social withdrawal and isolation. The rare woman who admits to negative feelings toward the baby and discomfort with the maternal role is usually reassured that she shares these emotions with the majority of new mothers without questioning further the extent of these feelings. Her poor self-image regarding her attractiveness, competence, and ability to manage her multiple roles may be legitimate concerns during the course of the adjustment but can also mean a sense of worthlessness typical for depression.

In other words, the distinction between the usual concomitants of the postpartum phase and a major depressive disorder does not readily present itself and many women often feel too embarrassed to disclose the intensity of their feelings. It is easier for them to refer to multiple vague somatic complaints, which may actually be a way of reaching out for help under the guise of socially more acceptable physical ailments. Half of the women with postpartum illness develop the affective disorder in the first month after delivery. The obstetrician at the six-week postpartum checkup has the opportunity to recognize postpartum illness early if he or she includes an evaluation of the woman's psychosocial adjustment.

Distinguishing indicators of postpartum psychiatric illness from normal concomitants of the postnatal period include:

1. *Worsening of sleep disturbances* and an inability to go back to sleep after feedings despite extreme fatigue.
2. Eating problems expressed as *hyper- or hypophagia.*
3. An increase in the *intensity and duration of depressed feelings* or irritability, particularly if unrelated to events. The mother's negative cognitive set frequently includes preoccupation with self-deprecatory thoughts (e.g., about her conduct during childbirth, her competence as a mother, and her body image) increasing discomfort with the maternal role, fears for the child and self-doubt, death wishes ("everybody would be better off without me"), and sometimes, suicidal or infanticidal fantasies.
4. *Lack of compensatory measures* to counteract the fatigue and exhaustion (e.g., taking naps or mobilizing emotional support) to the point that energy loss interferes with her functioning.
5. *Withdrawal and social isolation* while complaining about lack of emotional support, particularly by the father of the child.
6. *Faulty interaction* with the baby (e.g., misinterpretation of its cues or evident disinterest).

The mother's behavior with the child can be an important indicator for maternal depression. Symptomatology during the postpartum period differentiate the disorder from the "normal" concomitants after childbirth.

Early detection of postpartum illness will become easier if public education can lift the social stigma, thereby allowing the woman to admit to the symptoms as she would for a hemorrhage. But the education must also extend to the obstetrician. The prevalent biomedical approach focuses solely on the biochemical physical changes of pregnancy and childbirth. In reality, these changes are interacting dynamically with cognitive, affective, interpersonal, and social changes. A biopsychosocial approach is indispensable for comprehensive care. Early recognition of postpartum illness would be greatly facilitated if the intake checklist at the first prenatal visit would include the major potential predictors of depression. Alertness could be enhanced at prenatal visits by an occasional simple question such as, "How are things at home?" to gauge the marital situation and other stress factors. At the six-week postpartum checkup, the obstetrician could then more actively pursue any warning signs of this disabling and potentially fatal disorder.

The transition of her primary caretaker, the obstetrician, to the primary caretaker of the infant, the family physician or pediatrician, can be perceived by a woman as another personal deprivation and loss of support. The obstetrician who is concerned about the potential for postpartum psychiatric illness in a woman would add significantly to early detection by passing this information on to his or her colleague and by emphasizing to the patient that the door remains open to her for whatever problem she wants to discuss.

The use of *self-rating symptom checklists* pre- and postnatally has already been discussed; however, most psychological instruments for depression lack specificity and others are not tested for validity and reliability. Measures to detect answers influenced by social desirability would need to be included. Prospective research needs to first validate a reliable and simple questionnaire before the resistance of most obstetricians to use it could be addressed (Braverman and Roux 1978, Affonso and Arizmendi 1986, Vandenberg 1980).

Preventive Interventions

While potential risk factors can serve as valuable warning signals, many of them are not amenable to corrective measures. Additional support and adequate preparation for parenthood may act as a compensatory measure for the patient's vulnerability. Many studies show that prenatal psychosocial interventions can significantly help in the successful adjustment to the parental role, and thereby counteract the development of PPD. Exemplary research was done by Gordon and coworkers (1965). They reported a prenatal prevention experiment that included discussion periods in which the following points were stressed:

- The responsibilities of motherhood are learned, hence get informed.

- Get help from husband, dependable friends, and relatives.
- Make friends with other couples who are experienced with child-bearing.
- Don't overload yourself with unimportant tasks.
- Don't move soon after the baby arrives.
- Don't be overconcerned with keeping up appearances.
- Get plenty of rest and sleep.
- Don't be a nurse to relatives and others at this time.
- Confer and consult with husband, family, and experienced friends, and discuss your plans and worries.
- Don't give up outside interests, but cut down on responsibilities and rearrange schedules.
- Arrange for babysitters early.
- Get family doctor early.

Dr. Gordon reported that "as a result of the instruction, the experimental subjects took significantly more of these recommended steps than did controls and underwent significantly less subsequent emotional upset. In classes where husbands received special instructions with their wives, less than half as many women developed emotional problems as did wives who participated alone. Instructed mothers had greater success with their babies: their six-month-old infants were significantly less irritable and had fewer sleep and eating disorders than the control's babies."

The main points in the various studies about prenatal anticipatory guidance are the following:

1. To dispel the motherhood myth of the maternal instinct (i.e., an inborn knowledge of how best to take care of the baby), the myth of the unwavering limitless motherly love, and the myth of the total maternal fulfillment by the baby.
2. To strengthen the marital support by defining shared responsibilities and roles with realistic coping behavior during the parental adjustment.
3. To mobilize additional emotional support systems.
4. To reduce environmental stress factors.
5. To rearrange priorities.
6. To encourage a pregnant woman to become an apprentice to a new mother particularly if she has had no previous experience with an infant.

Ideally, this preventive mental health intervention would be undertaken by the obstetrician as part of the prenatal care for the high-risk patient. More realistically, counseling and anticipatory guidance could be an integral part of prenatal education classes in addition to teaching about the physical aspects of pregnancy, delivery, and the postpartum phase. Separate parental classes, self-help groups, warm lines for new mothers and fathers, media coverage of postpartum emotional disorders to dispel the social stigma, publications, teaching programs for the obstetrician-in-training may all be helpful and hopeful developments for women at risk for postpartum illness (Kumar 1986, Meeker 1984, Beattie 1978).

Special and additional attention has to be paid to patients with a *preexisting psychiatric disorder*. These women are at high risk for postpartum recurrence and require close collaboration between their obstetrician and psychiatrist for prevention. *Counseling* before conception should include information about the risk for both the mother and child, as well as an individually tailored management plan. Special concern is warranted for the psychiatric patient who is on *psychotropic medication*. Lithium, for instance, has a teratogenic effect in about 10 percent of the pregnancies, and other psychotropic medication, although not as clearly implicated as lithium, may have potential effects on the child's later development.

Ideally, any psychotropic medication should be discontinued before conception and, if at all possible, withheld during the first trimester. Medication should be reinstituted during the pregnancy only when the patient shows signs of decompensation. To avoid ill effects on the newborn, medication should be discontinued when the woman is getting close to labor. If the woman is near term and spontaneous labor has not begun after a few days, induction may be indicated. After delivery, the patient needs to be medicated at her previous maintenance level. Medication naturally has to be increased as required.

Different psychotropic medications reach different levels of concentration in breast milk. Opinions vary as to whether nursing should be generally discouraged or only for specific medications. After delivery, the emphasis is on the earliest possible correction of physiologic factors, such as electrolyte imbalance, anemia, and hypothyroidism, which might contribute to an imbalance. Some help with child care at home should be arranged before discharge, and frequent postpartum visits need to be scheduled.

Preventive measures to correct physiologic factors that may contribute to postpartum mental disorder are controversial. Progesterone, with or without estrogen, thyroid and cortisone medications, bromocriptine, tryptophan, and other drugs have been tried with varying results. Collaborative studies on a large scale are needed to determine the most effective way to prevent this debilitating postpartum disorder.

Research on the physiological aspects contributing to postpartum illness needs to be further explored. More emphasis needs to be placed on prevention based on our current knowledge of potential risk factors. Some of the risk factors may be corrected, while others may need compensatory measures. As many studies show, education and support have important roles in prevention of postpartum emotional disorders.

References

Affonso, D. D., and Arizmendi, T. G. (1986). Disturbances in post-partum adaption and depressive symptomatology. *J Psychosom. Obstet. Gynecol.*, 5(1): 15–32.

Beattie, J. (1978). Observations of post-natal depression, and a suggestion for its prevention. *Int. J. Soc. Psychiatr.*, 24:247–49.

Braverman, J., and Roux, J. F. (1978). Screening for the patient at risk for postpartum depression. *Obstet. Gynecol.*, 52:731–36.

Brockington, I. F., and Kumar, R. (Eds.) (1982). *Motherhood and Mental Illness.* Vol. 1. New York and San Francisco: Grune and Statton. Vol. 2, 1988.

Butts, H. F. (1969). Post-partum psychiatric problems. *J. the Nat. Med. Assoc.* (March) 61:136–40.

Chalmers, B. E., and Chalmers, B. M. (1986). Post-partum depression: A revised perspective. *J. Psychosom. Obstet. Gynecol.* 5(2):93–105.

Cox, J. L. (1983). Clinical and research aspects of post-natal depression. *Obstet. Gynecol.* 2(1):46–53.

Dalton, K. (1971). Prospective study into puerperal depression. *Br. J. Psychiatr.* 118:689–92.

———. (1980). *Depression After Childbirth.* London: Oxford University Press.

Gordon, R. E., et al. (1965). Factors in postpartum emotional adjustment. *Obstet. Gynecol.* 25:158–66.

Gordon, R. E., and Gordon, K. K. (1957). Some social psychiatric aspects of pregnancy. *J. Med. Soc. N.J.* 54:569.

Hamilton, J. A. (1962). *Postpartum Psychiatric Problems.* St. Louis: C. V. Mosby.

Hayworth, J., et al. (1980). A predictive study of postpartum depression: Some predisposing characteristics. *Br. J. Med. Psychol.* 53:161–67.

Inwood, D. G. (Ed.) (1985). *Postpartum Psychiatric Disorders.* Washington, DC: American Psychiatric Press.

Kendell, R. E. (1985). Emotional and physical factors in the genesis of puerperal mental disorders. *J. Psychosom. Res.*, 29:3–11.

Kumar, R. (1986). Motherhood and mental illness: The role of the midwife in prevention and treatment. *Midwives Chronical and Nursing Notes*, 2:70–74.

Kumar, R., and Robson, J. M. (1984). A prospective study of emotional disorders in childbearing women. *Br. J. Psychiatr.*, 144:35–47.

Meeker, C.A.H. (1984). *A Preventive Intervention for Postpartum Depression in Primiparous Women.* Dissertation.

Oakley, A., and Chamberlain, G. (1981). Medical and social factors in postpartum depression. *J. Obstet. Gynecol.*, 1:3.

O'Hara, M. W. (1987). Post-partum "blues," depression, and psychosis: A review (POG 00152). *J. Psychosom. Obstet. Gynecol.* 7(7):205–28.

O'Hara, M. W., et al. (1982). Predicting depressive symptomatology: Cognitive-behavioral models and postpartum depression. *J. Abnorm. Psychol.*, 91(6):457–61.

Paffenbarger, R. S. (1961). The picture puzzle of the postpartum psychoses. *J. Chron. Dis.* 13:161–73.

Paykel, E. S., et al. (1980). Life events and social support in puerperal depression. *Br. J. Psychiatr.*, 136:339–46.

Pugh, T. F., et al. (1963). Rates of mental disease related to childbearing. *N. Engl. J. Med.*, 268(22):1224–28.

Rosenwald, G. C. (1972). Early and late postpartum illnesses. *Psychosom. Med.*, 34(2):129–37.

Sandler, M. (Ed.) (1978). *Mental Illness in Pregnancy and the Puerperium.* London: Oxford University Press.

Stewart, D. E. (1985). Possible relationship of post-partum psychiatric symptoms to childbirth education programmes. *J. Psychosom. Obstet. Gynecol.*, 4(4).

Uddenberg, M., and Nilsson, L. (1975). The longitudinal course of para-natal emotional disturbance. *Acta Psychiatr. Scand.* 52(3):160–69.

Vandenbergh, R. L. (1980). Postpartum depression. *Clin. Obstet. Gynecol.* 23(4): 1105–11.

Weiner, A. (1982). Childbirth-related psychiatric illness. *Compr. Psychiatr.*, 23(2):143–54.

Chapter 6
Recent Clinical Management Experience

Ricardo J. Fernandez

Introduction

Are the clinical management and treatment of postpartum psychiatric disorders all that different? For that matter, do they really exist? Are they any different from the already recognized major psychiatric disorders?

The purpose of this chapter is twofold. The chapter first presents the reader with information which may persuade him or her to identify the uniqueness of these disorders. Then it describes some approaches currently in use by those who specialize in these problems. Other chapters in this book discuss the clinical presentations and symptoms unique to this group of disorders. The emphasis in this chapter is on the clinical approach. The material is from my clinical experience of six years working with postpartum women and from pertinent papers in the literature.

Postpartum Psychiatric Disorders—Fact or Fancy?

The existence of postpartum psychiatric disorders as separate entities is a matter about which opinions differ. There are those who think that psychiatric illness after childbearing is nothing more than a major psychiatric disorder occurring after the psychological and biological stress of pregnancy and delivery. Another group of colleagues believes that these disorders are distinctly different from other psychiatric illnesses and specific to the postpartum period and, as such, deserve their own diagnostic category or categories.

Regardless of orientation, there are clear differences in the clinical pictures of these women when they are compared with the signs and symptoms of recognized psychiatric disorders. Also, there appear to be treatment variations, both biological and psychological, which are especially effective for disorders in the postpartum period.

Population

Patients are women who are twenty to forty years old and are seen most frequently after their first delivery. Usually, there is no prior history of diagnosed psychiatric illness, and a review of their premorbid history reveals that most of them are highly functioning individuals. There is often a need to be organized and in control and a tendency to be a perfectionist. The patients often appear to have been the overfunctioning caretaking siblings in a dysfunctional family unit. With this experience they have been able to function very adequately in society and have been able to handle difficult and complex work situations. Usually, they have required no psychiatric or psychological treatment before the postpartum illness. Family history tends to be positive for alcoholism, affective illness, and thyroid disorder.

Differences in the Clinical Presentation

Certain clinical features are prominent in postpartum illness. Confusion is often part of the picture. The patient has difficulty with memory and concentration and has difficulty in thinking coherently. There is often bewilderment. Patients often complain of a vague mild sense of disorientation. "Fogginess" is a common complaint. These symptoms are recognized by the patient as distinctly different from her normal mental state. These symptoms have been noted in the literature and are often cited as an indication of a probable organic component in these disorders (Yalom et al. 1968, Dean and Kendell 1981, Brockington et al. 1981).

Another special characteristic is a high incidence of irritability and anxiety, when these cases are compared with women with major depression unrelated to childbearing. This is also true of feelings of guilt and inadequacy, which are increased in frequency in postpartum women (Pitt 1968).

Symptoms tend to fluctuate rapidly and unpredictably in postpartum cases. A patient's affect may go from euphoric to melancholic in a short period of time. This quality has been described as mercurial (Sneddon and Kerry 1985, Hamilton 1987).

A strong affective component is apparent in these disorders, with the psychotics often having a fairly clear manic flavor, often with religious delusions, psychomotor agitation, and occasionally, feelings of well-being (Brockington et al. 1981 and 1982, Dean and Kendell 1981). Patients with a postpartum psychosis often become depressed as the psychosis subsides.

The following are some additional observations from my clinical experience:

1. Among women with postpartum depression, a significant sub-group has severe, intrusive, and egodystonic obsessive rumina-tions of harming the infant. This is often accompanied by a severe agitated depression. This group tends to be particularly refrac-tory to most of the psychiatric medications currently available. In severe cases, electroconvulsive therapy (ECT) is an effective ap-proach.

2. Postpartum psychosis appears to respond to smaller doses of antipsychotics than psychosis unrelated to the postpartum pe-riod. Victims of postpartum psychosis also seem more prone to the side effects of psychotrophic drugs and usually require a shorter course of treatment.

3. There appears to be a high incidence of thyroid abnormalities, as well as low-normal or high-normal thyroid function in women with postpartum disorders. T. F. Nikolai and associates (1987) report an incidence of 11 percent of thyroid dysfunction in the postpartum group. This is supported by the position of Hamilton as well as recent articles in the obstetrics and gynecology literature addressing the growing recognition of postpartum thyroiditis of an autoimmune etiology (Hamilton 1987, Goldman 1986). In about 10 percent of women, thyrotoxicosis occurs in the first three months and lasts for one or two months. This is followed by a hypothyroid phase at two to six months, lasting three to five months and finally returning to the euthyroid state in about one year (Goldman 1986). About 40 percent of these women with abnormal thyroid function in the postpartum period go on to develop a permanent thyroid dysfunction (Nikolai et al. 1987).

4. An increasing incidence of alcoholism and compulsive gambling may be present in the families of postpartum depressives, and a past history of incest (involving the patient) in the postpartum psychotics. There appears to be a higher incidence of late luteal dysphoric disorder (previously called premenstrual syndrome) in women who have a postpartum psychiatric disorder.

5. Traumatic experiences of some postpartum cases relate to preg-nancy, delivery and the mother's ability to identify with the moth-ering role. The latter may have to do with the patient's own identity with her own mother, as well as role conflict related to the

many career and role options available to women today, choices that were less available in the past (Douglas 1963, Yalom et al. 1968, Brown and Shereshefsky 1972, and Markham 1961).

Biological Approaches to Postpartum Psychosis

Hospitalization is usually the preferred treatment setting for postpartum psychotic mothers, primarily because of the high level of dysfunction and the great risk of infanticide and suicide in this group (Inwood 1985). Other considerations in the choice of hospitalization versus outpatient care are prior history of response and the availability and extent of family and social support.

Mothers with postpartum psychosis respond well to the major tranquilizers at dosages which are usually lower than nonpostpartum psychotics. Postpartum patients seem much more sensitive to the side effects of these medications, particularly extrapyramidal symptoms such as pseudoparkinsonism, dystonia, akinesia, and akathisia. Anticholinergics are used as usual. Because of the manic quality, the sedating antipsychotics are preferred. I am particularly impressed with thioridazine because of its low incidence of extrapyramidal side effects. Lithium is often beneficial. The dose is titrated to therapeutic blood levels (around 1.0 mEq/L), carefully watching for side effects.*

Breast-feeding is usually discontinued because of the level of dysfunction and the potentially toxic doses of medication which may be used. This is particularly true for lithium which is known to be harmful to the nursing infant (Stile et al. 1984).

The duration of treated postpartum psychosis has been estimated at about five to six months (Sneddon and Kerry 1985). Antipsychotics should be tapered beginning in the second to fourth month, depending on the clinical picture. By five or six months, or shortly thereafter, the majority of patients no longer require any antipsychotics. This, however, is variable, and in some women, antipsychotic medication can be discontinued sooner.

As mentioned previously, depression often closely follows the psychotic state, sometimes presenting concurrently. With the emergence of depression, an antidepressant is added, generally following the guidelines for treatment of postpartum depressions. However, the depressions following psychosis usually do not have such a strong

---

*The effectiveness of lithium in postpartum mania is unquestioned. However, continued use of this substance should be balanced against its occasional toxic effects on the thyroid gland. This is of particular importance in the puerperium, when diminished thyroid-stimulating hormone and autoimmune thyroiditis may be having concurrent adverse actions on thyroid function.—Eds.

anxiety component, and anxiolytics are often not necessary. When agitation or anxiety is present in a depression following a psychosis, a small dose of a major tranquilizer is recommended along with the antidepressant. This may diminish the possibility of an exacerbation of psychotic symptoms.

Postpartum Depression

Postpartum depression cases can be subdivided into those preceded by a psychotic episode and those that are not. The former are easier to treat and respond well to a serotinergic antidepressant, often in conjunction with an antipsychotic. The "true" postpartum depressive (those with no postpartum psychosis preceding the depressive episode) present a spectrum of severity from mild to quite severe symptoms. The severe depressives present very often with marked obsessive thinking, usually of a nature destructive to the infant.

Patients with severe obsessive symptoms sometimes require antidepressants at a high dosage, for example, up to 600 mg of trazodone for control of the obsessive ruminations. Some of these patients respond to ECT.

Women with postpartum depressive disorders seem to do better on serotinergic antidepressants. Fluoxetine (Prozac), just recently available, a potent and exclusive serotinergic, seems highly effective in women with obsessive symptoms and appears to have a short onset of action.

One of the common characteristics of postpartum depression is sleeplessness and frequent awakenings. This problem can worsen initially with fluoxetine and may require concurrent administration of a sleep-inducing medication. Short-term use of hypnotics can be helpful. Another approach is the administration of a small dose of trazodone at bedtime, in conjunction with the fluoxetine.*

It is important to remember that insomnia is a symptom of the depression. As the fluoxetine diminishes the depression, the insomnia will resolve. Therefore, administration of a concurrent sleep-inducing medication is usually required only in the initial phase of treatment with fluoxetine.

When sleeplessness continues to be a problem, another serotinergic agent, such as doxepin or trazodone, may be preferable. Amitriptyline,

---

*As this book goes to press, the advantages of the drug are being balanced against its hazards, a debate which is taking place in court as well as in medical journals. When fluoxetine is initiated, patients should be under close observation. Some believe that this implies hospitalization.—EDS.

although a serotinergic, is less suitable because of its more severe side effects.

The use of fluoxetine is questionable in the breast-feeding mother. There is no research available at the time of this writing on the possible effects of fluoxetine on the nursing infant. Further, since it is a new medication, there is no long-term clinical experience as with the older drugs such as doxepin. Therefore, in breast-feeding mothers, doxepin may be the drug of choice.

Supporting the hypothesis that an abnormality of serotonin is involved in postpartum depression are studies that indicate a fairly clear relationship between progesterone and estrogen and serotinergic receptors (Biegon et al. 1983). The changes in these receptors seem similar to those found with chronic antidepressant administration and suggest that the high levels of estrogen and progesterone during pregnancy may have an antidepressant effect that is lost at the time of childbirth. Other studies have demonstrated a similar association between female hormones and changes in serotonin receptors (Ehrenkranz 1976, Peters et al. 1979).

Another useful serotinergic agent in treating these patients is the monoamine oxidase (MAO) inhibitor, phenelzine. Its effectiveness is supported by the finding of increased MAO activity in postpartum women and its significant correlation with depressed mood (George and Wilson 1981). Phenelzine is prescribed in the 45 to 60 mg per day range.

It is interesting to note the similarity between the severe postpartum depressive patient with obsessive ruminations and mild compulsive behavior (hiding knives, ritually avoiding the baby) and traditional obsessive-compulsive disorder. It is now fairly well recognized that there is a strong serotonin component in nonpostpartum obsessive-compulsive disorder, with reportedly good clinical response to serotinergic agents like clomipramine and fluoxetine.

Anxiety and agitation are often a component of the postpartum depressive picture. In the nonpsychotic postpartum depressive, these symptoms respond quite well to treatment with low to average doses of minor tranquilizers.

The possibility of a thyroid component in postpartum depression makes it imperative that a thorough thyroid screen be a part of any treatment plan. It is recommended that this include a thyroid-stimulating hormone (TSH) measurement. An interesting finding is that women with postpartum subclinical hypothyroidism seem to be particularly sensitive to the side effects of antidepressants, particularly fluoxetine.

Hamilton reports beneficial results in postpartum depressive patients upon administration of small amounts of thyroid hormone (Hamilton 1987). It is quite probable that many of these women were suffering from subclinical hypothyroidism during the puerperium and were not diagnosed as such.

If the diagnosis of subclinical hypothyroidism is conclusive, treatment can be initiated with thyroid replacement, such as L-thyroxine 50 to 150 mcg. per day, first obtaining then maintaining the patient within normal parameters. Depending on the clinical situation, the thyroid hormone can be given in addition to the antidepressant and the antidepressant discontinued at a later time.

When the patient is refractory to medications, or the severity of symptoms warrants it, electroconvulsive therapy (ECT) is the next choice. ECT has been used quite successfully in the treatment of postpartum disorders, particularly in Europe. In the United States, the aversion the public has to ECT may influence the patient to exclude this as a treatment choice in situations where it may be the most appropriate clinical approach.

The duration of treatment with medications depends on the clinical picture. Women who are treated early in the disorder and who have milder symptoms can usually be treated for shorter periods of time, perhaps up to four months. Those who come to treatment late in the disorder, who have severe affective symptoms and/or a significant obsessive component require longer periods of medication, perhaps six months to a full year after delivery.

Concerning breast-feeding and antidepressants, the mother's desire to nurse should always be considered. Generally, in the milder cases where lesser doses of tricyclic antidepressants are used, nursing seems to be clinically acceptable. To minimize effects on the infant, it is recommended that the patient take her medication after her last feeding and pump her breasts for the next few feedings, supplementing with bottled ones. Because of the lack of long-term clinical experience and research studies on trazodone and fluoxetine, it is recommended that a more established medication, such as doxepin, be used. When anxiolytics are prescribed, nursing is not recommended, since the minor tranquilizers have been associated with serious reactions in the baby, including jaundice and failure to thrive (Stile et al. 1984).

Decision regarding hospitalization of postpartum depressive patients requires a careful balance between possible disruption of the mother-child bond and imperative indications for the safety of the mother. Indications for hospitalization include definite suicidal thinking, severe dysfunction, and the severity of clinical presentation. These indications are increased in the absence of a strong home support system. In the severe depressive with obsessional features, the hospital can provide a setting for higher doses of medications and, if necessary, ECT.

As a result of the stigma our culture places on mental illness, as well as the fact that usually postpartum-impaired women have had no prior experience of significant emotional disorder, these patients sometimes exhibit marked difficulties in acceptance of their psychiatric illnesses. The denial of illness may interfere with compliance and may induce termination of medication before this is clinically appropriate.

Other Biological Treatment Considerations

Cortisol has been implicated as a possible etiological factor for postpartum disorders. It has been noted that cortisol levels are elevated during pregnancy and that it decreases soon after delivery (Hamilton 1987, Burke and Roulet 1970). A role for cortisol in these disorders is further suggested by the work of Ione Railton (1961). She administered prednisolone to women with postpartum symptoms early in the puerperium for a three- to four-week period with subsequent tapering of the medication. This was on the assumption that their postpartum symptoms were secondary to steroid withdrawal. She reported a shorter time to recovery and no recurrences in a small group of women with no active symptoms but with a prior history of postpartum disorders in previous pregnancies. Unfortunately, no one has followed up on this approach.

Many women with postpartum depression experience a significant worsening of the symptoms in the late luteal phase. Sometimes recognition and education is enough, and the patient will be able to tolerate a mild worsening for a few days. If the symptoms become severe, I usually institute progesterone premenstrually. This alleviates the symptoms in most cases. It is based on the work of Katharina Dalton (1984) in England.

Psychological Approaches

For the great majority of women with postpartum psychiatric illness, this is their first exposure to a significant mental illness, and it is often very difficult for them to accept. In order to alleviate excessive anxiety and to encourage trust, acceptance, and compliance with treatment, it is best to initially stress a biological understanding of their disorder. This disorder is comparable to other types of physical illness, particularly the possible hormonal etiologies of these disorders.

In conjunction with this, a strong educational approach is appropriate, and when clinically appropriate, the patient is encouraged to read literature available to the public on this subject (Dix 1985). The patient should also contact a local support group for postpartum disorders, if one is available. These groups are likely to reinforce biological concepts of the disorder, and the groups alleviate guilt and shame and increase compliance significantly.

Early in treatment, it is important to involve the family in assisting the patient with childrearing and arranging for the mother to have some time away from the infant. To assist in this, education of the husband and family with a biological orientation is imperative.

In the therapy hour, a supportive approach in terms of education and reassurance about her illness and basic childrearing is often quite helpful in the early stages of treatment. These patients often question their ability to care for their child. Reassurance is often very effective, along with basic guidance.

Empathy in the early phase of treatment is quite important in helping the patient deal with the severe narcissistic injury of her illness, together with the accompanying repressed rage. This rage is sometimes directed at herself, resulting in suicidal ideation. It may be directed at the child, resulting in infanticidal fantasies.

Suicidal risk is a matter for concern in both psychotic and depressed patients. It should not be taken lightly. Suicidal and infanticidal ideation can accompany postpartum illness and always requires clinical attention and concern.

Thoughts of harming the baby are often part of the obsessional rumination of the postpartum depressed mother, often without intent. However, careful assessment is imperative, particularly in the severe obsessive where judgment and reality testing begin to deteriorate.

Therapeutic intervention is often necessary in other areas. Environmental stressors have been shown to predispose to the condition (Gordon and Gordon 1967, Uddenberg and Nilsson 1975). Often there are recent and major changes in geographical location, employment, and financial status.

Cultural issues, including role conflict, are also quite common. Women in our society are caught in the double bind of attempting fulfillment in both motherhood and the career world. The woman needs to make some major decisions after childbirth, and this often ends in a no-win situation. If she decides on full-time mothering, there is often resentment about career and work opportunities relinquished. If the decision is to incorporate both, there may be guilt about the diminished time spent with the infant. The working mother's dilemma: quantity versus quality time.

The quality of the relationship with her own mother, her identity as a mother, and other material suggestive of premorbid psychological difficulties may be present. Some issues, such as inflexibility and control, may not have been a problem to the patient before her illness. In fact, these highly organized women do quite well in the working world. However, the demands of raising a child require patience and an acceptance of many things that cannot be rigidly controlled.

Unlike a job situation or a relationship with another adult, a parent is locked into the relationship with the infant. Once a parent, always a parent. Past coping mechanisms, such as removing herself from a toxic situation, are inappropriate and ineffective. The new mother may feel trapped, helpless, and out of control, and this may add significantly to her symptoms. She may present escape fantasies of running away from home, leaving the child and husband behind.

The patient should be made aware of these issues and reassured that they are not uncommon. Empathy with her emotional discomfort is imperative in conjunction with devising new methods for dealing with her child.

Once the therapeutic alliance has been established, based on biological, educational, and supportive approaches, and when the patient's symptoms have diminished, these social factors may be introduced for discussion and resolution. At this time, I usually see patients on a weekly basis.

As the acute disorder resolves and there is a return to normal patterns of thinking and functioning, these women may look retrospectively and reflectively at the episode, examining the impact the disorder has had on their lives. They may become appropriately saddened, perhaps even mildly depressed. This is an adjustment reaction to a major traumatic event and is best dealt with as such. It may be difficult to explain this adjustment reaction to a patient, and the concept of being depressed about being depressed may contribute to understanding.

The marital relationship may have suffered a degree of instability during the wife's postpartum depression (Kumar and Robson 1978, Robson and Kumar 1980, Nilsson and Per-Erik 1970, and Sosa et al. 1980). As the patient approaches full recovery, the husband may begin to go through his own adjustment reaction to the postpartum event. He may be disillusioned with the situation of having a child, and feel quite exhausted by the demands of an ailing wife and an infant child. The symptoms may be severe enough to require clinical intervention for the father. The possibility of an adjustment reaction in the father should be discussed with the couple, if possible, but certainly when the mother is in recovery. Her awareness may facilitate treatment for the husband, if this is indicated.

References

Biegon, A., Reches, A., et al. (1983). Serotinergic and noradrenergic receptors in the rat brain: Modulation by chronic exposure to ovarian hormones. *Life Sci.* 32:2015–21.

Brockington, I. F., Cernic, K., et al. (1981). Puerperal psychosis. *Arch. Gen. Psychiatr.,* 38:829–33.

Brockington, I. F., Winokur, G., et al. (1982). Puerperal psychosis. In I. F. Brockington and R. Kumar (Eds.), *Motherhood and Mental Illness.* London: Academic Press.

Brown, W. A., and Shereshefsky, P. (1972). Seven women: A prospective study of postpartum psychiatric disorders. *Psychiatry* 35(2):139–58.

Burke, C. W., and Roulet, F. (1970). Increased exposure of tissues to cortisol in late pregnancy. *Br. Med. J.* 1:657–59.

Dalton, K. (1984). *The Premenstrual Syndrome and Progesterone Therapy.* Chicago: Yearbook Medical Publishers.

Dean, C., and Kendell, R. E. (1981). The symptomatology puerperal illness. *Br. J. Psychiatr.,* 139:128–33.

Dix, C. (1985). *The New Mother Syndrome.* New York: Doubleday.

Douglas, G. (1963). Puerperal depression and excessive compliance with the mother. *Br. J. Med. Psychol.* 36:271–78.

Ehrenkranz, J.R.L. (1976). Effects of sex steroids on serotonin uptake in blood platelets. *Acta Endocrinol.* 83:420–28.

George, A. J., and Wilson, K.C.M. (1981). Monoamine oxidase activity and the puerperal blues syndrome. *J. Psychosom. Res.* 25:409–13.

Goldman, J. M. (1986). Postpartum thyroid dysfunction. *Arch. Int. Med.* 146: 1296–99.

Gordon, R. E., and Gordon, K. K. (1967). Factors in postpartum emotional adjustment. *Am. J. Orthopsychiatry* 37:359–60.

Hamilton, J. A. (1987). An integrated hypothesis regarding psychiatric illness after childbearing. Paper presented to Annual Meeting, Postpartum Support International, Santa Barbara, CA.

Inwood, D. G. (1985). The spectrum of postpartum psychiatric disorders. In D. G. Inwood (Ed.), *Recent Advances in Postpartum Psychiatric Disorders.* Washington, DC: American Psychiatric Press.

Kumar, R., and Robson, K. (1978). Neurotic disturbances during pregnancy and the puerperium. In M. Sandler (Ed.), *Mental Illness in Pregnancy and the Puerperium.* Oxford: Oxford University Press.

Markham, S. (1961). A comparative evaluation of psychotic and non-psychotic reactions to childbirth. *Am. J. Orthopsychiatry* 31:565–70.

Nikolai, T. F., Turney, S. L., et al. (1987). Postpartum lymphocytic thyroiditis: Prevalence, course and long-term follow-up. *Arch. Int. Med.* 147(2):221–24.

Nilsson, A., and Per-Erik, A. (1970). Para-natal emotional development. Part II. The influence of background factors. *Acta Psychiatr. Scand. (Suppl.)* 220: 63–141.

Peters, J. R., Elliot, J. M., et al. (1979). Effect of oral contraceptives on platelet noradrenaline and 5-hydroxytryptamine receptors and aggression. *Lancet* 2:933–36.

Pitt, B. M. N. (1968). Atypical depression following childbirth. *Br. J. Psychiatr.* 114:1325–35.

Railton, I. E. (1961). The use of corticoids in postpartum depression. *J. Am. Med. Women's Assoc.* 16:450–52.

Robson, K. M., and Kumar, R. (1980). Delayed onset of maternal affection after childbirth. *Br. J. Psychiatr.* 13:347–53.

Sneddon, J., and Kerry, R. J. (1985). The psychiatric mother and baby unit. In D. G. Inwood (Ed.), *Recent Advances in Postpartum Psychiatric Disorders.* Washington, DC: American Psychiatric Press.

Sosa, R., Kendell, J., et al. (1980). The effects of a supportive companion on perinatal problems. *N. Engl. J. Med.* 303(11):597–99.

Stile, I. L., Hegyo, T., et al. (1984). *Drugs Used in Neonates and During Pregnancy.* Orandell, NJ: Medical Economics.

Uddenberg, M., and Nilsson, L. (1975). The longitudinal course of para-natal emotional disturbance. *Acta Psychiatr. Scand.* 52(3):160–69.

Yalom, I. D., Lunde, D. T., et al. (1968). "Postpartum blues" syndrome. *Arch. Gen. Psychiatr.* 18:16–27.

Chapter 7
Maternity Blues: A Model for Biological Research

Jan L. Campbell

Maternity blues, also known as the baby blues, is probably the most common of the affective syndromes experienced by childbearing women. Its occurrence ranges from 27 to 80 percent of all deliveries (Pitt 1973, Hamilton 1962, Stein 1982). Onset is usually shortly after parturition, with variable symptoms, usually affective in nature. The syndrome is thought to be benign and self-limiting, resolving spontaneously within two weeks.

The etiology of the maternity blues is unknown. In general, published studies report no relationship with such factors as social class, marital status, economic condition, obstetric difficulties, or psychosocial stressors (for review, see Kennerly and Gath 1986). The syndrome has been described in Jamaican (Davidson 1972), African (Harris 1981, Ifabumuyi and Akindele 1985), European (Pitt 1973, Kendell et al. 1981), and North American (Hamilton 1962, Yalom et al. 1968) women and appears to occur without consideration of cultural or racial differences in populations.

The characteristics of common occurrence, across cultures, without relationship to social factors, suggests a biological etiology for maternity blues. That the affective symptoms also occur in relationship to a significant physiological shift in steroid hormones and neuroendocrine events suggests that maternity blues may be a heuristic model for effects of hormones on mood and mental status. Therefore, the purpose of this chapter is to briefly review areas in which there have been promising findings, and to suggest some possible directions for research.

One area receiving considerable investigation concerns what measurements can be used to establish a reliable and replicable evaluation of the blues. Most investigators have asked about the presence of symptoms such as tearfulness, depression, irritability, and anxiety. Some have included mood lability, occurring at short intervals such as one hour. Symptom and adjective checklists commonly used in the studies of affective disorder have been employed, although many of the symptoms may be confounded by the demands of infant care; insomnia is a good example of this problem. Some investigators have developed rating scales designed to evaluate postpartum blues for specific studies (Kennerly and Gath 1986, Hamilton 1962, Stein 1982, Cox et al. 1987). Kendell and coworkers (1981) have created analogue scales to rate similar symptoms. Such checklists and scales are more suitable for daily administration, in contrast to structured interviews which are lengthy and do not reflect *daily* changes in mental state. Two investigators have developed standardized scales with validity and reliability measures, designed specifically for women in the postpartum period (Cox et al. 1987, Kennerly and Gath 1986). Use of such measures would improve the ability to compare findings from various studies, which is currently a significant problem in interpreting the literature.

Of equal concern is the determination of a pattern of blues symptoms and the course of resolution, as this influences the timing of biological measurements. Most studies report symptoms at one or two times during the first two weeks after parturition. Those investigators who have reported daily rating of postpartum mood states, including symptoms of anxiety, tearfulness, irritability, depression, happiness, and lability, do not find a single predominant pattern. Yalom and associates (1968) studied women twice daily for ten days and described the sample as two groups, one with persistent crying and depression varying over the ten days; and the other with a relatively abrupt and usually brief episode of tearfulness and dysphoria at day three or four. Kendell and colleagues (1981) noted peaking of depression, tearfulness, and lability on Day five, and a gradual increase in irritability and decrease in anxiety. Stein (1982) recorded daily ratings for similar mood states, and found fourth- or fifth-day peaks for tearfulness, depression, restlessness, dreaming, and irritability. Patterns for concentration, headache, and fatigue did not fit the peaking pattern of other symptoms.

These findings suggest that the blues syndrome most often occurs within the first week following parturition and has a variable presentation with such core symptoms as tearfulness, depression, and mood lability. A useful next step might be comparison of those women with peaking or episodic blues to those with a more chronic and persistent course, to determine if there are differences such as previous personal or family history of psychiatric disorder or postpartum states, or neuroendocrine variables.

A related issue concerns those women with well-characterized blues whose symptoms persist beyond two or three weeks after parturition. Very little is known about the course of these women. Do they subsequently develop postpartum major depression? Findings are conflicting, with two studies suggesting that women with severe blues may have a more persistent course and two finding no relationship.

Kendell and coworkers (1981) found that the women with highest scores on lability and depression at day five were more likely to report persistent depressive symptoms through the 21-day rating period and at follow-up three to five months later. The day five peak did not, however, predict occurrence of postpartum depression. Cox and associates (1981) found that women with severe blues were particularly at risk of persistent depressive symptoms at subsequent evaluation three to five months postpartum. Yalom and colleagues (1968) noted that at eight-month follow-up, only one of twenty-two women had sought psychiatric care after prolonged blues symptoms, the others having resolved symptoms without significant difficulty. Kumar and Robson (1984) in their large prospective study of postpartum depression did not find any relationship between blues and depression three months after parturition. Hapgood and coworkers (1988) reported that the presence of depression, tearfulness, anxiety, and irritability ten to fourteen days postpartum predicted the occurrence of major depression at fourteen months follow-up but not at six months. History of psychiatric disorder also predicted depression at fourteen months, suggesting that late onset of depression in this sample may be unrelated to parturition.

The data from these prospective studies suggests that severe blues are associated with lengthier persistence of symptoms but are not sufficient to meet the criteria for diagnosable depression. Further research is clearly needed, and data regarding unusual course or severity of symptoms, family history of psychiatric disorder, or nonpostpartum depression would be useful in order to isolate subgroups for whom different biological or psychological factors may be pertinent.

Biological Research on Maternity Blues

Hypotheses regarding physiological and biochemical events that could be implicated as etiological factors in postpartum psychiatric disorders have primarily concerned the endocrine system. That affective symptoms occur postpartum, premenstrually, and at menopause suggests some relationship with the hypothalamic-pituitary-gonadal axis. Endocrine changes occurring during pregnancy and at parturition are unique in their magnitude and rapidity. During pregnancy, both estrogen and progesterone blood levels gradually increase, reaching the highest physiological levels to be experienced by the individual. At parturition, blood levels of both hormones fall precipitously, reaching baseline within two to five days (for review, see Deakin 1988). These striking changes have prompted hypotheses relating hormonal loss to postpartum mood changes. Bower and Altschule (1956) reported an apparent beneficial effect of progesterone administered to women with postpartum psychosis, and suggested that progesterone modulation of the anterior pituitary, and consequently of adrenal corticosteroids, might play a significant role in the etiology of the illness. Yalom and coworkers (1968) proposed that the sudden fall of progesterone at parturition might be related to maternity blues. Similarly, Dalton (1971) suggested an elated mood associated with prepartum rise in placental steroid output, followed by dysphoria associated with its loss. Smith (1975) has also suggested that abrupt loss of placental estrogen (estriol) might precipitate a withdrawal syndrome characterized by affective states.

Estrogen and Progesterone

There are four studies reporting blood levels of estrogen and progesterone during the first week following parturition, with conflicting findings. Nott and associates (1976) studied women selected for absence of psychiatric history or symptoms, obstetric or medical complications, or socioeconomic difficulties. Subjects were described using standardized measures, and blood samples were obtained at two- or three-day intervals for up to ten weeks postpartum. The subjects noted occurrence of blues symptoms and patterns similar to that described in other studies, but there were essentially no significant differences between blues and nonblues subjects in levels of progesterone or estrogen. There appeared to be a correlation between irritability and higher predelivery estrogen levels. The greater the progesterone drop the more likely were subjects to rate themselves depressed but less likely to report sleep disturbance, and the lower the estrogen level the more likely sleep disturbances were reported.

While these findings support the progesterone hypothesis, one should note that the symptoms were insufficient to establish a diagnosis of depression as late as ten weeks postpartum. These investigators also noted marked variability of progesterone and estrogen levels within individuals despite attempts to obtain samples in morning hours only. Feksi and colleagues (1984) studied salivary hormone levels in a similarly selected group of women using three symptom checklists given four times daily at the same time saliva samples were collected, for five days postpartum. In this group, women with higher maternity blues scores had higher levels of progesterone and estrogen than did those with lower blues scores. No information regarding patterns of hormones is given.

Results of these two studies are contradictory, although the patients samples are evidently similar and assessment of presence of blues is comparable. Timing of body fluid samples was somewhat different, and it is possible that the Nott study may have been compromised by limited technological sophistication in determination of hormone levels ten years earlier than the Feksi study. However, findings of Kuevi and coworkers (1983), using radioimmunoassay techniques showed that estrogen and progesterone blood levels were consistently lower among women with blues than those without blues and thus support the Nott study. Kuevi also noted marked across-subject variability in hormone levels and, to control for this factor, used subjects with a peaking pattern to determine if a significant change occurred on the day of peak symptoms. Change in estrogen or progesterone level did not occur on the peak day, although there was a significant change in circulating catecholamines.

Gard and associates (1986) also noted no difference in estrogen or progesterone levels in the first five postpartum days between women with or without maternity blues. The latter studies by Kuevi and Gard employed an unselected patient group and may have included some individuals with family or personal history of psychiatric disorder.

As noted by Nott and Kuevi, it is likely that the marked variability in estrogen and progesterone in the immediate postpartum period may obscure any significant differences in a small sample. The Kuevi finding that women with maternity blues have consistently lower estrogen and progesterone levels is tantalizing, and the study deserves replication in a larger sample. Because maternity blues is clearly heterogeneous, subjects should be chosen with careful attention to factors such as personal or family history of psychiatric disorder, socioeconomic status, and marital stability to reduce the number of possible confounding factors.

This work is important for two reasons. First, association of maternity blues with alterations in levels of progesterone or estrogen provides support for a hypothesized endocrine influence on mood disorders. The effects of estrogen and progesterone on neurotransmitters serotonin, norepinephrine, and dopamine have been reviewed by Deakin (1988) and by George and Sandler (1988). Considerable data suggests significant effects in animal models, but there is little available data in humans, and the common occurrence of maternity blues in women may offer a model for the study of brain and hormone interaction. Secondly, these findings would add impetus to evidence from treatment studies that estrogen and progesterone may be useful in management of postpartum depression (Hapgood et al. 1988, Dalton 1984). For these reasons, research on hormonal influences on mood and new treatment strategies may well be aided by employing maternity blues as a model.

Cortisol

Perhaps the best-known neuroendocrine function associated with affective disorders is the production of cortisol. Both hypercortisolemia and resistance to suppression with dexamethasone have been shown to be associated with major depression. That cortisol metabolism is altered during pregnancy and the postpartum period has prompted interest in a possible role for corticosteroids in postpartum affective disorders.

During pregnancy, plasma cortisol levels gradually increase, primarily in the bound (and presumably biologically inactive) fraction. Urinary free cortisol excretion is increased in late pregnancy, and this has been shown to be due to a decrease in the usual circadian variation of cortisol such that unbound levels remain elevated during the night. The result is tissue exposure that is two to three times normal (Burke and Roulet 1970). There is an additional surge of cortisol at labor, followed by a rapid decline to the second-trimester level in two or three days.

Handley and colleagues (1977 and 1980) have studied cortisol concentrations in two series of patients. The first series suggested a relationship between elevated mood and high concentrations of cortisol; in the second larger series, the finding could not be replicated as no patient experienced elated mood. A high cortisol level at 38 weeks gestation did, however, predict more severe postpartum blues.

Ballinger and coworkers (1982) reported an association between increased urinary excretion of 11-hydroxycortisol and mood elevation occurring during gestation but only reaching significance after delivery, when there appeared to be a delay in expected cortisol reduction, followed by a more acute fall than was seen in nonelated subjects. Kuevi and associates (1983) were unable to demonstrate a relationship between high cortisol blood levels and maternity blues, as were Gard and colleagues (1986). The latter studies did not report occurrence of elevated mood among patients.

Another approach to assessing alterations in cortisol production and the hypothalamic-pituitary-adrenocortical (HPA) axis following parturition in the dexamethasone suppression test (DST). Suppression of cortisol production in response to dexamethasone, a synthetic steroid, is thought to reflect normal HPA function, and nonsuppression has been associated with major depression. Two studies of recently delivered women suggest that the HPA axis may require more than a few days to return to normal function after parturition. Greenwood and Parker (1984) reported 82 percent of a sample of forty-five women three to five days postpartum were nonsuppressors, and the abnormal response was not correlated with mood change. Singh and coworkers (1986) reported an abnormal DST in 79 percent of postpartum women without maternity blues on Day five after parturition. The subjects had returned to normal suppressor status at one to five months later. Singh, therefore, concluded that the immediate postpartum period itself is a confounding factor for use of the DST is unlikely to be helpful by itself in studies of maternity blues.

These confusing results may occur in part because of differences in sensitivity and specificity of cortisol assays. Chemical measurements used by the Handley and Gard groups tend to be less sensitive than the radioimmunoassay techniques used by Kuevi, Feksi, and their colleagues. A second issue is the timing of cortisol sampling. Cortisol is secreted in pulses and demonstrates diurnal and seasonal variability, which are potential confounding factors. Individuals with hypercortisolemia tend to lose the diurnal variation in secretion, which has also been described in late pregnancy (Burke and Roulet 1970). Persistence of an unvarying pattern in the postpartum period could not be identified with a single daily sample. Simultaneous sampling of subjects at morning, evening, and late night time points would clarify the range and characteristics of cortisol secretion in the postpartum period and possibly demonstrate altered pattern or amount of cortisol secretion in women with mood changes. Further research seems warranted in light of the clinical report of Railton (1961) that low-dose prednisone was prophylactic for postpartum depression in a group of women with previous postpartum episodes.

Prolactin

Prolactin, a pituitary hormone required for lactation, reaches its peak at parturition and is maintained at high levels throughout lactation. A similar but less pronounced elevation occurs in the luteal phase of the menstrual cycle and has been associated with premenstrual syndrome (George and Sandler 1988). Carroll and Steiner (1978) hypothesized that prolactin may interact with the ovarian hormones to produce affective symptomatology. Specifically, premenstrually low progesterone associated with high prolactin may result in irritable hostility and anxiety; low estrogen associated with high prolactin may produce depressive symptoms.

This hormonal profile is, of course, present in the immediate postpartum period during which time prolactin levels are at the highest point. George and coworkers (1980) recently reported significant correlation of prolactin levels postpartum with symptoms of anxiety, tension, and depression among women with maternity blues and have suggested that prolactin or its central aminergic regulating system may be associated with the blues. Alder and associates (1986) were unable to find such an association, nor were Kuevi and colleagues (1983). In the latter two studies, samples were obtained with attention to suckling, but controls for stress and physical activity were lacking and may have confounded the findings.

Mastrogiacomo and coworkers (1982–83) compared women with idiopathic hyperprolactinemia and postpartum women with similar prolactin levels to normal controls. Postpartum women and hyperprolactinemic women were significantly more hostile than were controls; hyperprolactinemic women were more depressed and anxious than postpartum women. Since both hyperprolactinemic women and postpartum women had similar levels of prolactin and postpartum were no more depressed than controls, these data do not support the purported relationship between prolactin and depression or anxiety. There is evidence, however, that idiopathic hyperprolactinemia can be associated with affective symptoms that are diminished by administration of prolactin-lowering agents (Buckman et al. 1984). This suggests an interesting possibility to test the Carroll and Steiner (1978) hypothesis by administering bromocriptine, a drug that lowers prolactin, to women with maternity blues and obtaining blood levels of prolactin, estrogen and progesterone to determine any relationship with mood state both before and after bromocriptine is given. If the hypothesis were supported, one might wish to consider treating postpartum depression with bromocriptine, especially since this drug has been compared favorably as an antidepressant with imipramine (Waehrens and Gerlach 1981).

Tryptophan

Tryptophan is a dietary amino acid which is a precursor for brain serotonin, a neurotransmitter for which there is evidence of modulation by estrogen and progesterone (for review, see Deakin 1988). There has been considerable interest in the possibility that tryptophan supplementation might influence the course of affective disorder. Tryptophan crosses the blood-brain barrier by an active transport process that can be influenced by its plasma concentration. Since the rate-limiting enzyme in serotonin synthesis is not saturated by tryptophan, transport of this precursor into the brain may itself be the rate-limiting step (Fernstrom 1982). Tryptophan is, however, highly protein-bound, and factors that influence the ratio of free to bound tryptophan are not clear. Stein and coworkers (1976) obtained plasma tryptophan level for eighteen postpartum women and correlated these with mood determined daily for seven or eight days after parturition. A significant correlation occurred between severity of affective changes and free tryptophan, and levels were similar to those in a group of depressed nonpostpartum women.

Handley and associates (1977 and 1980) studied a larger series of seventy-one women, in which they were able to demonstrate lower free tryptophan in blues patients, but only during the season of the year when tryptophan is normally high. There was, however, a slower rise of blood tryptophan postpartum, significantly associated with occurrence of blues, and at six-month follow-up, with depression (Baker et al. 1984). In a subsequent multifactorial study, these investigators replicated the finding that a slower rise in total tryptophan predicted the blues, and especially a low blood level on Day one postpartum (Gard et al. 1986).

This suggests that tryptophan loading might avert the blues. One study reports three grams of L-tryptophan given daily did not reduce the incidence of blues (Harris 1980). While one might expect that tryptophan loading would uniformly increase blood levels, there may be a defect in tryptophan metabolism such as increased peripheral utilization that would reduce blood levels in some individuals. In addition, the cofactor pyridoxine is necessary for neuronal utilization of tryptophan, and it would be advantageous to provide supplemental pyridoxine in a tryptophan trial. That low blood tryptophan distinguishes blues in a total sample of 123 women in separate trials (Handley et al. 1977 and 1980) supports the contention that tryptophan and possibly serotonin may be linked to maternity blues. A therapeutic trial should include tryptophan blood levels in the week prior to delivery, on Day one postpartum, and at least twice during tryptophan and pyridoxine supplementation for ten days.*

*While tryptophan, a common amino acid, has generally been regarded as nontoxic, experimental and clinical trials should be held off until clarification of reports in late 1989 to the U.S. Food and Drug Administration that certain preparations of the amino acid had been found to be toxic.—Eds.

Conclusion

This brief review has focused on some aspects of research on maternity blues that suggest a direction for future investigation. Emergence of rating scales constructed specifically for measurement of blues will facilitate comparison of findings from different studies and may define a more reliable rate and pattern of occurrence. Prospective studies with daily ratings of mood states for at least two or three weeks, and postpartum follow-up for at least three months may clarify the question of a predictive relationship between blues and postpartum depression which could be clinically useful.

The utility of maternity blues as a model for hormonal influence on mood states can be improved by careful delineation of characteristics such as personal or family history of psychiatric illness which suggest a biological predisposition. Obviously, maternity blues is likely to be highly heterogeneous in etiology with considerable variation in the influence of sex hormones on mental status. Recognition of clinical subgroups may possibly facilitate attempts to correlate neuroendocrine factors and altered mood states.

Endocrine studies are complicated by lack of information regarding expected fluctuation of hormones, both diurnal and seasonal, in parturient and nonparturient women. It is essential, therefore, that controls be carefully selected and conditions within groups be held constant. For example, women who are breast-feeding must not be compared with those who are bottle-feeding, and nonparturient controls must be matched for age, parity, and other factors known to influence hormone production. Neuroendocrine studies ideally would incorporate sampling at multiple time points for determination of differences in patterns of secretion.

Clinical trials of various agents such as progesterone might suggest an etiology for blues and are benign in effect. Study designs, blinded with regard to the administered agent, with frequent sampling for blood levels of appropriate hormones or tryptophan are most likely to be informative. A similar trial of prednisolone is suggested by the clinical report of prednisolone prophylaxis of postpartum blues (Railton 1961).

In summary, maternity blues may be a heuristic model useful in the study of endocrine and other biological factors in mood states. The frequency and predictability of maternity blues in a relatively large population accessible for prospective studies and the availability of appropriate instruments for measurement of clinical states and known biochemical correlates provide the potential for fruitful research.

References

Alder, E. M., Cook, A., Davidson, D., West, C., and Bancroft, J. (1986). Hormones, mood and sexuality in lactating women. *Br. J. Psychiatry*, 148:74–79.

Baker, J. M., Handley, S. L., Waldron, G., et al. (1984). Seasonal variation in plasma tryptophan in parturient women. *Progress in Neuropsychopharmacol. Biol. Psychiatry*, 5:515–18.

Ballinger, C. B., Kay, D.S.G., Naylor, G. J., et al. (1982). Some biochemical findings during pregnancy and after delivery in relation to mood change. *Psychol. Med.*, 12:548–56.

Bower, W. H., and Altschule, M. D. (1956). Use of progesterone in the treatment of postpartum psychosis. *N. Engl. J. Med.*, 245:157–60.

Buckman, M. T., Kellner, R., Mattox, J., et al. (1984). Psychological distress in hyperprolactinemic women. Fourth International Conference on Prolactin. Charlottesville, Virginia.

Burke, C. W., and Roulet, F. (1970). Increased exposure of tissues to cortisol in late pregnancy. *Br. Med. J.* 1:657–59.

Carroll, B. J., and Steiner, M. (1978). The psychobiology of premenstrual dysphoria: The role of prolactin. *Psychoneuroendocrinology*, 3:171–80.

Cox, J. L., Connor, Y., and Kendell, R. E. (1981). Prospective study of the psychiatric disorders of childbirth. *Br. J. Psychiatry*, 140:111–17.

Cox, J. L., Holden, J. M., and Sagovsky, R. (1987). Detection of postnatal depression: Development of the ten-item Edinburgh Postnatal Depression Scale. *Br. J. Psychiatry*, 150:782–86.

Dalton, K. (1984). Progesterone prophylaxis for postnatal depression. Proceedings of the Biennial Conference of the Marcé Society.

———. (1971). Prospective study into puerperal depression. *Br. J. Psychiatry*, 118:689–92.

Davidson, J.R.T. (1972). Postpartum mood change in Jamaican women: A description and discussion on its significance. *Br. J. Psychiatry*, 121:659–63.

Deakin, J.F.W. (1988). Relevance of hormone—CNS interactions to psychological changes in the puerperium. In R. Kumar and I. F. Brockington (Eds.), *Motherhood and Mental Illness*, 2nd ed. London: Butterworth.

Feksi, A., Harris, B., Walker, R. F., Riad-Fahmy, O., and Newcombe, R. G. (1984). Maternity blues and hormone levels in saliva. *J. Affective Disord.*, 6:351–55.

Fernstrom, J. D. (1982). Acute effects of tryptophan and single meals on serotonin synthesis in the rat brain. In B. T. Ho, J. C. Schoolar, and E. Usdin (Eds.), *Serotonin in Biological Psychiatry*. New York: Raven Press.

Gard, P. R., Handley, S. L., Parsons, A. D., and Waldron, G. (1986). A multivariate investigation of postpartum mood disturbance. *Br. J. Psychiatry*, 148: 567–75.

George, A. L., Copeland, J.R.M., and Wilson, K.C.M. (1980). Prolactin secretion and the postpartum blues syndrome. *Br. J. Pharmacol.*, 70:102.

George, A., and Sandler, M. (1988). Endocrine and biochemical studies in puerperal mental disorders. In R. Kumar and I. F. Brockington (Eds.), *Motherhood and Mental Illness*, 2nd ed. London: Butterworth.

Greenwood, J., and Parker, G. (1984). The dexamethasone suppression test in the puerperium. *Aust. N.Z. J. Psychiatry*, 18:232–84.

Hamilton, J. A. (1982). The identity of postpartum psychosis. In I. F. Brockington and R. Kumar (Eds.), *Motherhood and Mental Illness*. New York: Academic Press.

Hamilton, J. A. (1962). *Postpartum Psychiatric Problems.* St. Louis: C. V. Mosby.

Handley, S. L., Dunn, T. L., Baker, J. M., et al. (1977). Mood changes in the puerperium and plasma tryptophan and cortisol concentrations. *Br. Med. J.,* 2:18–22.

Handley, S. L., Dunn, T. L., Waldron, G., et al. (1980). Tryptophan, cortisol and puerperal mood. *Br. J. Psychiatry,* 136:498–508.

Hapgood, C. C., Elkind, G. S., and Wright, J. J. (1988). Maternity blues: Phenomena and relationship to later postpartum depression. *Aust. N.Z. J. Psychiatry,* 22:299–306.

Harris, B. (1981). Maternity blues in East African Clinic Attenders. *Arch. Gen. Psychiatry,* 38:1293–95.

———. (1980). Prospective trial of L-tryptophan in maternity blues. *Br. J. Psychiatry,* 137:233–35.

Ifabumuyi, O. I., and Akindele, M. O. (1985). Postpartum mental illness in northern Nigeria. *Acta Psychiatr. Scand.* 72:63–68.

Kendell, R. E., McGuire, R. J., Connor, Y., and Cox, J. L. (1981). Mood changes in the first three weeks after childbirth. *J. Affective Disord.,* 3:317–26.

Kennerly, H., and Gath, D. (1986). Maternity blues reassessed. *Psychiatric Developments.* 1:1–17.

Kuevi, V., Causon, R., Dixson, A. F., Everard, D. M., Hall, J. M., Hole, D., Whitehead, S. A., Wilson, C. A., and Wise, J.C.M. (1983). Plasma amine and hormone changes in "postpartum blues." *Clin. Endocrinol.,* 19:39–46.

Kumar, R., and Robson, J. M. (1984). A prospective study of emotional disorders in childbearing women. *Br. J. Psychiatry,* 144:35–47.

Mastrogiacomo, I., Fava, M., Fava, G. A., et al. (1982–83). Postpartum hostility and prolactin. *Int. J. Psychiatr. Med.* 12:289–94.

Nott, P. M., Franklin, M., Armitage, C., et al. (1976). Hormonal changes and mood in the puerperium. *Br. J. Psychiatry,* 128:379–83.

Pitt, B. (1973). Maternity blues. *Br. J. Psychiatry,* 122:431–33.

Railton, I. E. (1961). The use of corticoids in postpartum depression. *J. Am. Med. Women's Assoc.,* 16:450–52.

Singh, B., Gilhotra, M., Smith, R., Brinsmead, M., Lewin, T., and Hall, C. (1986). Postpartum psychosis and the dexamethasone suppression test. *J. Affective Disord.,* 11:173–77.

Smith, S. L. (1975). Mood and the menstrual cycle. In E. F. Sachar (Ed.), *Topics in Psychoneuroendocrinology.* New York: Grune and Stratton.

Stein, G. (1982). The maternity blues. In I. F. Brockington and R. Kumar (Eds.), *Motherhood and Mental Illness.* London: Academic Press.

Stein, G., Milton, F., Bebbington, P., et al. (1976). Relationship between mood disturbances and free and total plasma tryptophan in postpartum women. *Br. Med. J.,* 2:457.

Waehrens, J., and Gerlach, J. (1981). Bromocriptine and imipramine in endogenous depression: A double-bind control trial on outpatients. *J. Affective Disord.,* 3:193–202.

Yalom, I. D., Lunde, D. T., Moos, R. H., and Hamburg, D. A. (1968). "Postpartum blues" syndrome. *Arch. Gen. Psychiatry,* 18:16–27.

Chapter 8
The Mother and Baby Unit: An Important Approach to Treatment

Joan Sneddon

This is a personal study of my seven years' experience in a psychiatric mother and baby unit, first as a junior lecturer then later as consultant in charge of the unit. Treatment of severe puerperal illness is very rewarding, since if the patients are treated correctly and for long enough the prognosis is very good.

Fifty-five mothers with severe puerperal illness were treated during the first five years. By the end of seven years, eight had been readmitted with a second puerperal illness. It became clear that the second illness was similar to the first in presentation and response to treatment. Careful history-taking disclosed a recurrence rate of 50 percent with the next baby.

Because no more than two psychiatrists were involved with the care of puerperal women in the city, liaison between obstetricians, general practitioners, and ourselves was very good and admission to the unit could be quickly arranged. This liaison was especially important when looking after a woman pregnant for the second time who had had a previous puerperal illness. She was seen at her request and reassured that we were available and willing to see her if it became necessary.

It has long been recognized that the ordinary psychiatric ward is not a suitable or safe place for a puerperally ill mother and her baby. Many wards refuse to accept the baby, as they feel the child would be at risk among disturbed patients. At the same time, mothers are often not willing to accept admission without their baby, and it is not always possible to find someone to care for the baby at home.

The conjoint admission of a child to a psychiatric hospital with his or her mentally ill mother was pioneered by Y. F. Main at Cassek Hospital, Surrey, England, in 1948 (Main 1958). Originally, only neurotic women were admitted, but by 1955, patients with puerperal depression and anxiety were also admitted, though those with puerperal psychosis were excluded.

Douglas (1956) found that joint admission of mother and baby prevented the psychotic mother from relapsing after discharge. Baker and coworkers (1961) opened a mother and baby unit in 1959 for what was called "puerperal schizophrenia." They accepted any patient, however severe the maternal illness. Treatment was with chlorpromazine and electroconvulsive therapy (ECT), and the results were reported as very good. At the same time, the Massachusetts Mental Health Center was beginning to admit babies with their mentally sick mothers (Van der Walde et al. 1968). The authors described how the initial anxiety and resistance among nurses, doctors, patients, and relatives was gradually replaced by an increase in confidence. Bardon and associates (1968) reported admitting mothers with several children. Patients who were believed to be infanticidal were not admitted, but one case of infanticide occurred and one mother was found drowned in the bath. Two mothers committed suicide during a relapse out of hospital, accentuating the need for long-term follow-up.

In 1977, our Mother and Baby Unit was opened in Sheffield for the treatment of mothers with postpartum psychosis and major postpartum depression. The unit also accepted patients with chronic schizophrenia to assess their coping abilities with their baby and women who were neurotic or had personality disorders and whose babies were considered at risk owing to the mother's behavior.

Our main aims were to provide a haven where both mother and baby would be safe, however severe the maternal illness, and to make the unit as much like home as possible, so that families felt welcome when they visited and therefore were less likely to press for early discharge of the mother (Sneddon et al. 1981). As a result of good relationships with these families throughout the illness, they have cooperated with us in helping our clinical research. We continually reassured those with postpartum psychosis of the good prognosis.

If a woman had a psychiatric breakdown during the puerperium and needed admission, mother-baby bonding could continue if we also admitted the baby. Although at first she might be unfit to look after her child, she would be able to see and touch him or her and, as she began to recover, to care for him or her under the unobtrusive but careful observation of the nursing staff. She was more likely to agree to being admitted if she was able to bring her baby, particularly when no alternative arrangements were possible for his or her care. Knowing that she could care for her child, she was more confident in her role as a mother before discharge, especially when the baby was her first.

The importance of the whole family in the management of postpartum illness needs to be stressed, as many husbands blamed themselves and needed constant explanation and reassurance about the good prognosis. They were encouraged to visit at any time and to help care for and feed the baby. Grandparents were also welcome. Seeing the family together gave us a chance to assess the family problems and to help.

Having the unit enabled follow-up of our patients with postpartum illness. This is vital for recognition of relapse and its early treatment. It can be lifesaving.

The Mother and Baby Unit consisted of single rooms, a milk kitchen, and a laundry situated at one end of an acute admission ward. Such a ward has the most skilled nursing staff. This is vital to provide adequate care for patients subject to rapid changes of mood and behavior and also to offset the risk of injury to the baby from other disturbed patients. Very disturbed puerperal psychotic patients were not admitted to the ward that has the Mother and Baby Unit. In practice, it was the acutely disturbed mother who was the greatest risk to her baby. We admitted any mother and baby referred to us from a hospital, general practice, or other psychiatrist, taking mothers as early as three days postpartum, with a midwife visiting until the twelfth day. We tried to avoid admitting older babies who were crawling, due to lack of space. As the mothers are usually well by six months postpartum, this was not often a problem.

There are great advantages in having a psychiatric unit as part of a district general hospital in that there is 24-hour obstetric and pediatric care available. The midwife visits both mother and baby until the twelfth day. Equipment such as cots, prams, bedding, and changing units are provided and used specifically for individual babies, and disposable diapers are used. Prepared formula is delivered direct from the manufacturers and stored in a refrigerator in the nursery. We had no serious outbreak of infection. Mothers are encouraged to use their own baby clothes.

Some of the babies were breast-fed on admission, but few successfully. The depressed were too agitated or lethargic, the manic too impatient, and the depressed or deluded often thought the baby was dead. Almost invariably, bottle feeding became necessary. As the mothers were usually not drinking or eating well, problems with engorged breasts were few. Firm binding of the breasts was all that was necessary.

It cannot be overemphasized how much the daily management of these patients depends on dedicated and skilled nursing at all times. We also depend on the skills of the obstetric nurses to recognize early signs and symptoms and also think it is very important to impart our knowledge to obstetricians, midwives, and health visitors.

Postpartum Psychosis

Presentation

It was possible to be exact about this as patients were often seen in the maternity hospital within a few days of the birth. After the birth the mother is well for the first few days. This is the latent interval. Then, after one to two sleepless nights, she becomes acutely disturbed and requires admission to a psychiatric ward. Insomnia not caused by pain or a crying baby is an alerting sign in the first few weeks; 75 percent of these patients were admitted within two weeks of delivery.

The earlier the onset, the more dramatic the presentation. Many early cases present with elements of affective, schizophreniform, and organic features. The organic signs include clouding of consciousness, disorientation, perplexity, and visual hallucinations. The clinical picture fluctuates daily or even hourly. Patients seem to slip in or out of psychosis while you watch. They require extremely skilled nursing, as inexperienced nurses may be lulled into a sense of false security. In some patients manic symptoms were most prominent. An example of postpartum psychosis is the following:

> A girl of nineteen had been perfectly well throughout her pregnancy, and her previous health was good except for minor epilepsy for which she was taking sodium valproate (Epilim) as an anticonvulsant. This was stopped early in the pregnancy. On the sixth day postpartum she said that she had had an epileptic attack, which she recognized in retrospect because she had bitten the inside of her mouth. After that she went into a dreamy state. However, as she was to be discharged that day, she told no one. She was admitted from home by the general practitioner on the day after her discharge—withdrawn, dreamy, unwilling to speak, incontinent, and experiencing auditory, visual, and olfactory hallucinations. Her condition deteriorated, she became mute and lay in bed refusing food and water. She was treated with a phenothiazine and ECT and made a complete recovery in three to four weeks.
>
> When she was able to speak to us after three treatments with ECT, she told us that she was going to hell, that the devil was controlling her and that he had been licking her and was now going to blow her up. She thought that people put thoughts into her head telling her to kill herself, and that the baby was dead. She made a full recovery, was

an inpatient for six weeks and was followed up until six months after delivery. Her grandmother had had a psychiatric illness at meno-pause.

Following the birth of her second baby, she realized she was be-coming ill again and went to see her doctor, who (she says) did nothing and didn't believe her. So she had to admit herself via the Emergency Department. By the time she was admitted, she was again speechless, refused to be undressed or examined, and refused medication. She walked up and down the corridor, every 100 yards or so falling to the floor and after a few moments picking herself up and walking on. As her response to ECT had been so good last time, it was started again. After the first treatment she returned to normal for half an hour before drifting backward into her dreamy state. After the second treatment, she was sufficiently improved to be sitting knitting when I visited her.

She then told me that the reason she had kept falling down was because the devil had been pushing her. She also said that she had been in touch with dead relatives and that she could read the news in the next day's newspapers in advance. All these odd ideas dis-appeared with further treatment, and she made a full recovery. Incidentally, she also changed her doctor.

Treatment

1. Nursing observation must be constant as the clinical picture in this illness changes rapidly. The mother's feelings for the baby during the acute stage include total rejection, wishes to injure him or her, and unwillingness to be separated for even brief moments. Seven mothers tried to injure their babies, and five took overdoses, three prior to admission and two while on leave.

2. Phenothiazines are the most useful drugs irrespective of the pre-senting symptoms (Sneddon and Kerry 1985). Chlorpromazine 25 mg three times a day is safe if the baby is breast-fed. If the dosage needs to be increased the mother should stop breast-feeding. Tricyclic anti-depressants are not helpful and may make the early confusional symp-toms worse. The effect of ECT is dramatic. With experience, we use it early to reduce the length of illness so that mother-baby bonding can be restored as quickly as possible. Treatment with ECT avoids the need to give large doses of phenothiazines to nursing mothers.

Postpartum illness is particularly sensitive to ECT in that even the first treatment may change a catatonic mute woman into one who will eat, drink, and communicate. She must be very carefully assessed before each treatment and never given a course of treatments without review. After three to four months, when the mother is recovering but not yet well, the tricyclic antidepressants in combination with Stelazine and an antiparkinsonian drug can be helpful in relatively small doses; e.g., imipramine, 25 mg t.i.d., Stelazine, 3 mg t.i.d. and an antiparkinsonian drug.

3. The mother goes home for a trial weekend as soon as possible; at first without her baby, as we feel it important for the patient and her husband to be alone together at home. Later, she takes the baby and the length of leave is increased, but she is not formally discharged.

4. The mother and baby return to the ward at regular intervals until the baby is at least six months old. This gives doctors and nurses a better chance to assess progress than the more formal outpatient appointment, and the mothers are pleased to see nurses who had looked after them. Seeing the patients now well is very encouraging for other mothers not yet well enough to leave.

Relapse is common and almost to be expected. The relapse is often premenstrual, even in those who have never suffered from premenstrual tension. It is rarely as severe as the initial illness. Some patients reach a plateau at four months, not ill enough for inpatient care but feeling that they will never fully recover. Again, reassurance given to the whole family at this stage is important. It is noticeable how many describe "something clicked into place" or "the cloud suddenly lifted" between five and seven months postpartum.

5. Each mother is also seen on the ward by the health visitor who is to visit her regularly after discharge and who will bring her back to the ward if it seems necessary. A social worker is sometimes involved.

6. We discuss contraception as soon as possible with the couple to ensure that the woman does not become pregnant again within the next one to two years. This does not reduce the risk of recurrence but allows the first baby mothering time.

The majority of patients with this type of puerperal psychosis are well by six or seven months postpartum, but close follow-up is vital. Many disasters such as suicide and infanticide occur after the mother has been discharged presumably well.

Discussion

The author believes that puerperal, steroid, and postoperative psychoses are similar in presentation and prognosis. They may all present with a mixture of affective, schizophreniform, and organic symptoms in the same patient at different times. There is a latent interval of several days between the event and the onset of psychosis. The psychosis responds to treatment, and recovery is nearly always complete. There is an increased risk of recurrence compared with controls, but a patient may have another baby, another operation, or another course of steroids without developing psychosis. In all three conditions, there is a sudden change in circulating adrenal steroids, which suggests that it is the speed of change in the genetically predisposed that may be the trigger.

This syndrome, the so-called spectrum psychosis, has been described by Hall and associates (1979). The described psychotic reactions in patients with medical conditions not involving the nervous system, who were given more than 40 mg of prednisolone daily. The latent period, average 5.9 days, was followed by the acute onset of symptoms. The authors stress that there is no stable characteristic presentation of spectrum psychosis.

All of the cases described by Hall responded well to phenothiazines. They were made worse by tricyclic antidepressants even when the symptoms were depressive.

Stengel and associates (1958) described postoperative psychosis and noted the latent interval and the frequent occurrence of perplexity and bewilderment in the clinical picture. They described the similarity between postoperative and puerperal psychosis. Three of their patients had had both. There were fewer patients diagnosed as schizophrenic than might have been expected from the numbers.

From our observations of puerperal psychoses, the presentation is similar to Hall's description, and the organic signs and symptoms differentiate this syndrome from functional psychoses. Also relevant is the fact that patients with puerperal psychoses respond to phenothiazines better than to tricyclic antidepressants.

Many writers have described the wide variation in presentation of puerperal psychosis. Paffenbarger (1961) inferred that the findings in his epidemiological study suggested the likelihood of organic factors in causation. Jarrahi-Zadeh and his coworkers (1969) suggested that puerperal and steroid psychoses were similar.

Brewer (1977) found the incidence of postabortion psychosis to be much lower than that of postpartum psychosis. He considered the excess of puerperal psychosis may indicate that hormonal, biochemical, and other physiological changes after childbirth are the major precipitating factors in puerperal psychosis.

There is an increase of estrogens and both free and bound cortisol in the plasma toward the end of pregnancy. At term there is a 2½ fold increase in corticosteroids at the tissue level, similar to the level found in Cushing's disease. Gyermek and colleagues (1967) wondered if the maternity blues was due to sudden withdrawal of progesterone which has been shown to be a tranquillizer in animals. Keeler and coworkers (1964) described a woman who developed an acute psychosis following the sudden withdrawal of Enovid (an estrogen-progestogen combination), which had been given for endometriosis. The psychosis was similar to a previous puerperal episode she had had and was relieved when progesterone was reintroduced and withdrawn more slowly.

Something important must be happening during the latent interval between birth, steroids, or surgery and the onset of psychosis. Is it the *speed* of change in circulating hormones in genetically predisposed individuals? If this is the cause, these illnesses are organic in origin, and this explains not only the variability of symptoms but the similarity between presentation within the three groups. It explains why Stengel and coworkers (1958) found fewer cases of schizophrenia than expected in their postoperative psychoses, why Hays's statistical analysis (1978) indicated that patients with a diagnosis of schizophrenia following childbirth formed a separate entity from classical schizophrenia, and why Kadrmas and associates (1979) found that patients with puerperal mania had more first-rank symptoms of acute schizophrenia than nonpuerperal manic patients. It explains the occurrence of symptoms usually associated with organic psychosis—the disorientation, perplexity, and memory difficulties—and the variability of symptoms over time. It simplifies the diagnosis to postpartum psychosis, and treatment is symptomatic, as in steroid and postoperative psychosis.

Major Postpartum Depression

This is the most dangerous illness for both mother and child because suicide and infanticide may occur. It may present acutely in the first few weeks, but more commonly, the onset is insidious and the diagnosis missed by the patient, family, and doctor. One of the difficulties is that the new mother may be ashamed to admit to being depressed and determined not to tell anyone. The so-called smiling depression occurs and may mask suicidal thoughts. It is therefore very important to inquire about symptoms of depression, the mother's feelings for the baby and whether they have changed. It is equally important to get a good history from the father. No woman is immune to postpartum depression but professional women may be too proud to admit it and their husbands too busy to notice. Special care must be taken with mothers who are doctors, nurses, teachers and other professionals as they seem to be especially at risk and it is in them that the diagnosis can be easily missed.

There is initially a latent interval which may be several weeks or months. Sometimes, there has been a temporary elation for the first few weeks known as the "baby pinks," to distinguish it from the baby blues. It is important that this is asked about, and hopefully it has been written in the obstetric notes. It is a help in diagnosis in difficult cases.

Loss of love for the child, which the mother finds painful, is also an important symptom.

It is difficult to know exactly when the condition starts. Often it is between six weeks and three months. Four mothers out of fifty-five were admitted to the unit later than six months postpartum, but the depression had started between six weeks and three months postpartum. The diagnosis had been missed or the patient had not been treated with full doses of antidepressants or for a long enough period. Sometimes, these patients were seen after an overdose or an attempt to injure the child. Three were nurses.

Some patients present with what sounds like a neurotic depression caused by family problems. Experience has shown that most had an endogenous depression presenting in a neurotic manner which often failed to respond to tricyclic antidepressants but responded well to ECT.

Another hazard is that mothers may present with anxiety and irritability that is more prominent than their depression, but the correct diagnosis is that of postpartum depressive illness presenting atypically.

Treatment

The general management of the patient is the same as for postpartum psychosis.

These patients, often six weeks to three months postpartum, are less likely to have organic and schizophreniform symptoms. They may respond to full doses of tricyclic antidepressants. Usually by the time these patients are admitted to the unit, the condition is severe and the mother is unable to bond or look after her baby. Response to tricyclics in these cases is slow and often poor. It is kinder to use ECT, which is usually successful and decreases the time in which the mother cannot bond with her baby. Again, assessment must be made before each ECT treatment, but depressed patients may need more treatments than those with postpartum psychosis.

After a course of ECT, the patient can commence antidepressant treatment. This seems more likely to be effective after ECT, and it must always be remembered that this is a relapsing illness. It is interesting that mothers fully realize the benefits of ECT and often come back to the unit relapsing and asking for more ECT. If the relapse is premenstrual, the patient often improves when the period starts.

Mothers often reassure inpatients about the value of ECT and the good prognosis, and this raises morale in the unit.

Depressed patients must not be treated exclusively with benzodiazepines. They are contraindicated in breast-feeding mothers as they are excreted in the milk and make the baby drowsy and slow to feed. It is also known that diazepam (Valium), by its disinhibiting effect, can be reponsible for potential baby batterers becoming actual batterers. Benzodiazepines can also make depression worse.

Recovery may take a year or more postpartum. An example of this type of patient is the following:

> A woman age 30, a competent, confident school teacher in line for deputy head and happily married, had a planned pregnancy. The baby, a boy, was normal, but after a few weeks she found she was becoming unable to cope with the baby and rejected him. She was referred to a Mother and Baby Unit in the north of England and, whilst there, was given antidepressants and told she had not learnt how to be a good mother and that she should get a nanny and return to work. This distressed her so much she ran away from the unit and tried to jump from a bridge but was fortunately rescued by a passing lorry driver and returned to the unit. A few weeks later, she was discharged but referred to another psychiatrist in another city, who continued the antidepressants and saw her weekly. She smiled during all this time, and the depth of her despair was therefore masked.
>
> One morning she decided that she would never recover and was no use to her husband or the baby. She drove her car to Sheffield, booked into a hotel and took a massive dose of antidepressants. The manageress fortunately broke down the door, the patient was admitted to intensive care and recovered. By the time I saw her, her suicidal intent was revealed, but she was still smiling and bitterly ashamed that she, of all people, should have got to this state. I'm delighted to say she made a rapid recovery with ECT, and the happy, bossy schoolteacher came back with delight to show us her much beloved baby who nearly lost his mother.

The lessons from this case are important to learn. She had all the symptoms of severe postpartum depression and she nearly died.

The continuum from mild depression responding to antidepressants to severe depression that responds to ECT is a slippery slope. If in doubt it is safer to admit the mother and baby for observation.

Lessons to Be Learned

The lessons learnt about the treatment of puerperal illness have been very helpful to us and our staff:

The premorbid personality is often competent and confident.
It is important to recognize the latent interval and then insomnia ushering in the acute illness.

The diagnosis of depressive illness is usually not made early enough.
The response to ECT is usually excellent.
Continual family reassurance of the good prognosis is important.
Relapse is common.
A long follow-up is necessary to prevent disaster.

Patients with Chronic Schizophrenia and Neurotic and Personality Disorders

Some of the chronic schizophrenic patients had been psychiatric in-patients throughout pregnancy, were delivered in the obstetric hospital and then admitted to the Mother and Baby Unit. Others were admitted from outside. Their condition did not usually deteriorate during the puerperium; in fact, some did not realize that they had had a baby. Marriages tended to break down, and the children were often brought up by the father or adopted away. Watching these women, it seemed as though they did not have the emotional sensitivity to bond with their baby.

Mothers with neurotic and personality disorders bonded with their babies, but because of their low frustration levels and disorganized life-styles, they often lost patience with their babies and the children were at risk of injury.

In the foregoing groups, the baby continues to be at risk compared with those with puerperal psychotic illness or depression, who after recovery, are usually loving, competent mothers.

Problems in Running a Mother and Baby Unit

However carefully the mothers are observed, there are always hazards in admitting a very disturbed mother and her baby. However, some mothers would refuse informal admission if they could not bring the baby, and the child could be more at risk at home.

Despite every possible precaution, seven mothers attempted to injure their babies while on the ward; e.g., one tried to suffocate twins, one hit the child on the head with a heavy ashtray, one tried to feed her medication to the baby. Five women took overdoses, three before admission and two while on leave. One young mother killed her baby three months after discharge. A particularly tragic incident occurred:

A young mother with postpartum psychosis was at times very depressed. Within a period of ten days, she set fire to herself and the burns prohibited the use of ECT. She took an overdose of medication, told no one until it was too late to treat her, and finally ran away from the ward and threw herself in front of a passing lorry and was killed. At the time, she was under special observation, but even this did not prevent her from escaping the vigilant eye of the watching nurse.

With all these problems, nurses enjoy working on a mother and baby unit and feel very strongly that the baby should be admitted with the mother.

The unit is expensive. The per patient cost of caring for mother and baby has been calculated at three times as much as the care of the ordinary psychiatric patient. However, one must consider this does not include the cost of alternative care for the baby. Because many of our patients are on extended leave but not discharged, with a bit of juggling it is possible to look after six mothers and babies in three beds.

Above all, we aim to keep mother and baby together to encourage bonding and to allow leave as soon as possible, hoping that the family by then has enough confidence in us to bring the mother back if she starts to relapse.

The Loss of the Unit

With short notice and very little discussion, the Sheffield Mother and Baby Unit was closed on the grounds of economy. The loss of the unit has destroyed a large infrastructure under one umbrella.

The doctors, nurses, and ancillary staff of the unit supported the city obstetricians and general practitioners. They could call for advice as well as to request admission. Nurses in the unit enjoyed the challenge, morale was high, and results were good.

Community midwives and health visitors felt more confident knowing that the unit was available if problems arose. Pediatricians felt reassured that the unit was looking after the baby of the disturbed mother. The unit provided a unique teaching facility for doctors and medical students, and was a source of much clinical research on puerperal illness.

What happens now to our mothers and babies?

Sheffield psychiatry became sectorized, and a mother is treated by the psychiatrist for the area in which she lives. This psychiatrist usually has no facilities for the care of the baby, and the baby is either left at home or admitted to the pediatric ward with all the attendant risks of infection.

This situation may lead to the premature discharge of the mother who may not have learned to bond or care for the baby in those early critical weeks.

Closure of the Mother and Baby Unit is a retrograde step that has wasted a lot of expertise in this very important field. At this time, our best service may be to train those looking after mothers and babies, and especially midwives and health visitors, to pick up the early signs of illness before tragedy has ocurred. We hope that the mothers will receive good treatment on ordinary psychiatric wards.

References

Baker, A. A., Morison, M., Game, J. A., et al. (1961). Admitting schizophrenic mothers with their babies. *Lancet* 2:237–39.

Bardon, D., Glaser, Y.I.M., Prothero, D., et al. (1968). Mother and baby unit: Survey of 115 cases. *Br. Med. J.,* 2:755–58.

Brewer, C. (1977). Incidence of post-abortion psychosis: A prospective study. *Br. Med. J.* 1:476.

Douglas, G. (1956). Psychotic mothers. *Lancet* 1:124–25.

Gyermek, L., Genther, G., and Fleming, N. (1967). Some effects of progesterone and related steroids on the central nervous system. *Int. J. Neuropharmacol.* 6:191.

Hall, R.C.W., Popkin, M. K., Stickney, S. K., et al. (1979). Presentation of steroid psychosis. *J. Nerv. Ment. Dis.* 167:229–36.

Hays, P. (1978). Taxonomic map of schizophrenics with special reference to puerperal psychosis. *Br. Med. J.* 2:755–57.

Jarrahi-Zadeh, A. J., Kane, F. J., et al. (1969). Emotional and cognitive changes in pregnancy in early puerperium. *Br. J. Psychiatry,* 115:797–805.

Kadrmas, A., Winocur, G., and Crowe, E. (1979). Postpartum mania. *Br. J. Psychiatry* 135:551–54.

Keeler, M. H., Kane, T., and Daly, R. (1964). An acute schizophrenic episode following abrupt withdrawal of Enovid in a patient with previous postpartum psychiatric disorder. *Am. J. Psychiatry* 120:1123–24.

Main, T. F. (1958). Mothers with children in a psychiatric hospital. *Lancet* 2:845–47.

Paffenbarger, R. S. (1961). The picture puzzle of the postpartum psychoses. *J. Chron. Dis.* 13:161–73.

Sneddon, J., and Kerry, R. J. (1980). Letter. *Br. J. Psychiatry,* 136:520.

Sneddon, J., Kerry, R. J., and Bant, W. (1981). Psychiatric mother and baby unit. *The Practitioner,* 225:1295–1300.

Sneddon, J., and Kerry, R. J. (1985). The psychiatric mother and baby unit: A five-year study. In D. G. Inwood (Ed.), *Recent Advances in Postpartum Psychiatric Disorders.* Washington, DC: American Psychiatric Press.

Stengel, E., Zeitlyn, B. B., and Rayner, E. H. (1958). Post-operative psychoses. *J. Ment. Sci.* 104:389–402.

Van der Walde, P. H., Meeks, D., Grunebaum, H. U., et al. (1968). Joint admission of mothers and children to a state hospital. *Arch. Gen. Psychiatry* 18:706–11.

Chapter 9
The Integrated Care of Hospitalized Women with Postpartum Psychiatric Illness

Deborah A. Sichel and Jeanne Watson Driscoll

The postpartum period is known for being the highest risk period in a woman's life for psychiatric illness (Paffenbarger and McCabe 1966, Kendell et al. 1981, Brockington et al. 1982). Therefore, a full evaluation of the risk factors of an individual patient is mandatory during pregnancy. The obstetrician, nurse, and midwife should note any unusual depressive symptoms during previous postpartum periods, even if spontaneous remission occurred. A brief family history of postpartum psychiatric illness in the patient's mother, sisters, and grandmothers should also be taken (Thuwe 1974). Early referral for further psychiatric evaluation needs to follow a positive history.

Once a psychiatric illness is recognized in a postpartum patient, a critical decision regarding home care or hospitalization must be made. Hospitalization is mandatory in a severely depressed woman or if a psychosis is present. Less frequently, a severe postpartum panic disorder may require the more rigorous care of an inpatient unit* (Metz et al. 1988).

Moderately depressed patients represent a dilemma, since the intrinsic lability of this illness cannot be underestimated. We cannot impress upon clinicians too strongly the mercurial nature of these illnesses and the rapidity with which they can deteriorate and suicidal ideation acted upon. The clinician needs to realize that one is dealing with a woman

---

*Panic disorder appears to be a significant syndrome occurring postpartum. The incidence is not known. We have admitted some patients to our unit who have had a rapidly deteriorating panic disorder with significant intervening anxiety. We continue to investigate the possible link and biological correlates of this syndrome with the other postpartum syndromes.

who, along with the inherent suicidal dangers of a depressive or psychotic illness, has a severely devastated ego. These women believe themselves to be failures at what they perceive to be the most fundamental of tasks—mothering. Also, at this point in their illness, they do not have the capacity to sustain patience with themselves or objectivity around anticipating recovery. Guilt and shame at their "loss of control" are major issues in current and future treatment. Patients may feel undeserving of their babies. Some women feel "punished" for previous events in their lives, e.g., abortions and/or family conflicts.

Because of the prominence of these feelings, professionals need to be extremely careful about statements that might fuel these myths and heighten the patient's guilt. All too often, misguided and untimely comments about the patient's previous family conflicts and past problems increase the patient's distress around personal responsibility for the illness.

Postpartum depressions are sometimes refractory to treatment and require skilled and aggressive psychiatric and pharmacological treatment. The physician must maintain an atmosphere of concern and openness and avoid judgmental statements. One of the authors (D.S.) has known many physicians to express irritation with statements like, "Isn't it time you gave all this stuff up now?" when what was needed was some skillful pharmacological maneuvering. These countertransference issues must be contained and never projected into the patient's area of care. This is a crucial issue and must be imparted to all levels of caregivers.

This chapter only focuses on the integrated care of hospitalized patients. Suffice to say that patients should never be left alone in the early stages of treatment. Family and friends have to be educated regarding the risks of suicide and harm to the baby. The patient should not have access to her own medication until the physician is sure that she is well into recovery. If these parameters for home care cannot be established, hospitalization is mandatory.

Hospitalization

Hospitalization is only the beginning of the treatment plan. Many issues need to be addressed during the hospitalization of women with postpartum psychiatric disorders. Education of the family and staff is a vital, ongoing element in the care of the patient. Maternal self-esteem, the mother-baby relationship, family dynamics, and the husband-wife relationship need thorough evaluation before any discharge is made.

Hamilton (1985) eloquently points to the importance of the initial interview for subsequent treatment success. At this juncture, the patient and her family need to be told that she is not defective and that this illness is acute and that she can anticipate recovery. Reassurance that the illness does not imply poor mothering ability nor retribution for any past problems is important.

The illness must be named—postpartum depression, postpartum psychosis, or postpartum panic attacks. Patients are markedly relieved to have their distressing set of symptoms given a name. Although these specific names are not in the current *DSM-III-R*, the authors use them and encourage the staff to use them, since we believe that these illnesses are specific to the postpartum period.

Treatment is divided into acute and long-term issues. A multidisciplinary, problem-oriented treatment plan is developed on admission. This allows for the full integration of care and for each member of the treatment team to know what the active problems are on a daily and/or weekly basis, what is being done, and who is specifically responsible.

Table 9.1 is a sample of a multidisciplinary treatment plan that accounts for the various medical, psychiatric, and nursing diagnoses. We have found this the best way to provide integrated care. It also allows for an extended time frame, addressing long-term treatment issues when the mother has returned home and is coping on a daily basis. The plan is a clinically applicable tool that lists problems and target symptoms in psychosocial, medical, and mother-infant categories. For each problem, there is an expected outcome by discharge, together with specific interventions to achieve this. The responsible clinician is listed in the fourth column. The plan is somewhat different for each patient, depending mainly on the diagnosis, e.g., depression, psychosis, or panic attacks.

The problem list presented below covers all three diagnoses. Psychosocial, medical, and mother-infant issues indicate the multitude and depth of the problems to be resolved.

Discussion

We believe that the ideal hospitalization situation for women with postpartum psychiatric illness is a Mother and Baby Unit, as is done in England (Sneddon and Kerry 1985). (See Chapter 8.) However, because of the current climate of third-party reimbursement and financial constraints, coupled with litigation risks, this does not appear to be a realistic option for the United States in the near future. Therefore, we have constructed a treatment plan aimed at the best utilization of resources within the U.S. health care system.

This plan integrates the psychiatric, medical, nursing, and psychosocial diagnoses serving to clarify the multiple levels at which treat-

TABLE 9.1. Problems, objectives, interventions, and responsibilities.

Problem	Expected outcome	Interventions	Responsible
Postpartum psychosis	See under specific symptom/nursing diagnosis	• Antipsychotic medications: high potency are preferable to avoid sedative effects (Trifluoperazine, Perphenazine, Thiothixene) Monitor for Parkinsonism, dystonia (treat with Benztropine or Diperhydramine)	Psychiatrist, clinical nurse specialist, primary and associate nurses
Postpartum depression; postpartum panic disorder	See under specific symptomatology/nursing diagnosis	• Antidepressant medications: Tricyclic or Fluoxetine. Increase doses as rapidly as the patient can tolerate (also used for panic disorder) • Start anti-anxiety medications: Clonazepam in doses of 0.5 mg. BID or TID until antidepressant response is achieved (also used for panic disorder) • Adjunct use of Lithium or L-Triiodothyronine to augment antidepressant response if necessary • Monitor blood levels and potential side effects • ECT for severe suicidal depression or treatment resistance on medications	Psychiatrist, clinical nurse specialist, primary and associate nurses
R/O Sheehan's syndrome; R/O thyroid dysfunction	Diagnosis confirmed or ruled out	• Lab work: Prolactin; ACTH; GH; TSH; T3; T4; antimicrosomal antibodies • Consult endocrinologist	Psychiatrist, primary nurse, endocrinologist

Nursing Diagnosis	Expected Outcomes	Interventions	Team Members
R/O medical contribution to panic disorder; Alteration of thought processes (hallucinations, delusions, paranoid ideation)	Diagnosis confirmed or ruled out; Patient will verbalize the absence of hallucinations, delusions, and/or paranoid ideation	Consult internist; • Establish trust/rapport; • Provide safe, supportive environment; • Individual therapy; • Milieu therapy; • Reality test; • Medicate as prescribed; • Monitor side effects	Psychiatrist, primary nurse, internist; Psychiatrist, psychologist, primary nurse, associate nurse, social worker
Potential of violence to self and/or others	• Patient will verbalize and agree to a suicide contract; • Patient will verbalize absence of suicidal thoughts	• Develop suicide contract; • Encourage verbalization of feelings with health-care provider; • Suicide precautions as needed	Psychiatrist, psychologist, primary nurse, associate nurse, social worker
Diminished self-esteem secondary to: self-blame, hospitalization, impaired cognitive functioning	• Patient will verbalize positive feelings regarding self; • Patient will verbalize an understanding that she is not responsible for this illness	• Individual therapy; • Group sessions; • Journal keeping; • Family sessions	Psychiatrist, psychologist, clinical nurse specialist, social worker, primary and associate nurse, group leaders
Lack of coping repertoire	• Patient will list two personal strengths; • Patient will list two coping mechanisms that have been successfully utilized during the hospitalization	• Individual therapy; • Group sessions; • Relaxation techniques; • New parents' group; • New mothers' group	Psychiatrist, psychologist, clinical nurse specialist, social worker, primary and associate nurse, group leaders
Unrealistic expectations of self and role performance	• Patient will ask for and accept help from caretakers; • Patient will display patience with temporarily diminished capacities; • Patient will verbalize beginning realistic expectations of self in maternal role	• Individual therapy; • Milieu therapy; • Group sessions	Psychiatrist, psychologist, clinical nurse specialist, social worker, primary and associate nurse, group leaders

TABLE 9.1. *Continued.*

Problem	Expected outcome	Interventions	Responsible
Potential for altered family development	• Couple will demonstrate constructive communication and mutual understanding with partner	• Couples' therapy • Family meetings • Observe communication styles during visiting hours	Psychiatrist, psychologist, clinical nurse specialist, social worker, primary/associate nurse, couples' therapist
Alteration in nutritional status	• Patient will maintain weight • Patient will select and eat foods from menu	• Engage in community dining • Encourage nutritional intake (six small meals per day) • Consult: dietician	Psychiatrist, psychologist, clinical nurse specialist, social worker, primary/associate nurse, dietician
Sleep dysfunction	• Patient will verbalize feeling rested upon wakening • Patient will verbalize that she had two to three nights of uninterrupted sleep	• Explore sleep rituals • Encourage use of relaxation/meditation techniques (learned in childbirth classes) • Sleep medication as needed (Fluorazepam or Temazepam for first week)	Psychiatrist, psychologist, clinical nurse specialist, social worker, primary/associate nurse
Anxiety	• Patient will verbalize a decrease in anxiety symptoms • Patient will verbalize identification of anxiety feelings	• Encourage identification of anxiety symptoms • Establish trusting rapport • Encourage verbalization of anxiety and coping style • Anti-anxiety medication PRN	Psychiatrist, psychologist, clinical nurse specialist, social worker, primary/associate nurse
Delayed (altered) maternal role attainment secondary to illness and hospitalization	• Patient will verbalize a desire to care for her infant • Patient will verbalize feelings of attachment to her infant • Patient will verbalize and demonstrate comfort with infant care skills	• Baby will visit for progressively longer periods (supervised) • Encourage patient to provide care to infant • Reinforce maternal knowledge of caretaking skills	Primary/associate nurse, social worker, clinical nurse specialist (Psych and MCN), developmental specialist

Nursing Diagnosis	Expected Outcomes	Interventions	Caregivers
Potential for impaired infant growth (emotional and/or physical) secondary to maternal psychiatric illness	• Patient will verbalize support networks for follow-up with infant • Patient will verbalize comfort with established relationship with pediatrician and/or nurse practitioner	• Consult: developmental specialist, maternal-child clinical nurse specialist • Inform pediatrician and/or nurse practitioner for maternal admission for infant follow-up • Refer to home health care for after discharge • Refer: developmental specialist	Primary/associate nurses, clinical nurse specialist, pediatrician, family physician, nurse practitioner, home health agencies
Contraception/family planning	Patient and her partner will verbalize an understanding of the need to prevent pregnancy while on psychotropic medications	• Individual therapy • Couples' therapy • Discuss contraceptive options • Refer to OB/GYN	OB/GYN, psychiatrist, psychologist, primary nurse
Breast engorgement secondary to separation of mother/baby	• Patient will verbalize breast comfort • Patient will maintain milk supply with expression during hospitalization if this is her desire • Patient will breast-feed her infant during visits if pharmacologically safe	• Ice packs PRN if abrupt weaning • Analgesics PRN • Manual/electric pump to facilitate regular expression of milk • Store or discard milk depending on safety of medications being used • Refer to lactation consultant	Primary/associate nurse, MCN clinical specialist, lactation consultant
Potential for relactation depending on the psychopharmacological status at discharge	Establish relationships with lactation consultant to initiate relactation process after discharge	• Manual/electric pump to facilitate milk expression • Refer to lactation consultant	Primary/associate nurses, MCN clinical specialist, lactation consultant
Alteration of skin integrity secondary to: episiotomy, caesarean incision, lochial drainage	• Patient will demonstrate healthy wound-healing (episiotomy, caesarean incision, placental site) • Patient will verbalize signs and symptoms of infection	• Assess wound healing • Peri care PRN • Sitz bath as per orders	Primary/associate nurses, obstetrician, certified nurse midwife

ment is administered. In our clinical experience, it is vital that outcomes for each problem are met prior to discharge. Failure to reach these goals may mean the patient is not ready to transfer home.

There must be ongoing evaluation of suicidal risk and potential for harm to the infant, even after discahrge.

Antidepressant medications should be used in therapeutic dosages, with therapeutic blood levels achieved. We have found that the tricyclics (imipramine, desipramine, or nortriptyline) have been the most effective because of their minimal sedative qualities. Occasionally, a sleep disorder can persist even though other target symptoms have been relieved. Small bedtime doses of amitryptiline (10 to 25 mg) or trazodone (50 mg) have been useful adjuncts in these situations. Physicians are ill-advised to send patients home on sedatives or hypnotic sleep medications, since their effectiveness can diminish, and ongoing symptomatology can be masked.

We are now using fluoxetine (Prozac) extensively and have found it to be highly effective in dosages of 40 to 60 mg every morning. Negotiating the first few weeks on fluoxedine may be somewhat difficult. Patients sometimes report transient nausea, headaches, and anxiety. Symptomatic treatment with prochlorperazine (Compazine), acetaminophen (Tylenol), and clonazepam (Klonysin) usually allows patients to adjust to the fluoxetine, and symptoms subside.*

Clonazepam is a highly potent benzodiazepine, and it is extremely useful in managing the extreme anxiety and agitation often seen in these syndromes. Doses of 0.5 mg two to four times a day quickly alleviates distressful symptoms. Slow tapering of one 0.5 dose daily, every week of clonazepam is easily accomplished, once the depression has lifted. Use of antipsychotics should be limited to the less sedating derivatives, since difficulty is experienced in rehabilitation and bonding behavior if mothers are sedated.

Electroconvulsive therapy (ECT) should always be considered a viable option for treatment-resistant patients. A specific course of six to twelve treatments should not be prescribed, since frequently only two or three treatments are necessary for symptom abatement. However, the authors have also seen relapse after two to three months and further treatments may be necessary at that time.

Full thyroid evaluation, including antimicrosomal antibodies, should be done, as well as a work-up for the uncommon Sheehan's syndrome.

---

*As this book goes to press, the advantages of the drug are being balanced against its hazards, a debate which is taking place in court as well as in medical journals. When fluoxetine is initiated patients should be under close observation. Some believe that this implies hospitalization—Eds.

Many cases of postpartum thyroid syndromes pass undetected since physicians often do not suspect problems. The most common syndrome is a thyroiditis with an initial thyrotoxic phase, followed by a hypothyroid phase. Most often these symptoms are transient, but occasionally permanent thyroid disease persists, and long-term follow-up of patients is necessary (Jansson et al. 1988). These disorders have been correlated with poor concentration, carelessness, depression and somatic complaints (Hayslip et al. 1988).

The need for adequate contraception should be addressed thoroughly, and our patients are counseled that further pregnancies should not be attempted for at least eighteen months or even two years after the current episode.

The possibility of relactation for a breast-feeding woman, at a later time, has been raised by some of our patients. We have been successful in promoting relactation in one patient who, when weaned from antipsychotics and benzodiazepines, reestablished breast-feeding through the utilization of the Supplemental Nutrition System.* Breast-feeding was stopped at two months postpartum and reestablished at five months, when the patient was being maintained only on desipramine (175 mg at bedtime). Monitoring of breast milk levels and baby's serum levels of desipramine revealed that the drug was not detectable, a result that has been reported previously (Stancer and Reed 1986).

As the woman's mental status normalizes, the infant is brought in to visit for increasingly longer periods of time. Staff have found the collaboration of a developmental specialist and a maternal child clinical nurse specialist to be assets in assessing and intervening with the issues of maternal-infant caretaking skills.

Discharge Planning

Ongoing family and individual therapy is vital. The length of treatment may continue up to eighteen months after discharge. Additional discharge plans include referral to "Depression After Delivery" support groups, maternal-child home health nurses, and communications with the pediatrician regarding the progress of maternal recovery.

A postpartum psychiatric illness frequently ushers in the first stages of the breakdown of a marriage. It was noted many years ago by Karnosh and Hope (1937) that "many women are not the same after the birth of a baby," and we believe that the havoc wreaked by post-

---

*Supplemental Nutrition System available from Medela Co., 457 Dartmoor Dr., Box 386, Crystal Lake, IL 60014.

partum illnesses in families has not yet been accurately assessed. In our clinical work, we often see the early unraveling of relationships in high-risk families. We have found that group support for couples aimed at addressing the issues of personal and parental development helps mutual tolerance and understanding, while also encouraging the grieving process from the loss of the "normal" postpartum adjustment period.

We need to pay close attention to the mother-infant unit, since a woman who is cognitively and affectively impaired cannot interact with her infant in the usual attentive way and may need significant help in this area. Intellectual deficits have been noted in children whose mothers were depressed in the first year of life (Cogill et al. 1986). Hence, the role of the developmentalist may be important in the rehabilitation of these cases.

Conclusions and Recommendations

The design of a plan for integrated care of the woman hospitalized with postpartum psychiatric illness is only one part of the overall treatment plan. Preparedness for the possibility of these illnesses begins during pregnancy with education, support, and understanding. When a woman has had a prior experience of a postpartum psychiatric illness, she should be counseled about the availability of pharmacological prophylaxis in future pregnancies (Dalton 1980). (See Chapter 17.)

Through the efforts of the authors, information regarding depression, psychosis, and panic disorders that may occur after the birth of a baby is now being provided in the Boston area in childbirth education classes. Increasing numbers of health care providers are becoming informed regarding the diagnosis and treatment of postpartum psychiatric illnesses via in-service education, grand rounds presentations, and conferences in the area.

Our goal is that through these educational processes, the voices of women in pain will be heard and responded to during the nineties. Early detection and rapid treatment will, hopefully, delay the time spent "hiding" and promote the ongoing, healthy development of the maternal role and family integration during the postpartum period.

References

Brockington, I. F., Winokur, G., et al. (1982). Puerperal psychosis. In I. F. Brockington and R. Kumar (Eds.), *Motherhood and Mental Illness*. London: Academic Press.

Cogill, S. R., Caplan, H. L., et al. (1986). Impact of maternal postnatal depression on cognitive development of young children. *Br. Med. J.* 292:1165–67.

Dalton, K. (1980). *Depression after Childbirth.* New York: Oxford University Press.

Doenges, M., Townsend, M. C., et al. (1989). *Psychiatric Care Plans: Guidelines for Client Care.* Philadelphia: F. A. Davis.

Hamilton, J. A. (1985). Guidelines for therapeutic management of postpartum disorders. In D. G. Inwood (Ed.), *Recent Advances in Postpartum Psychiatric Disorders.* Washington, DC: American Psychiatric Press.

Hayslip, C. C., Fein, H. G., et al. (1988). The value of serum antimicrosomal antibody testing in screening for symptomatic postpartum thyroid dysfunction. *Am. J. Obstet. Gynecol.* 159(1):203–9.

Hurt, L. D., and Ray, C. P. (1985). Postpartum disorders: Mother-infant bonding on a psychiatric unit. *J. Psychosoc. Nursing,* 23:15–20.

Jansson, R., Dahlberg, P. A., et al. (1988). Postpartum thyroiditis. *Clin. Endocrinol. Metabol.,* 3:619–35.

Karnosh, L. J., and Hope, J. M. (1937). Puerperal psychoses and their sequelae. *Am. J. Psychiatry* 94:537–550.

Kendell, R. E., Rennie, D., et al. (1981). The social and obstetric correlates of psychiatric admission in the puerperium. *Psychol. Med.* 2:340–50.

Metz, A., Sichel, D. A., and Goff, D. C. (1988). Postpartum panic disorder. *J. Clin. Psychiatry* 49:278–79.

Paffenbarger, R. S., Jr., and McCabe, L. J., Jr. (1966). The effect of obstetric and perinatal events on risk of mental illness in women of childbearing age. *Am. J. Pub. Health,* 56:400–407.

Sneddon, J., and Kerry, R. J. (1985). The psychiatric mother and baby unit: A five-year study. In D. G. Inwood (Ed.), *Recent Advances in Postpartum Psychiatric Disorders.* Washington, DC: American Psychiatric Press.

Stancer, H. C., and Reed, K. L. (1986). Desipramine and 2-hydroxydesipramine in human breast milk and the nursing infant's serum. *Am. J. Psychiatry* 143:1597–1600.

Thuwe, I. (1974). Genetic factors in puerperal psychosis. *Br. J. Psychiatry* 125:378–85.

Chapter 10
The Provision of Services for Postpartum Mental Illness in the United Kingdom

Ian Brockington

Conditions in the National Health Service (NHS) have favoured the development of services for mental illness in recently delivered mothers. Although they leave much to be desired, and are only at the stage of a few innovative schemes, our services seem to be more advanced than in other countries. Development has occurred in two phases: first, the opening of units for joint admission of a mentally ill mother with her baby, and secondly, the deployment of resources in the community so that treatment can be delivered to the home.

Psychiatric Mother and Baby Units

It was Tom Main who, in 1948 at the Cassel Hospital, pioneered the admission of healthy children with their mentally ill mothers. He specifically drew attention to the dangers of disrupting the mother-infant relationship by admitting the mother without her child and to the opportunity that joint admission gave for studying disturbances of mothering. He worked out with nurses and administrators the special arrangements which had to be made for play areas, laundry services, mealtimes, and sleeping, and he occasionally admitted a whole family (Main 1958). Dr. Main's patients suffered from depression and neuroses, and treatment was with psychotherapy, but in 1959 Baker and his colleagues (1961) at Banstead Hospital opened a ward for mothers with puerperal psychosis and showed that patients admitted with their babies were more likely to take full care of them when they returned home. The Banstead unit was followed by a handful of other units opened at Shenley Hospital near St. Albans, Barrow Gurney Hospital in Bristol, Withington Hospital in Manchester, St. John's Hospital in Lincoln, Springfield Hospital in South London, and the Bethlem Royal Hospital in Kent. These are all specialized wards with no other function except to care for joint admissions, but many other hospitals took up Main's original idea of admitting mothers and babies to general psychiatric wards, designating certain side rooms for joint admission.

The proliferation of joint inpatient facilities in Britain has been documented by Aston (1989), who wrote to all the British psychiatric hospitals in 1987 to find out what provision they made for joint admission. He found that 147 of 305 hospitals made some provision, of which 125 provided inpatient care, 7 day-care, and 15 both. There was one unit with twelve beds (Hull), one with ten beds (Lincoln), one with nine (Manchester), and four with eight beds (Shenley, Bethlem Royal, Bristol, and Springfield), all of these being self-standing specialized units. Below this size almost all the units were attached to general psychiatric wards. There were seven with six beds, three with five beds, eight with four beds, ten with three beds, forty-four with two beds, and eighteen with only one, the remainder having no designated rooms but occasionally admitting babies. It is clear from these figures that the practice of joint admission is widespread, but the distribution of facilities is haphazard, and few of the big cities have specialized units: London has only three specialized units for 8 million inhabitants, and the next two biggests cities (Birmingham and Glasgow) have none. The national average is 5.8 beds per million, with a total of 1,179 admissions per year (four admissions per year per bed), i.e., 1.9 per thousand live births.

The Manchester unit, where I worked from 1975–80, is a good example of the strengths and weaknesses of specialized mother and baby units. It provided nine beds nominally serving the North Western Regional Health Authority (population 4.4 million). However, distance prevented patients being admitted from most of the region, and in fact 81 percent came from Manchester, Salford, and the neighboring boroughs to the south of the city (Stockport, Trafford, and Tameside), an effective catchment area of 2 million. Those familiar with the geography of this conurbation, which is an area of dense population and has a good road network including an orbital motorway, will note that patients were rarely admitted from the contiguous boroughs to the north of the city (e.g., Bury, Bolton, Rochdale, and Oldham). Evidently a distance of more than ten miles is a strong deterrent to joint admission. With such a catchment area the unit was rarely full, and average bed occupancy was only about six beds—this in spite of the fact that we had no deployment of community services for postnatal mental illness at the time. The average admission rate per year was about 50, for which ten staff were required (three nursery nurses, two night nurses, and five day nurses), providing two nurses and one nursery nurse on duty during the day and one nurse by night. The number of staff was not much below that required for a 28-bed general psychiatric ward, admitting 200 patients per year, so the cost was about three times as much per patient as a general ward.

At the same time the advantages for teaching and research were considerable. Advances in knowledge follow specialization as regular as clockwork. So long as psychiatrists see no more than the occasional patient with puerperal psychosis, and psychiatric nurses the occasional mother with a "bonding" disorder, the level of theory and practice is bound to remain rudimentary. When there is a flow of patients with the same disorder, minds can begin to see new patterns, to identify problems, to ask questions, and crystallize hypotheses. It is likely that the major factor in the progress made in our understanding of postpartum disorders in recent years has stemmed from the opening of specialized mother and baby units. The specialized unit, dedicated to the care of pregnancy-related psychiatric illness, fosters the development of the highest standards of diagnosis and treatment, as well as clarifying diagnosis and classification thus leading to innovations in treatment and prevention. It enables the nursing staff to become expert in the assessment of the mother-infant relationship, in the teaching of mothering skills, and in helping mothers with disruptions of the "bonding" process. A specialized unit can play a valuable part in training general psychiatrists, general practitioners, psychiatric nurses, midwives, and health visitors and thus can influence the level of skill that future practitioners and nurses will have in this area.

The disadvantage of the Manchester unit was that it had nothing else to offer except inpatient care. A natural extension of such an inpatient service is to provide day-care as well. Indeed, day-care is particularly appropriate for postnatal mental disorders because almost all the positive elements of inpatient care can be provided (especially the stimulating and supportive social environment) without disrupting family life. It is a great advantage to have an attached day nursery so that the elder siblings of the newly arrived baby can also be admitted, thus further minimizing the disruption caused by mental illness. Professor John Cox of Keele University has developed a service based entirely on day-care (the "Parent and Baby Day Unit," a name which emphasizes the service provided to the whole family). He took over a building adjacent to the central bus depot in Hanley, which is one of the six towns of the "potteries," a conurbation of about 400,000 inhabitants. The location is ideal to provide access, and the referral rate is about 300 patients per year, one-third of the referrals coming from health visitors.

Development of Community Services for Postnatal Mental Illness

A more radical approach to the provision of care is that pioneered by Dr. Margaret Oates in Nottingham. It is highly disruptive to a family for the mother to be removed in the postnatal period, and Dr. Oates (1988) has demonstrated that it is possible to treat severe postpartum illness at home. In 1982 she appointed her first community psychiatric nurse in postnatal mental illness. In that year she carried out a home treatment pilot study of two patients with manic and schizoaffective illness. The community psychiatric nurse spent a number of hours each day in the patients' homes, and health visitors and midwives visited daily on a rota basis. Links were maintained with midwives and with the patients' general practitioners who also visited frequently. In 1984 a second community psychiatric nurse and full-time psychiatric social worker were added to the team, which also included Dr. Oates herself (devoting all her clinical work to the service), a senior registrar, a registrar, and a psychologist (these last three devoting about half their time to the service). It is important to add that the team also had the services of a group of six Homestart volunteers; Homestart is a national voluntary organization of mothers who support other mothers at home, after a six-week period of training, under supervision of a trained social worker. During the twelve-month period from March 1983, eleven patients were seen initially on a domiciliary visit and managed at home throughout the course of their illness, and twenty other patients were initially admitted, but discharged home before full recovery. To deal with such patients, three levels of care were worked out:

1. The nurse spent eight hours per day in the home, leaving only when a responsible adult took over the care, and the psychiatrist visited on alternate days. This level of care could only be maintained for one patient at any one time.
2. The nurse visited at least twice daily, for at least two hours per visit, and during her absence another responsible adult was present. The psychiatrist visited twice weekly.
3. The nurse visited on alternate days and the psychiatrist weekly.

It was not possible to treat all the patients at home. Home treatment could only be maintained if the family wished it and another responsible adult lived with the patient, if the general practitioner, health visitor, and midwife agreed, and if the patient lived within twenty minutes of the hospital. Patients who could not be treated at home were admitted to the six-bed mother and baby unit, situated in the academic psychiatry department in Queens University Hospital.

We in Birmingham have had some experience with the home treatment of puerperal psychosis. We at present lack an inpatient mother and baby unit, and can only with difficulty admit mothers and babies at all. With a three-person medical team and two part-time community nurses, we have treated several patients at home and can confirm that this form of care is not only feasible, but greatly appreciated by the patients and their families. There are all sorts of problems about home treatment, but Stein and Test (1980) and Hoult and coworkers (1984) have demonstrated that it is greatly preferred by patients and their families as an approach to the management of all kinds of psychiatric illness. It is necessary to insist that standards of case-taking and investigation are maintained up to the level practiced on inpatient units. In Birmingham we do this by involving our medical students who take the histories and then present the facts to the senior registrar or consultant visiting the home. Then in most instances, the community psychiatric nurse is brought in to supervise drug therapy and provide psychotherapeutic and psychological treatment for as long as necessary. This involves a great deal of traveling over an area of about 100 square miles. The service is coordinated by a secretary who keeps in telephone contact with patients and staff.

Dr. Oates used the Nottingham Case Register to estimate the frequency of referral of mental illness related to pregnancy and the need for services. From March 1983 to February 1984, there were 87 women referred within twelve months of childbirth from a catchment area of 390,000 with 5,200 births, i.e., 1.6 percent of all women delivered. The total number of patients referred to the service, including other postnatal women from neighboring areas of Nottinghamshire and women who became ill during pregnancy, was not far below the average number (200 per year) of referrals received by consultant colleagues managing catchment areas of 50,000 inhabitants, and the severity of the illness was, if anything, greater.

One cannot help noticing, however, that referral rates even to an exemplary high-profile service are surprisingly low. There is a major discrepancy between these referral rates and the often quoted figures for the frequency of postnatal depression in the community. It is said that 10 to 15 percent of women suffer from postnatal depression, though (in the author's opinion) too low a threshold has been used to define this disorder. Only one study (Watson et al. 1984) has provided data on duration, and no study has reported adequately the effect on functioning. Even so, Watson and colleagues showed that 6 percent had a depressive disorder lasting at least six months developing after childbirth, and an equal number had a continuous depression totalling six months starting before childbirth and continuing into the postnatal period. Even the best developed services are not reaching more than about 1.5 percent of all women delivered.

To put this in perspective, one has to remember that Britain has a complete family doctor service, and many or most general practitioners would consider themselves competent to diagnose and treat postnatal depression. In evaluating that competence one would take note of the fact that up until ten years ago most general practitioners received only four to eight weeks undergraduate training in psychiatry; since vocational training was made mandatory, a substantial number (perhaps half) of the trainees in general practice have included six months of psychiatry in their rotational training, but often that training is in the care of acute and chronic psychosis, and few training schemes include adequate training in psychotherapy and counseling.

It is not very clear exactly what is happening in Britain, but one would guess that the majority of women with postnatal depression do not refer themselves to any doctor; patients will tolerate depression for several weeks before they recognize that something is wrong and overcome a natural reluctance to admit to psychiatric complaints. Those who do refer themselves will mostly be treated by a doctor with minimal training in psychiatry. Thus we have a major problem with outreach to the patients who need our help.

Obstetric Liaison Services

The logical extension of the deployment of services for postnatal illness is the development of links with the obstetric services, providing psychiatric advice for women who become depressed or disturbed during pregnancy and also seeking early warning of psychiatric vulnerability in pregnant mothers, using for this purpose the high level of supervision of future mothers in the antenatal clinics. The earliest example of this form of service is probably that of Ounsted in Oxford. Margaret Lynch and Jacqueline Roberts, working with him, showed that midwives were often able to detect problems in the mother-infant relationship in the early postpartum period. In fact, twenty-two of fifty mothers who later threatened to abuse their babies, or actually did so, and only three of fifty control mothers had documented evidence of the midwives' concern, as shown by remarks like "she cannot stand her baby's cry," or "she does not know how to respond to the baby's needs" (Lynch and Roberts 1976 and 1977).

Recently, Kumar in London and Riley in Buckinghamshire have reported their experience of setting up an obstetric liaison service.

Appleby and associates (1989) (working with Kumar) reported on their experiences of providing such a service for Kings College Hospital (2,500 deliveries per year) in the eighteen-month period from April 1985. A registrar spent two sessions per week in the maternity hospital with the intention of seeing women with a history of depression; however, most of the women referred had actual symptoms, and 42 percent were referred after delivery (29 percent becoming ill during the first week after delivery). Ninety-two patients were assessed in eighteen months (about 2 percent of all pregnant women).

Riley (1986) has reported her experience in Aylesbury, High Wycombe, and Milton Keynes in Buckinghamshire (population 530,000), where in 1982 she was appointed as the first NHS consultant with a special responsibility for pregnancy-related psychiatric disorder. In 1984, 133 new referrals were seen, of whom fifteen were admitted; eighty-one were referred by general practitioners, forty-nine by obstetricians or gynaecologists, and three by psychiatrists. During this period there were about 5,000 births. The commonest reason for referral was postnatal depression (thirty-nine patients), but antenatal depression (twenty-six patients) was not far behind. Thirty-five patients were referred from the antenatal clinics because they were considered to be at risk of postnatal illness. The remaining thirty-two referrals were with premenstrual syndrome (14), puerperal psychosis (3), postabortion depression (3), maternity blues (3), gynaecological problems (3), poststerilization depression (2), bereavement counseling (2), and others (2).

We in Birmingham have also had experience of providing an obstetric liaison service to three maternity hospitals: the Queen Elizabeth Maternity Hospital from April 1988 and Dudley Road Hospital and Sorrento Hospital from October 1988 (total deliveries about 11,000). In a six-month period we received twenty-nine referrals from all sources. Most of these were women with current psychiatric symptoms. As in the course of postnatal illness, these referral rates seem low. Diana Riley's referral rate of about 60 patients from Buckinghamshire antenatal clinics dealing with about 5,000 pregnant women is similar to Appleby's referral rate of about fifty patients from 3,800 pregnant women at Kings College Hospital, and both are higher than the referral rates we have had in Birmingham, and they lie between 1 and 1.5 percent of all pregnant women. This seems a low rate of referral when it is borne in mind that Kendell and coworkers (1987) reported that 486 of 54,087 (about 1 percent) of Edinburgh women pregnant for the first time had already been admitted to a psychiatric hospital. If we can accept survey results such as those of Watson and associates (1984), at least 5 percent of multiparous women will have had a prolonged postnatal depression after their last pregnancy, and another 5 percent will be depressed during pregnancy. To them can be added women with alcoholism and other addictions, and those with severe social problems. It is evident that the problem of reaching those in need is not solved simply by setting up a service and inviting referrals. There is a reluctance on the part of either the midwifery services or the pregnant mothers themselves to specify factors that should lead to referral.

Progress Toward the Ideal Service

We can begin to see the shape of an ideal service for pregnancy-related mental illness which is slowly emerging. Such a service should aim to *prevent* psychiatric disorder in those who are vulnerable, make an early diagnosis when it occurs, and treat it rapidly and effectively with minimal disruption of family life. It should include:

1. A specialist team treating the most severe and intractable cases, providing training, and undertaking research.
2. Inpatient facilities and associated day-care.
3. A community service providing home treatment.
4. A preventive service.

It is not generally accepted that there should be a specialist team for this area of psychiatry which is not highly specialized. We can distinguish between different levels of specialization in psychiatry: forensic psychiatry, child and adolescent psychiatry, drug dependence, and some forms of psychotherapy are considered to be so specialized that most general psychiatrists do not feel competent to take on work in these areas and refer all patients to those with more specialized training. However, there are other areas, of which the best example is alcoholism but which also includes neuropsychiatry, eating disorders, and resistent affective disorders, in which all psychiatrists claim some expertise, but which nevertheless are enhanced by the input of specialized teams who advise, train, research, and take on intractable patients. Pregnancy-related disorders fall into this group.

The team should have skills in assessment (diagnosis) and treatment. Assessment includes the diagnosis of puerperal psychosis in all its forms, its distinction from disorders of the mother-infant relationship, teasing out the factors responsible for depression during pregnancy and the postnatal period, and diagnosing the obsessional neuroses which are not infrequent in the puerperium (obsessions of infanticide). On the nursing side, the diagnostic skills are particularly concerned with the quality of the mother-infant relationship and of mothering skills. The professional nursing team should be experienced in managing psychotic illness, and this is an area that requires more research because some of these postpartum psychoses are too prolonged. Nursing skills, including various forms of counseling and helping a depressed mother to cope with the maternal role, are most important and should include treating the patient at home, as well as working with the husband who suffers from his wife's depression and is potentially the main source of emotional support. For the most difficult patients, especially with obsessional and "bonding" disorders, a clinical psychologist can make a useful contribution.

An inpatient unit is an essential part of the service, since Dr. Oates has made it clear that home treatment is not always feasible. But the number of beds required is low, perhaps as few as five per million population. This means that a large city or conurbation should have a specialized unit, and smaller cities require only side-room facilities. Such small units are expensive, and the staff providing inpatient care should also be caring for day patients. It seems a great advantage, from every point of view including the economic, that the inpatient staff should be involved in the community service. Thus staff move easily from the ward to the home in respond to demand. Inpatient staff assess the patient at home to determine the need for admission, and the psychotherapeutic relationship developed on the ward is continued at home after discharge.

When planning a community service, one should bear in mind that a specialized mental health team is only one of many agencies dealing with the problem of postnatal mental illness. Apart from the general psychiatric services and sometimes the child psychiatry services, there are the primary care teams (general medical practitioners and health visitors), the obstetric services (providing antenatal care, inpatient care at the time of delivery and a domiciliary midwifery service), the social services, and voluntary agencies, especially the National Society for the Prevention of Cruelty to Children, which deals particularly with the problem of child abuse and neglect. The team of specialists is the health authority's contribution to a social problem of considerable magnitude. It should establish links with all the other services and try to ensure that those in need do not fall between the gaps in the network.

Voluntary organizations can play a very important aprt in the support of the depressed mother. The teams in Nottingham, Birmingham, and Buckinghamshire have all found it invaluable to work with voluntary agencies. While Homestart has been the main agency in Nottingham and the National Childbirth Trust in Buckinghamshire, we have used the Association for Postnatal Illness, a national organization started by Claire Delpech. Our local organizer, Debbie Lloyd, is an integral member of our team. One of the main contributions voluntary organizations can make is to provide social support for the isolated mother.

Prevention is the great challenge of postnatal illness because this is one of the few areas of psychiatry in which primary prevention is feasible. Conditions are optimal for prevention because antenatal care has been so highly developed by the obstetric services. However, although a start has been made with obstetric liaison, no one in Britain has yet been able to develop an effective preventive service.

In summary, we have made some progress in the last thirty years. The National Health Service has allowed the proliferation of inpatient mother-and-baby admission, which is a great advance on the unaccompanied admission of the sick mother, but very little funding is available to evaluate the service, and we do not know even the most elementary facts about these units, such as the risks to babies admitted to general psychiatric wards. Apart from this wholesale introduction of joint admission to a high proportion of psychiatric hospitals, we have only a few experimental schemes to boast of. There have been a handful of specialized inpatient and day units, and some pioneering efforts to develop community services. I believe that during the next ten years these innovative clinical developments and associated research will transform the core of the mentally ill mother and set an example of a psychiatry which is expert in diagnosis and treatment, community-based, and preventive in outlook.

References

Appleby, L., Fox, H., Shaw, M., and Kumar, R. (1989). The psychiatrist in the obstetric unit. *Br. J. Psychiatry* 154:510–15.

Aston, A. (1989). Personal communication.

Baker, A. A., Morison, M., Game, J. A., and Thorpe, J. G. (1961). Admitting schizophrenic mothers with their babies. *Lancet* 2:237–39.

Hoult, J., Rosen, A., and Reynolds, I. (1984). Community oriented treatment compared to psychiatric hospital orientated treatment. *Soc. Sci. Med.* 18:1005–1010.

Kendell, R. E., Chalmers, J. C., and Platz, C. (1987). Epidemiology of puerperal psychosis. *Br. J. Psychiatry* 150:662–73.

Lynch, M. A., Roberts, J., and Gordon, M. (1976). Child abuse: Early warning in the maternity hospital. *Develop. Med. Child Neurol.* 18:759–66.

Lynch, M. A., and Roberts, J. (1977). Predicting child abuse: Signs of bonding failure in the maternity hospital. *Br. Med. J.* 1:624–26.

Main, T. F. (1958). Mothers with children in a psychiatric hospital. *Lancet* 2:845–47.

Oates, M. (1988). The development of an integrated community-orientated service for severe postnatal mental illness. In R. Kumar and I. F. Brockington (Eds.), *Motherhood and Mental Illness*, Vol. 2. Cambridge: Cambridge University Press.

Riley, D. (1986). An audit of obstetric liaison psychiatry in 1984. *J. Reprod. Infant Psych.* 4:99–115.

Stein, L. I., and Test, M. A. (1980). Alternative to mental hospital treatment. *Arch. Gen. Psychiatry* 37:392–97.

Watson, J. P., Elliott, S. A., Rugg, A. J., and Brough, D. I. (1984). Psychiatric disorder in pregnancy and the first postnatal year. *Br. J. Psychiatry* 44:453–62.

Chapter 11
Rituals and Support: An Anthropological View of Postpartum Depression

Laurence Dean Kruckman

The Role of Medical Anthropology

Major changes in the life cycle such as puberty, pregnancy, childbirth, illness, and death have long attracted the interest of anthropologists. This is because they typically are socially dramatized, e.g., rites of passage and healing ceremonies—and hence stimulate ethnographic description. Also, these events illustrate the interactive nature of biological and cultural processes.

The demonstration that biological and cultural systems are interdependent may be one of anthropology's most important contributions to the understanding of human behavior. The development of medical anthropology reflects the elaboration of these traditional interests. The study of health phenomena as they are affected by cultural and social factors encompasses the notion that such phenomena may contribute to the understanding of sociocultural systems. Health and disease are related not only to biological factors but also to cultural resources and the social organization governing them. In viewing biological and cultural systems as interactive, mechanistic, and symbolic, modes of explanation are integrated. While we may postulate or even have objective measures of underlying biological processes, we know that the experiences of those mechanisms are filtered, mediated, and directed by culturally constituted frameworks.

Postpartum Depression as Disease and Illness

A. Kleinman (1978) has attempted to conceptualize this process in terms of the distinction between "disease" and "illness." Disease in the

Western medical paradigm is the malfunctioning or maladaptation of biologic and psychophysiologic processes in the individual, while illness represents personal, interpersonal, and cultural reactions to disease or discomfort. It includes factors governing perception, labeling, explanation, and validation of the discomforting experience. These processes are embedded in a complex family, social, and cultural basis. Because the experience of illness is an intimate part of the social system of meanings and rules for behavior, it is strongly influenced by culture.

Recent cross-cultural studies of childbirth have emphasized that while childbirth is universally similar from a physiological perspective, it is conceptualized, structured, and experienced differently in every culture (Cosminsky 1977, Harkness 1987, Jordan 1980, Pillsbury 1978, Upreti 1979).

One clearly negative outcome of the perinatal period in the West is postpartum depression. However, the nature of this phenomenon, as a disease and as an illness, and its correlation with behavior remain unclear. The very term used to describe the disease, "depression," has deep experiential and emotional connotations in Western culture, and the word has been applied rather imprecisely to both mild and transient forms of depression which are quite common in the first postpartum days, as well as to the more severe psychotic reactions which are relatively rare. Most of the research on postpartum depression has looked to the biological and/or psychosocial etiologies such as hormonal shifts, maternal age and parity, psychiatric history, and so on. Little consideration has been given to the impact of the cultural patterning of the postpartum period as it relates to the etiology of postpartum depression. This includes factors such as the structure of the family and social group and role expectations of the new mother.

Changes in our management of childbirth have resulted in a definition of the perinatal period which virtually excludes any notion of a postpartum period after hospitalization. As a result we have social and public policy which fails to provide necessary social support and assistance to the new mother, and it provides no social recognition for the change in her status. While we recognize no formal social structuring of the puerperium once the mother has returned home, there is a popular or folk notion of this period as being emotionally draining, stressful, and fatiguing. Elsewhere it has been suggested that midlevels of depression may represent a culture-bound syndrome of the West resulting in part from modern birthing practices and the lack of clear role definition and provision of social support to the new mother (Stern and Kruckman 1983).

Rituals and Support: Cross-Cultural Research

Cross-cultural research reveals that birth is almost universally treated as a traumatic life crisis event. As such, this period is usually a candidate for consensual shaping and social patterning. In most societies, birth and the immediate postpartum period are considered a time of vulnerability for mother and child—indeed, frequently a time of ritual danger for the entire family or community. In order to deal with this danger and the uncertainties associated with birth, most cultures have produced sets of internally consistent practices and beliefs designed to manage the physiologically and socially problematic aspects of parturition in a way that makes sense in that particular cultural context.

Cultures, over a period of hundreds or thousands of years, have developed "policy" in the form of myth and rituals concerning the stressful event of birth. The perinatal period, conception through childbirth and the puerperium, is differently defined in terms of its behavioral, social, and experiential content. Perinatal events are not merely physiological sequences, but they reflect what Jordan has termed "biosocial" phenomena, in which the behavior and feelings of the women, as well as those around her, are differentially patterned, emphasized, and ritually marked. This patterning of perinatal events represents each society's "policies" about the perinatal period for the mother, child, and family and as such reflects theories about the nature and implications of these events for the wider social system.

It has been assumed by anthropologists that events in the life cycle are structurally or ritually marked because they are problematic or mark a transition in social roles. The recognition of these transitions assists the individual to pass through them and assume a new role. Specifically referring to childbirth, A. V. Van Genepp (1960) notes, "It is apparent that the physiological return from childbirth is not the primary consideration, but that instead there is a social return from childbirth."

A review of the ethnographic literature on childbirth shows remarkably little evidence for postpartum depressions in non-Western settings. For example, researching the influence of native customs on obstetrics among the Ibibio in Nigeria, Kelly (1967) states, "Postpartum depressions are rare. This may be due to the postpartum customs of the Ibibio people." D. V. Hart's study (1965) in Southeast Asia found "no unusual anxieties or apprehensions" in the postpartum period. In a study of eighty women from four castes in Nepal, N. S. Upreti (1979) notes that, "postpartum 'blues' or depression seems to be less prevalent among Nepalese than among many Westerners." The psychosocial support system available to Nepalese women may account for this discrepancy in mother's feelings and behaviors. In research on the postpartum period ("doing the month") in China, B. Pillsbury (1978) found no evidence of postpartum depression, and suggests the importance of social support in the puerperium. S. Harkness (1987) found that among mothers in Kenya where close support and care are provided by the husband, parents, and relatives, postpartum depression is uncommon.

Before interpreting these findings, there are several methodological caveats. First, the absence of evidence for postpartum depression cross-culturally may reflect the lack of attention given to pregnancy by anthropologists until recently. Secondly, in cross-cultural research, comparisons and assessments are difficult because of the unique Western conceptualization of "depression," which is not often compatible with other cultures. This mixture of behavioral manifestations and internal feeling or emotional state is difficult to define even within a strict Western context. Finally, the ethnographic descriptions available tend to be vague about method, sample size, elicitation techniques, and informant characteristics, all of which contribute to the difficulty of evaluating statements about postpartum depression.

The term "culture-bound syndrome" was coined by P. M. Yap (1951) to define so-called bizarre behaviors in non-Western settings which he believed to be essentially psychogenic in origin. These syndromes are culture-bound in that certain systems of implicit values, social structure, and obviously shared beliefs produce unusual forms of psychopathology that are confined to special areas. Social and cultural factors bring about special forms of mental illness, although these are viewed by Yap to be variations of generally distributed psychogenic disorders.

The apparent lack of postpartum depression cross-culturally may be explained by one of several alternatives:

1. Postpartum depression cannot claim a hormonal etiology or we would see its expression globally.
2. Cultural factors may cushion or prevent its expression in traditional cultures.
3. In other cultures it is masked or labeled in such a way as to escape easy detection by Western observers.

Along with Gwen Stern, the author of this chapter examined several cultural patterns that may be present in cultures where postpartum depression, as such, is not reported. These cultural patterns may be subdivided into:

1. Patterns of structural change in standard life activities.
2. Patterns that regard the new mother as vulnerable or polluted.
3. Patterns that recognize a change of status of the new mother (Stern and Kruckman 1983).

Structural Changes

In China and Nepal, relatively little attention is paid to pregnancy. However, when Jiminez and Newton (1979) reviewed the literature on 202 societies, they found many elaborate postpartum rituals. The normal duties of women were interrupted in all cultures, but in half of them women returned to normal activities within two weeks.

While the length of time allocated to special activities varies considerably, D. Rafael (1976) has suggested that it coincides frequently with time units used for other activities. For example, the notion of a 40-day postpartum period is common in Spain, Latin America, and the Caribbean, as well as among Moslems. This coincides with the length of various religious observances. Our own six-week period prior to the postnatal checkup corresponds to this interval as well. The important point is that the period is conceptualized as finite and different from normal life. In almost all societies it is a period viewed as being recuperative, during which care is given to the new mother, her activities are limited, and her needs are taken care of by (typically) female relatives.

Views of Vulnerability or Pollution

In their view of practices in the Far East, Jiminez and Newton found that the stated reasons for restrictions on activities in the postpartum period related to two views: (1) that it was a time of ritual impurity (49 percent of examined societies) and (2) that it was a time to enable the new mother to rest, regain strength, and care for the baby (41 percent of examined societies).

Many of the recognitions of the postpartum period are aimed at reestablishing identity. For example, S. Cosminsky (1977) describes an eight-day period in rural Guatemala, where the new mother's activities are restricted and special efforts are made to keep her warm. "During this period the mother is considered *muy delicada* ("very weak") and she is susceptible to cold and *aire* ("wind") which will make her milk cold and thin and thus make the child sick."

C. and C. M. Frake (1957) note that among the Eastern Subanum of Mindanao (Philippines), successful birth indicates a time of fear and concern. In this society, during a seven- to eight-day period following childbirth the new mother is subjected to a regime of confinement, rest, special diet, heat treatment, and elaborate medication. The purpose is to prevent the woman from getting sick and to protect her from supernatural beings who are thought to be attracted by the blood of childbirth. The infant is also considered at risk, and rituals enacted to protect the child include the spreading of chicken blood to alleviate any loneliness he might have after removal of the hearth which has been heating mother and child.

Related to the notions of vulnerability and pollution are widespread patterns of seclusion for the new mother wherein she is directed to rest. For example, Punjab women are strictly secluded from everyone except female relatives and the midwife for five days. In the Yucatan, relatives come to greet the new baby only after the eight-day seclusion of the mother and baby.

It has been suggested that this seclusion functions to promote successful lactation and nursing. In addition, it absolves the new mother of her normal duties which are typically taken over by female relatives, thereby ensuring rest.

Among the Ibibio of Nigeria, J. V. Kelley (1967) reports that the new mother and infant are secluded in the "fattening room," a special hut in the family compound. They are cared for by older women. The new mother's only functions are to eat, sleep, and care for her baby.

Requirements of strict rest, usually for a minimum of one week, correspond to former practices in the United States, where a week's hospitalization following childbirth was the rule. Still-existing social policy reflects a need for seclusion, rest, and recuperation in the concept of "maternity leave" for female employees. (The simple factor of mandated rest after childbirth as a factor in promoting postpartum well-being has not been subjected to research.)

Seclusion and rest are typically facilitated by functional assistance from family members, especially female relatives. M. Mead and N. Newton (1967) note several kinds of help which women receive: (1) help in the sense of protection from injury; (2) economic assistance and food; and (3) personal assistance. This third type of help involves the care of any older children, household help such as cooking, and personal attendance during labor. In most societies a great deal of help is provided by many individuals. Frequently, pregnant women return to their home of origin when birth is imminent to ensure that this assistance is available.

Social Recognition

In addition to the social support which results from functional assistance with the household and child care tasks, considerable recognition is often given to the new mother. As early as 1884, George Engelmann noted the frequency of ceremonies marking the return of the mother from her isolated state, when cleansed and purified, to her home and family. Many of the rituals, dietary regulations, seclusion and rest, and solicitude from husband and female relatives accomplish what D. Rafael (1976) has termed "Mothering the Mother."

H. Gideon's description (1962) of childbirth in the Punjab documents a sequence of events in which friends come to congratulate the new mother, the maternal grandmother places protective objects around the bed (to remain there for forty days), the nipples are ceremoniously washed on the third day postpartum, the "stepping out" ceremony is performed on the fifth day when the new mother is given wheat and holy water, and a purification ceremony is performed on the ninth day in which she is bathed and her hair washed by the midwife and she is served a ceremonial meal. After three months of rest, the new mother returns to her husband's family, having been given many gifts (*shushak*) for herself and the baby.

Kelley (1967) notes that among the Ibibio, following seclusion in the "fattening room," the mother and baby emerge to a feast in their honor, the mother is given a new dress by the husband, and a palm tree is planted for the baby.

A high percentage of women in the United States seem to experience nonpsychotic postpartum depression compared with third-world settings where explicit rituals are practiced. This finding should stimulate research on postpartum depression in the United States as a form of legitimate social deviance resulting from perceptions of role helplessness. Stern and Kruckman (1983) suggest that a relationship exists between the strategies typically employed cross-culturally in the postpartum period, which serve to mobilize social support for the new mother, and postpartum mental health. Our hypothesis states that the negative outcomes of baby blues and depression in the United States result from the relative lack of (1) social structuring of postpartum events, (2) social recognition of role transition, and (3) meaningful assistance to the new mother including the provision of information regarding child and self care. Conversely, explicit cultural recognition of new social status and assistance in fulfilling former role expectations as well as caring for the newborn may serve to mask, prevent, or cushion the experience of negative postpartum emotional states.

The Role of Postpartum Rituals

The cross-cultural research on postpartum rituals suggests that they may cushion or prevent the expression of what in the West is designated as depression. This may be accomplished in several ways:

1. Fried and Fried (1980) have suggested that they are a set of evocative devices for rousing, channeling, and domesticating powerful emotions such as hate, fear, affection, and grief.
2. Transition rituals function to enhance and solidify social roles. This is not simply, as Meyer Fortes (1962) has argued, a matter of giving the stamp of legitimacy to the structural positions of a society but rather giving recognition to an essential human bond, without which there could be no society.
3. Rituals serve as a learning process. Through ritual, the responsibilities, attitudes, and techniques of motherhood are revealed to the younger members of the group.
4. Rituals are also a form of support. Rituals marshall regular, reliable and predictable physical support from family members and the community. Rituals also stimulate attention concerning the emotional needs of new mothers, reassuring them of their physical and emotional health and celebrating with them their new status.

An examination of the anthropological literature on childbirth and the postpartum period. Further, the anthropological perspective offers a cultural mirror that allows comparison of supportive measures, or "policies," in the United States and those in the third world, as the following example illustrates.

La Cuarentena

The traditional Mexican *cuarentena*, or "postpartum rest period" (or "quarantine"), is a typical ritual that has structured the postpartum period. The term *cuarentena* refers to a forty-day rest period. The specific details vary but usually include rest and seclusion; assistance from female relatives in caring for the house and baby; eating of special foods, especially chicken and fried tortillas, and avoidance of other foods, especially pork, citrus fruits, and chile; and restrictions on bathing and washing of the hair which are believed to protect the new mother from exposure to cold or *mal aire* ("evil air"). Visits by selected kin occur only on specified days. These individuals are thought to neutralize spiritual impurity, attract sorcery to themselves, and become cultural links or bridges to the community. A. V. Van Genepp (1960) argues that the visits of the selected relatives facilitate the changes in social and physical condition without abrupt disruption of living patterns. These postpartum rituals act to reintegrate the mother into her family, neighborhood and society.

Research reported by G. Stern and Kruckman (1983) compared Chicana women in Chicago who practiced *la cuarentena* with those who did not. The former were found to have a more positive response to pregnancy and a lower rate of postpartum depression than the women who did not practice the ritual. This finding supports the conjecture about the relationship between cultural patterning of the postpartum period with an emphasis on rest, seclusion, assistance from relatives, and explicit recognition of changed social status and the experience of postpartum depression.*

The focus on the new mother or mother and infant in non-Western settings contrasts with the pattern in the United States which tends to focus on the baby. It appears that cultures that still retain postpartum rituals such as *la cuarentena* do not consider the physiological return from childbirth as its primary consideration. Rather, there is an equal or greater concern for a mother's social return from childbirth. The idea of a dual return to some approximate state of normalcy, first expressed by Van Genepp, has profound implications for current postpartum research, treatment, and prevention.

The Role of Support

The relationship between rituals and the expression of postpartum depression seems obvious, given what we know in the West about depression and support. During the past twenty years, scholars from several disciplines have suggested that social support promotes mental and physical well-being, especially in the face of stressful experiences (Cohen and Wills 1985, Sarason and Sarason 1985, Cassell 1976).

The lack of social support and marital intimacy have long been linked with psychological distress (Caplan 1974). Barton Hirsch (1986) correlated lack of support with mental health problems among widows, and Lenz and coworkers (1986) found a relationship between "instrumental" support and physical illness. Nuckolls and associates (1972) found that mothers scoring high in "favorable psychosocial assets" had one-third the birth complications of those scoring low on these items. The importance of having a confidant during the postpartum period

*The investigative work on which this conclusion is based consists of retrospective inquiry regarding the experience of "postpartum depression." The inquiry was conducted among what appears to have been a random sample of mothers. The "postpartum depressions" reported, therefore, would appear to have been comparable to those derived from questioning of random samples of obstetrical populations, where about 10 percent are found "depressed." In Chapter 3 this group was designated as "test-derived depressions" and distinguished from "clinically derived depressions," who are from a population that presents for medical treatment. The latter, designated as "major postpartum depression, moderate and severe," have a rate of occurrence which is one to two orders of magnitude less frequent than "test-derived depression." Evidence or inferences regarding organic etiological factors in clinically derived depressions do not necessarily obtain for test-derived depressions.—EDS.

was said to be a preventive of mental illness (Sosa et al. 1980). Robertson (1980) found that the relationship to the husband was a critical factor in postpartum illness. Bull and Lawrence (1985) found that emotional support was a matter of concern to most new mothers. C. Cutrona (1982) found that prolonged postpartum depression is closely linked to the lack of social support.

It is obviously not feasible to return to a rural extended-family social environment to achieve better postpartum support. Mutual self-help groups are probably a realistic alternative albeit a partial one. An effective model of a mutual self-help volunteer organization would make its own policy, especially regarding the kind of help offered. Members control the resources; the help offered is based on veteran members' own experiences in solving particular problems; organizational structure is governed by consensus, and the group size is small and intimate. Mutual support groups of this kind function to provide information, material help if necessary, and emotional and physical support. This concern has a special meaning because it emanates from mothers who have had similar experiences. As new mothers realize that they share a common series of concerns and problems, they discover that what seemed unusual is common. Mutual self-help groups replicate many of the components of support found cross-culturally, and they have the potential to cushion or prevent expression of moderate depression.

Conclusion

Despite the increasing national awareness of postpartum events such as child abuse and neglect, failure to thrive, sudden infant death syndrome, divorce, infanticide, and suicide, there is currently little field research on how people organize and experience their lives in this critical period. We know very little about what occurs when new mothers return home after giving birth in hospitals. Determining the behavioral sequences and social components that contribute to negative outcomes requires research on both the biochemical and psychosocial aspects of the postpartum period. Observational and ethnographic studies should be completed both in the United States and cross-culturally so that we can understand what actually transpires in the home, where the onset of depression usually occurs today. Although the biological and psychological models of etiology place the origins of this disorder in different domains, they are similar in that both consider the origin as an internal process. To gain a more precise picture of the complex picture puzzle of postpartum illness, we must also study external social and cultural factors. Only then will we begin to unravel the confusion and develop appropriate and effective prevention and treatment strategies.

Acknowledgments

A special thanks is owed to Gwen Stern, who played a major role in conceptualizing many of the ideas expressed above, some of which were published in *Social Science and Medicine,* Volume 17, 1983. Many of the thoughts concerning postpartum rituals were stimulated by Chris Asmann-Finch. I am grateful to both for their assistance.

References

Bull, M., and Lawrence, D. (1985). Mothers' use of knowledge during the first postpartum weeks. *J. Obstet. Gynecol. Nursing,* 14:315–20.

Caplan, G. (1964). *Support Systems and Community Health.* New York: Behavioral Publications.

Cassell, J. (1976). Social support as moderator of life stress. *Psychosom. Med.,* 38:300–14.

Cohen, S., and Wills, T. (1985). *Social Support and Health.* New York: Academic Press.

Cosminsky, S. (1977). Childbirth and midwifery on a Guatemalan finca. *Med. Anthropol.,* 1:69–104.

Cutrona, C. (1982). Nonpsychotic postpartum depression: A review of recent research. *Clin. Psychol. Rev.* 2:487–503.

Engelmann, G. (1884). *Labor Among Primitive Peoples,* 3rd ed. St. Louis: J. H. Chambers and Company.

Fortes, M. (Ed.) (1962). *Marriage in Tribal Societies.* Cambridge: Cambridge Papers in Social Anthropology.

Frake, C., and Frake, C. M. (1957). Post-natal care among the eastern Subanum. *Silliman Journal,* 4:207–15.

Fried, M. N., and Fried, M. H. (1980). *Transitions: Four Rituals in Eight Cultures.* New York: Norton.

Gideon, H. (1962). A baby is born in Punjab. *American Anthropologist* 64:1220–34.

Harkness, S. (1987). The cultural mediation of postpartum depression. *Med. Anthropol. Quart.,* 1:194–209.

Hart, D. V. (1965). *Southeast Asian Birth Customs: Three Studies in Human Reproduction.* New Haven: Human Relations Area Files.

Hirsch, Barton (1986). Natural support systems and coping with major life changes. *Am. J. Community Psychol.,* 8:159–71.

Jimenez, M., and Newton, N. (1979). Activity and work serving pregnancy and the postpartum period: A cross-cultural study of 202 societies. *Am. J. Obstet. Gynecol.* 135:171–76.

Jordan, B. (1980). *Birth in Four Cultures: A Cross-Cultural Investigation of Childbirth in Yucatan, Holland, Sweden, and the United States.* Quebec City: Eden Press Women's Publications.

Kelley, J. V. (1967). The influence of native customs on obstetrics in Nigeria. *Obstet. Gynecol.* 30:608–12.

Kleinman, A. (1978). Culture, illness and care: Clinical lessons from anthropological and cross-cultural research. *Ann. Intern. Med.* 88:251–58.

Lenz, E., et al. (1986). Life changes and instrumental support as predictors of illness in mothers of six-month olds. *Research in Nursing and Health*, 9:17–24.

Mead, M., and Newton, N. (1967). *Childbearing: Its Social and Psychological Aspects.* Baltimore: Williams and Wilkins.

Nuckolls, K., Cassel, J., et al. (1972). Psychological assets, life crisis and the prognosis of pregnancy. *Am. J. Epidemiol.,* 95:431–41.

Pillsbury, B.L.K. (1978). Doing the month: Confinement and convalescence of Chinese women after childbirth. *Soc. Sci. Med.* 12:11–112.

Rafael, D. (1976). *The Tender Gift: Breastfeeding.* New York: Schocken Books.

Robertson, J. (1980). A treatment model for postpartum depression. *Canada's Mental Health,* 28:16–17.

Sarason, I., and Sarason, B. (Eds.) (1985). *Social Support Theory: Research and Applications.* Boston: Martinus Nijhoff.

Sosa, R., Kennell, J., et al. (1980). The effect of a supportive companion on perinatal problems, length of labor and mother-infant interaction. *N. Engl. J. Med.* 303:597–99.

Stern, G., and Kruckman, L. (1983). Multi-disciplinary perspectives on postpartum depression: An anthropological critique. *Soc. Sci. Med.* 17(15):1027–41.

Upreti, N. S. (1979). *A study of the family support system: Child bearing and child rearing rituals in Kathmandu, Nepal.* Ph.D Diss., University of Wisconsin—Madison.

Van Genepp, A. V. (1960). *The Rites of Passage.* Chicago: University of Chicago Press.

Yap, P. M. (1951). Mental diseases peculiar to certain cultures. *J. Ment. Sci.* 97:313–27.

Part III
The Organic Matrix

The American Civil War was in its second year when L. V. Marcé's second book, a textbook of *maladies mentales,* was published. In this book Marcé placed postpartum psychiatric disorders unequivocally among *les causes physiques,* the organic psychiatric conditions, along with the delirium of typhoid fever and malaria, and the occasional madness which followed the use of alcohol, opium, and hashish. He suspected a *connexion* between postpartum illness and the organs of generation, but his inference could not have been exploited until information about the endocrine system developed around the turn of the century.

As another century winds down into its last decade, it is time for a review of organic connections with the mental symptoms that occur occasionally, as the endocrine system recedes from the accelerated activity of pregnancy.

In Chapter 12, Dr. Robert Filer presents a review of endocrine changes from pregnancy through the puerperium. He finds in the psychiatric literature no single paper with indisputable evidence of a systematic connection between serum hormonal levels in the puerperium and the appearance of specific psychiatric syndromes. In Chapter 13, two Australians, Roger Smith and Bruce Singh, narrow and deepen the discourse to the falling hormone levels and disturbed equilibria of the hypothalamic-pituitary-adrenal axis, and they note the circumstances and possibilities of adverse influences on mental processes. Chapter 14, by Junichi Nomura and Tadaharu Okano, reports positive results in which hormone therapy appears to have had strikingly beneficial effects in longitudinally studied patients.

The distinguished endocrine pathologist, Professor H. L. Sheehan, devoted his life to the study of postpartum hypopituitarism. Frequently associated with this often fatal disease were syndromes of psychosis and depression. These psychiatric conditions disappeared very quickly when medication for the hypopituitarism, cortisone and thyroxine, were administered. The resemblance of these psychiatric syndromes to those which present themselves in psychiatric practice, often without overt evidence of hypopituitarism, did not escape Professor Sheehan's attention. In Chapter 15, Liverpool colleagues of Professor Sheehan, J. C. Davis and M. T. Abou-Saleh, describe the psychiatric symptoms seen in postpartum hypopituitarism.

The use of single laboratory values to define or exclude a diagnosis carries the implicit assumption that a value in the "normal" range is reason to exclude that variable from complicity in an illness. It has become apparent that some laboratory values may be associated with symptoms at one time, while there may be no such association at another time. A mechanism to account for this in reproductive-related mental states is discussed by Barbara Parry in Chapter 16.

Obstetrical patients who are at high risk for postpartum psychiatric illness, including those who have had such an illness before, are candidates for the prophylactic measures described in Chapter 17. While absolute certainty of prevention cannot be assured, there are fairly good indications that estrogen, administered at the time of delivery and continued for a few days may produce effective prophylaxis. Other approaches to prophylaxis are discussed. The likelihood that diminution of the rate of fall of these hormones lessens the probability of a postpartum psychiatric disorder is one more indication that these illnesses have important organic and hormonal factors in their etiology.

Chapter 12
Endocrinology of the Postpartum Period

Robert B. Filer

The female endocrine system undergoes tremendous changes during the course of pregnancy with increases in production, secretion, and serum levels of many hormones. These elevations continue through the pregnancy. At delivery, there is an abrupt alteration in the endocrinological milieu brought about by the many physiological changes that occur with parturition. The endocrine changes that occur during the postpartum period are secondary to three major changes. The first of these is delivery of the fetus and placenta removing a large source of hormone production during pregnancy. The second source of changes is the withdrawal of estrogen which leads to lowering serum-binding protein. These changes result in lower serum levels of many of the circulating hormones. The third change that occurs in the postpartum period leading to alterations in hormone production is the elevation of prolactin that occurs with delivery and with breast-feeding. Prolactin is a potent inhibitor of many endocrine systems.

The association between the endocrine changes after delivery and postpartum depression has never been well established. Although it would be rewarding to be able to isolate an endocrine cause for the depression, no such association has been delinated to date. All reports of the correlation between postpartum depression and hormonal changes have been anecdotal and not the result of prospective controlled studies. The goal of this chapter is to summarize the endocrine changes that take place during the puerperium and hypothesize potential areas for research.

Steroid Hormones

With removal of the fetus and placenta, all hormones normally produced by these two during the pregnancy begin to disappear. The rate of clearance of these hormones is dependent on the half-life of the hormones in the bloodstream and disappearance occurs in two phases. The first phase is a rapid clearance that results from removal of the hormone from the blood compartment. The second phase takes much longer time and results from removal of the hormone from any extra-vascular compartment (hormone present outside the blood compartment) (Tulchinsky and Ryan 1980). In discussing the changes that occur with these hormone levels postpartum; reference will be made to a first half-life (rapid clearance) and a second half-life (clearance from the extravascular compartment).

Estrogens

Estrone (E_1) and estradiol (E_2) are synthesized throughout the pregnancy in the placental tissue by conversion of dehydroepiandrosterone sulfate (DHEAS) (Siiteri 1963). DHEAS is secreted into both maternal and fetal circulatory systems providing this substance to the placenta. An active sulfatase enzyme within the placenta removes the sulfate from DHEAS and allows further conversion to androstenedione and subsequent aromatization to estrone (Warren and Timberlake 1962). Estrone is easily reduced to estradiol, and these are secreted into both maternal and fetal circulation. The majority of estrogen secretion is into the maternal circulation (Tulchinsky 1973). Estriol (E_3), a compound normally seen to any extent only during pregnancy, is produced by 16-alpha hydroxylation of fetal DHEAS in the fetal liver. The 16-alpha hydroxy DHEAS is then transported to the placenta where the sulfate group is removed by the sulfatase enzyme (Siiteri and Mac-Donald 1966). Again, the majority of this is secreted directly into maternal circulation. Maternal serum levels of E_1, E_2, and E_3 continue to rise throughout pregnancy until they peak at term (Fuchs and Klopper 1983). With delivery of the placenta, there is a rapid decline in serum levels of all estrogen compounds. Serum estradiol has a first half-life of approximately twenty minutes and a second half-life of six to seven hours (Tulchinsky and Kounman 1971). Because of this short time span, there is a rapid disappearance of estradiol from circulation, its concentration reaches less than 2 percent of the prepartum levels within twenty-four hours of delivery. Estradiol levels reach levels compatible with early menstrual cycle within one to three days after delivery (Tulcinsky and Kounman 1971). Both estrone and estriol have similar declines in their plasma levels and are in prepregnancy range within three days of delivery. These changes in estrogen levels are a direct result of removal of the placenta, the largest producer of estrogen during pregnancy.

Progesterone

Synthesis of progesterone takes place in the placenta by conversion of maternal cholesterol into pregnenolone and subsequently into progesterone (Winkel et al. 1980). The placenta does not have the capacity to synthesize cholesterol from acetate and depends on maternal supply of cholesterol for progesterone production (Hellig et al. 1970). The placenta also does not require a functioning fetal circulation in order to maintain progesterone production; therefore, fetal cholesterol is not a regulating factor in progesterone production. Serum progesterone levels rise through about the second week after ovulation where it remains relatively unchanged until the placenta takes over production at ten weeks (Yoshimi et al. 1969, Henzl and Segre 1970). From the tenth week on, progesterone levels rise until term at which time they are approximately 170-fold higher than follicular phase levels (Tulchinsky et al. 1972).

With removal of the placenta at delivery, there is a dramatic fall in the progesterone levels. The half-life of serum progesterone is extremely rapid. The first half-life has not been documented, and the second half-life is approximately twenty minutes (Lin et al. 1972). Plasma concentrations of progesterone do not reach follicular levels as quickly as estradiol because of continued hormone-producing activity of the corpus luteum of pregnancy during the first few days in the postpartum period. Progesterone levels normally reach luteal phase levels within one day of delivery (Zarate et al. 1974, Weiss and Rifkin 1977, Llauro et al. 1968) and follicular phase levels within three to seven days after delivery (Yannone et al. 1968, Friedman et al. 1976, Said et al. 1973, Weiss and Rifkin 1977).

Androgens

There are three primary androgens that exist in the female: testosterone, dehydroepiandrosterone (DHEA), and DHEAS. Serum levels of testosterone increase dramatically throughout pregnancy and are significantly elevated in the third trimester as opposed to the nonpregnant state. These increases begin early in pregnancy at approximately thirteen to sixteen weeks and continue until term. The levels drop precipitously at delivery (Demish et al. 1968). The primary reason for increase in testosterone production is secondary to the high estrogen levels. Estrogen stimulates the liver to synthesize a binding protein that binds both estrogen and testosterone in the blood. This binding protein is called testosterone estradiol–binding globulin (TeBG) (formerly called sex hormone–binding globulin). As more TeBG is secreted, more testosterone is secreted so that the nonbound fraction, which is the active hormone, remains constant. In essence, although the total testosterone level increases during pregnancy, the unbound, and therefore the active, portion of the testosterone remains normal (Mizuno et al. 1968, Belisle et al. 1977). With the precipitous drop in estrogen levels after delivery, the TeBG levels also drop causing a secondary drop in the total testosterone level (Tulchinsky and Chopra 1973).

DHEA and DHEAS levels in pregnant women are actually much lower than in the nonpregnant state (Gandy 1968). This is unusual for steroid hormones because of the massive production of these hormones by the placenta. Unlike the others, DHEA and DHEAS are constantly being utilized by the placenta to create estrogens. As explained in the section on estrogen levels during pregnancy, DHEA and DHEAS are the substrates needed to form estrone, estradiol, and estriol during pregnancy. Because of this, the total level of DHEA and DHEAS drop during pregnancy. In addition, because of the increase in TeBG and subsequent increase in binding of these androgens, the unbound or active portion of these compounds is dramatically decreased during pregnancy. With removal of the placenta during delivery, there is a gradual rise in these levels to baseline levels.

Cortisol

Plasma cortisol levels increase throughout pregnancy (Cohen et al. 1958). Once again, this appears to be secondary to the hyperestrogen state existing in pregnancy. As estrogen levels increase throughout pregnancy, they stimulate the liver protein synthesis capability causing an increase in secretion of all liver proteins. This includes transcortin which is the binding protein for cortisol. Nonpregnant levels of transcortin are 3.5 mg/dl. These increase throughout pregnancy to a level of approximately 7 to 10 mg/dl in the third trimester (DeMoor et al. 1966, VanBaelen and DeMoor 1974). These changes in the transcortin level are secondary to the estrogen stimulation of the liver and can be seen in women on estrogen replacement therapy. Secondary to this rise in transcortin, there is a concomitant rise in cortisol levels. Cortisol levels double during the first trimester over nonpregnant levels and demonstrate a threefold increase by the third trimester. Interestingly, the diurnal variation (normal fluctuation during the day) is preserved during pregnancy (Cohen et al. 1958).

Free cortisol, the unbound active fraction, also increases throughout pregnancy. Levels reach a 2.5-fold higher level at term than in the nonpregnant state. The reason for this rise in free cortisol is twofold. Higher estrogen levels in pregnancy seems to stimulate an increased free cortisol level. This rise in the free cortisol plasma level can be seen in women on estrogen replacement therapy as well as in pregnancy (Plager et al. 1964). In addition, the higher progesterone levels force cortisol to be displaced from its binding globulin thereby increasing the amount of free cortisol (Laatikainen et al. 1980). Both progesterone and cortisol are bound in the serum to transcortin. Therefore, if more progesterone is present, more progesterone will be bound with transcortin, displacing more of the cortisol. It is felt that this accounts only minimally for the increased plasma-free cortisol during pregnancy.

Thyroid Hormones

As with the other hormones previously discussed, thyroid physiology changes during pregnancy. With the increase estrogen levels, the liver is stimulated to increase all protein synthesis. Thyroid-binding globulin (TBG) is a liver protein released into the circulation to bind and transport thyroid hormone. Levels of TBG increase throughout pregnancy (Skjoldebrand et al. 1982).

The thyroid secretes primarily two hormones. These are thyroxine (T_4) and triiodothyronine (T_3). T_3 is the more active of the two compounds and is the primary activator of the thyroid hormone function. The majority of thyroid hormone is secreted as T_4 from the thyroid and subsequently converted to T_3 in the peripheral cells. Because of the increase in binding globulin levels during pregnancy, there is a concomitant increase in total T_4 and T_3 levels of circulation. The free, or active, portion of each of these hormones remains constant (Fuchs and Klopper 1983). Therefore, there is no overall increase in thyroid hormone activity in the body during pregnancy. At the time of delivery, there is a drop in protein synthesis secondary to the removal of the placenta and lowering of estrogen levels in the circulation. During this time, total T_3 and T_4 levels also drop back to the nonpregnant levels, but the free T_4 and T_3 remain constant.

Protein Hormones

Prolactin

Prolactin is a protein hormone secreted by the pituitary gland to stimulate lactation in breast tissue. Prolactin secretion increases in early gestation and continues to rise throughout the second and third trimester (Friesen et al. 1976). The level remains elevated for two to eight weeks in the postpartum period whether or not nursing takes place. Spurts of prolactin release are seen in response to suckling (Jeppson et al. 1976, Noel et al. 1974) and gradually disappear over the same time period. Elevation in prolactin is felt to be secondary to the hyper-estrogenic state seen during pregnancy.

Human Chorionic Gonadotropin

Human chorionic gonadotropin (hCG) is a glycoprotein hormone, which means it contains a 30 percent carbohydrate and 70 percent protein moiety. It consists of a hormone nonspecific alpha subunit and a hormone specific beta subunit. The alpha subunit of hCG is almost identical to the alpha subunit of the luteinizing hormone (LH) (Belli-sario et al. 1973). The beta subunits are similarly homologous (Carlsen et al. 1973). Owing to the striking structural similarities between the two molecules, hCG has very similar biological properties to LH. During the perimplantation phase, hCG is secreted by the developing pregnancy (Levin et al. 1975) and stimulates the corpus luteum to continue progesterone secretion. This progesterone is necessary for continued growth of the fetus and for preparation in the endometrium for implanation. The serum levels of hCG rise rapidly during the first trimester and peak at approximately forty to ninety days of pregnancy (Braunstein et al. 1973). During the second trimester, the levels drop significantly and remain constant until delivery. With delivery and removal of the placenta, the hCG levels drop dramatically and return to zero within two weeks of parturition.

Endocrine Changes as Related to Postpartum Depression

Because of the major changes in serum levels of so many hormones during the immediate postpartum period, it is very tempting to search for a hormonal cause of postpartum depression.* In theory, it makes a great deal of sense to imagine that one of these hormones triggers postpartum depression during the massive shifts that are occurring at this time. Unfortunately, very little has been done to truly evaluate this notion. All the data previously presented are hormonal shifts that occur in all women during the postpartum period. No testing has been done to differentiate various levels between patients with postpartum depression versus normal subjects. Desire to find a medical cause for this emotional disorder has led to several attempts at treatment, none

---

*Doctor Filer often uses the word "depression" for all psychiatric illnesses after child-birth, including the agitated syndrome of early onset, postpartum psychotic depression (postpartum psychosis).—EDS.

of which have demonstrated a direct association between the medication and the results.

The rapid drop in progesterone levels has suggested the use of progesterone as a treatment for postpartum depression. Katharina Dalton (1971) first reported the effect of progesterone in treating postpartum depression. Subsequently, she published data in which the progesterone prophylaxis was standardized (Dalton 1982). Treatment comprised of intramuscular injection of progesterone, 100 mg per day for the first seven days following delivery. Subsequently, 400 mg progesterone suppositories were utilized daily for two months or until the onset of menstruation. Use of progesterone did lower the incidence of postpartum depression. Unfortunately, there were no controls in this study, and nothing was done to eliminate the placebo effect so common in any medical treatment, In 1985, Dalton published another study using this progesterone regimen in what was reported as a "control study." Again, she demonstrated a reduced risk of postpartum depression recurrence in her population as compared with her controls. Unfortunately, the controls in this study consisted of five women whose obstetricians refused to treat them and one woman who refused treatment during labor. Again, these "controlled" patients received no treatment at all. This study fails to eliminate the placebo effect. In addition, some of her data is compared with controls from previous studies, a group of patients under an entirely different set of circumstances.

Railton (1961) also reported the use of prednisolone in the treatment of postpartum depression. Her study compared sixteen women who were placed on 5 to 10 mg of prednisolone with sixteen women who received no treatment. The main finding in this study was that the treated patients shortened their depression period from eight months to two to five months. Again, although this study reportedly had controls, this was not a double-blind study, and the placebo effect cannot be eliminated. These are the only studies to date that have been published concerning hormonal treatment in postpartum depression, and both failed to eliminate the placebo effect as a possible contributing factor. Of interest is the fact that no study has been published comparing the change in hormonal levels between patients who develop postpartum depression and those who do not. An absolute difference in this change would help identify both patients prone to postpartum depression and the hormonal changes that cause it. I doubt the absolute difference in levels will ever be identified between these two groups. Better designed studies are necessary to truly correlate hormonal treatment with prevention of postpartum depression.

One interesting area of study is in the field of endorphins. These are opioid-like compounds created in the body by the enzymatic cleavage of a larger precursor that are released in response to stress and pain. They have analgesic and euphoric action within the body. Administration of the narcotic antagonist naloxone has been shown to have a dysphoric effect on the body (Schull et al. 1981). Several studies have demonstrated an elevation in the plasma concentrations of endorphins during pregnancy and particularly during labor (Facchinetti et al. 1982, Browning et al. 1983). A drop in these levels during the postpartum period might account for many of the symptoms seen in postpartum depression. Brinsmead and coworkers (1985) published a study measuring beta endorphin levels in the antepartum, intrapartum, and postpartum period. They demonstrated a significant rise in beta endorphins during labor followed by a postpartum drop. No significant difference could be seen between the antepartum and postpartum levels. They theorize that postpartum depression was not related to absolute levels of beta endorphin but rather to the change from high levels intrapartum to the normal levels postpartum. Again, no cause and effect is clearly demonstrated by this study, but this theory does warrant further evaluation.

In summary, the hormonal environment of the postpartum period is one of tremendous change. The removal of the fetus and placenta during delivery causes a rapid drop in many of the hormones produced during pregnancy. Labor and parturition also contribute to changes in hormonal levels. These massive shifts in serum hormonal levels coincide with the onset of postpartum depression making it very easy to look to these compounds as precipitators of this disorder. Unfortunately, treatment of a hormonal cause for postpartum depression consists mostly of anecdotal findings and a few poorly controlled studies. There still exists a vast array of areas available for study and consideration in this field.

References

Belisle, S., Osathanondh, R., and Tulchinsky, D. (1977). The effect of constant infusion of unlabelled dehydroepiandrosterone sulfate on maternal plasma androgens and estrogens. *J. Clin. Endocrinol. Metab.*, 45:544.

Bellisario, R., Carlsen, R. B., and Bahl, O. P. (1973). Human chorionic gonadotropin: Linear amino acid sequence of the a subunit. *J. Biol. Chem.*, 248: 6796.

Braunstein, G. D., Grodin, J. M., Vaitukaitis, J. L., and Ross, G. T. (1973). Secretory rates of human chorionic gonadotropin by normal trophoblast, *Am. J. Obstet. Gynecol.*, 115:447.

Brinsmead, M., Smith, R., Singh, B., Lewin, T., and Owens, P. (1985). Peripartum concentrations of beta endorphin and cortisol and maternal mood states. *Aust. N.Z. J. Obstet. Gynaecol.*, 25(3):194–97.

Browning, A.J.F., Butt, W. R., Lynch, S. S., and Shakespear, R. A. (1983). Maternal plasma concentrations of β-lipotrophin, β-endorphin and α-lipotrophin throughout pregnancy. *Br. J. Obstet. Gynaecol.*, 90:1147.

Carlsen, R. B., Bahl, O. P., and Swamenithan, N. (1973). Human chorionic gonadotropin: Linear amino acid sequence of the b subunit. *J. Biol. Chem.*, 248:6810.

Cohen, M., Stiefel, M., Reddy, W. J., and Laidlaw, J. C. (1958). The secretion and disposition of cortisol during pregnancy. *J. Clin. Endocrinol.*, 18:1076.

Dalton, K. (1971). Puerperal and premenstrual depression, *Proc. R. Soc. Med.*, 64:1249.

———. (1982). Depression after childbirth. *Br. Med. J.*, 284:1332.

———. (1985). Progesterone prophylaxis used successfully in postnatal depression. *The Practitioner*, 229:507.

Demish, K., Grant, J. K., and Black, H. (1968). Plasma testosterone in late pregnancy and after delivery. DeMoor, P., Steeno, O., Biosens, I., and Hendiilex, A.:Data on transcortin activity in human plasma by gel filtration. *J. Clin. Endocrinol.*, 42:477.

DeMoor, P., Steeno, O., Biosens, I., and Hendiilex, A. (1966). Data on transcortin activity in human plasma by gel filtration. *J. Clin. Endocrinol.*, 26:71.

Facchinetti, F., Centini, G., Parrini, D., et al. (1982). Opioid plasma levels during labour. *Gynecol. Obstet. Invest.*, 13:155.

Friedman, C., Gaeke, M. E., Fang, V., and Kim, M. H. (1976). Pituitary responses to LRH in postpartum periods. *Am J. Obstet. Gynecol.*, 124:75.

Friesen, H. G., Fourmier, P., and Desjardins, P. (1976). Pituitary prolactin in pregnancy and normal and abnormal lactation. *Clin. Obstet. Gynecol.*, 124:75.

Fuchs, F., and Klopper, A. (1983). *Endocrinology of Pregnancy*. Philadelphia: Harper and Row.

Gandy, H. M. (1968). Concentration of testosterone, androstenedione, dehydroepiandrosterone, dehydroepiandrosterone sulfate, pregnenolone and progesterone in maternal venous and umbilical venous and anterial plasma. *Excerpta Med. Int. Congr. Ser.*, 157:172.

Hellig, H. D., Gattereau, D., Lefevbre, Y., and Bolte, E. (1970). Steroid production from plasma cholesterol: I. Conversion of plasma cholesterol to placental progesterone in humans. *J. Clin. Endocrinol. Metab.*, 30:624.

Henzl, M. R., and Segre, E. J. (1970). Physiology in human menstrual cycle and early pregnancy. A review of recent investigations. *Contraception*, 1:315.

Jeppsson, S., Nilsson, K. O., Rannevik, G., and Wide, L. (1976). Influence of suckling and of suckling followed by TRH or LH-RH on plasma prolactin, TSH, GH and FSH. *Acta Endocrinol.*, 82:246.

Laatikainen, T., Pelkonen, J., Apter, D., and Ranta, T. (1980). Fetal and maternal serum levels of steroid sulfates, unconjugated steroids and prolactin at term pregnancy and in spontaneous labor. *J. Clin. Endocrinol. Metab.*, 50:489.

Levin, R. M., Rao, C. V., and Yassman, M. A. (1975). The measurement of human chorionic gonadotropin-lutenizing hormone levels in plasma by means of radioreceptorassay. *Fertil. Steril.* 26:190.

Lin, T. J., Lin, S. C., Erlenmeyer, F., Kline, I. T., Underwood, R., Billiar, R. B., and Little, B. (1972). Progesterone production rates during the third trimester of pregnancy in normal women, diabetic women and women with abnormal glucose tolerance. *J. Clin. Endocrinol. Metab.*, 34:287.

Llauro, J. L., Runnebaum, B., and Zander, J. (1968). Progesterone in human peripheral blood before, during and after labor. *Am. J. Obstet. Gynecol.,* 101:867.

Mizuno, M., Labotsky, J., Lloyd, C. W., Kobayashi, T., and Murasawa, Y. (1968). Plasma androstenedione and testosterone during pregnancy and in the newborn. *J. Clin. Endocrinol.,* 28:1133.

Noel, G. L., Suh, H. K., and Frantz, A. G. (1974). Prolactin release during nursing and breast stimulation in postpartum and nonpostpartum patients. *J. Clin. Endocrinol. Metab.,* 38:413.

Plager, J. E., Schmidt, K. J., and Staubitz, W. J. (1964). Increased unbound cortisol in the plasma of estrogen-treated subjects. *J. Clin. Invest.,* 43:1066.

Railton, I. E. (1961). The use of corticoids in postpartum depression. *J. Am. Med. Women's Assoc.,* 16:450–52.

Said, S., Johansson, E.D.B., and Gemzell, G. (1973). Serum œstrogens and progesterone after normal delivery. *J. Obstet. Gynaecol. Br. Comm.,* 80:542.

Schull, J., Kaplan, J., and O'Brien, C. P. (1981). Naloxone can alter experimental pain and mood in humans. *Physiological Psychology,* 9:245.

Siiteri, P. K., MacDonald, P. (1963). The utilization of circulating dehydroepiandrosterone sulfate for estrogen synthesis during human pregnancy. *Steroids,* 2:713.

Siiteri, P. K., and MacDonald, P. C. (1966). Placental estriol biosynthesis during human pregnancy. *J. Clin. Endocrinol.,* 26:751.

Skjoldebrand, L., Brundin, J., Carlstrom, A., and Pettersson, T. (1982). Thyroid associated components in serum during normal pregnancy. *Acta Endocrinol.,* 100:504.

Tulchinsky, D. (1973). Placental secretion of unconjugated estrone, estradiol and estriol into the maternal and fetal circulation. *J. Clin. Endocrinol. Metab.,* 36:1079.

Tulchinsky, D., and Chopra, I. J. (1973). Competitive ligand-binding assay for measurement of sex hormone binding globulin (SHBG). *J. Clin. Endocrinol. Metab.,* 37:873.

Tulchinsky, D., Hobel, C. J., Yeager, E., and Marshall, J. R. (1972). Plasma estrone, estradiol, estriol, progesterone and 17-hydroxyprogesterone in human pregnancy. I. Normal pregnancy. *Am. J. Obstet. Gynecol.,* 112:1095.

Tulchinsky, D., and Kounman, S. G. (1971). The plasma estradiol as an index of fetal placental function. *J. Clin. Invest.,* 50:1490.

Tulchinsky, D., and Ryan, K. (1980). *Maternal-Fetal Endocrinology.* Philadelphia: W. B. Saunders, p. 145.

VanBaelen, H., and DeMoor, P. (1974). Immunochemical quantitation of human transcortin. *J. Clin. Invest.,* 39:160.

Warren, J. C., and Timberlake, C. E. (1962). Steroid sulfatose in the human placenta. *J. Clin. Endocrinol. Metab.,* 22:1148.

Weiss, G., and Rifkin, I. (1977). Progesterone and estrogen secretion by puerperal human ovaries. *Obstet. Gynecol.,* 46:557.

Weiss, G., O'Byrne, E. M., Hochman, J. A., Goldsmith, L. T., Rifkin, I., and Steinetz, B. G. (1977). Secretion of progesterone and relaxin by the human corpus luteum at mid pregnancy and at term. *Obstet. Gynecol.,* 50:697.

Winkel, C. A., Snyder, J. M., MacDonald, P. C., and Simpon, E. R. (1980). Regulation of cholesterol and progesterone synthesis in human placental cells and culture by serum lipoproteins. *Endocrinology,* 106:1054.

Yannone, M. E., McCurdy, J. R., and Goldfien, A. (1968). Plasma progesterone levels in normal pregnancy, labor and the puerperium. *Am. J. Obstet. Gynecol.*, 101:1058.

Yoshimi, T., Strott, C. A., Marshall, J. R., Lipsett, M. B. (1969). Corpus luteum function in early pregnancy. *J. Clin. Endocrinol. Metab.*, 29:225.

Zarate, A., Canales, E. S., Soria, J., Leon, C., Garrido, J., and Fonseca, E. (1974). Refractory postpartum ovarian response to gonadal stimulation in nonlactating women. *Obstet. Gynecol.*, 44:819.

Chapter 13
The Hypothalamic-Pituitary-Adrenal Axis and Mood Disorders Related to Pregnancy

Roger Smith and Bruce Singh

Endocrinology and Mood Disorders

From a biological point of view, mood can be seen as the result of a pattern of neuronal activity within the limbic system and hypothalamus. This is clearly a dynamic situation, and shifting balances in the activity of different neuronal groups in this area are affected by many different influences. The limbic system and hypothalamus are an important integration site for input from the external environment, the higher centres, the brain, and the afferent neurones containing information on the internal environment.

This constantly changing input from multiple sources has a profound effect on the activities of the mood-related neuronal groups. The activity of these neurones is also substantially influenced by the hormonal environment in which they find themselves. Neurone-to-neurone communication is modulated by many different hormones and transmitters. The importance of the hormonal environment is illustrated by the many endocrinopathies that can present with, or are characterised by, disturbances of mood and behaviour such as the aggression that may be seen with hypoglycemia, the paranoia seen in some disturbances of thyroid function, and the mania and depression observed with high-dose steroid therapy and Cushing's syndrome. Psychiatric pharmacotherapy aims to influence the balance of neuronal activity within the limbic and hypothalamic system by the use of drugs that modify neuronal activity such as the dopaminergic antagonist.

Pregnancy and Mood Change

Pregnancy is a time of many changes: in social circumstance, physical appearance, and internal hormonal environment. Placed in this context, it is not surprising that pregnancy is also a time of alteration in mood and that mood changes are common both antepartum and postpartum. The crucial aspect of pregnancy is, of course, delivery of the infant. This is a time of maximal change in physical appearance, social environment, and once again, hormonal environment. This dramatic change is followed in the majority of women by an alteration in mood, commonly known as the postpartum blues, and in a substantial minority of women by later depression. While the primary event in mood alterations is not yet elucidated, it is evident that a full understanding of the alterations in the hormonal environment that pregnant and parturient women experience are important.

Hypothalamic-Pituitary-Adrenal Axis in Nonpregnant Humans

In the past decade major changes have occurred in our understanding of the functioning of the hypothalamic-pituitary-adrenal axis, and a review of this is required to appreciate the even more profound changes that have occurred in our understanding of the endocrinology of pregnancy.

The hypothalamic-pituitary-adrenal axis functions to regulate the plasma levels of cortisol. Cortisol itself has functions throughout the body where its lipid-soluble nature allows it to penetrate into every tissue compartment. While a full biochemical understanding of the role of cortisol is still awaited, a substantial advance is the appreciation that many cortisol actions are mediated by the production of a peptide substance, lipocortin, which inhibits phospholipase A_2, an important enzyme required to release arachidonic acid and allow production of leukotrienes, thromboxanes, and prostaglandins (Fowler 1986). It is thought that lipocortin mediates many of the immunosuppressive actions of cortisol, but the mechanism of action of cortisol in altering behaviour remains unknown.

Major changes have also occurred in our understanding of how the plasma concentrations of cortisol are regulated. Classical endocrinology attributes control of cortisol to a hypothalamic-releasing factor operating on the corticotrophs of the anterior of the pituitary and stimulating production of adrenocorticotropic hormone (ACTH) which in turn stimulates cortisol release from the adrenal cortex. Cortisol, in turn, has a negative feedback effect on the production of

ACTH and the corticotropin-releasing factor of the hypothalamus. Variations in cortisol level that occur with time of day and during stress are due to alterations in the secretion of the corticotropin-releasing factors from the hypothalamus.

While the broad picture remains unchanged, some potentially important details have been added recently. It is now understood that ACTH is produced from a large precursor molecule known as proopiomelanocortin. This molecule is synthesised by the corticotrophs of the anterior pituitary and can be cleaved into a number of bioactive fragments of which ACTH is but one. ACTH is still the most important stimulator of cortisol production by the zona fasiculata and reticularis of the adrenal cortex, but the fragments of proopiomelanocortin that flank the ACTH molecule have received increasing attention in the last ten years. On the carboxy terminal side of ACTH, lies a 31–amino acid fragment known as beta-endorphin, this is one of the endogenous opiates and is of particular interest because it is cosecreted with ACTH and rises during stress. A role for it as a stress-related analgesic has been proposed although not conclusively demonstrated (Smith et al. 1989). On the amino terminus of the proopiomelanocortin molecule is a segment known as gamma-MSH (melanocyte stimulating hormone). Fragments including gamma-MSH have been shown to stimulate the growth of the adrenal cortex and to potentiate the cortisol secretory response of the adrenal cortex to ACTH (Owens and Smith 1987).

Changes have also occurred in our understanding of how the activity of the corticotrophs producing ACTH and beta-endorphin are regulated. It is now appreciated that there are at least two regulators of corticotroph function. First, corticotropin-releasing factor has been identified (Vale et al. 1981) and is now known to be a 41–amino acid polypeptide produced in cells of the paraventricular nucleus of the hypothalamus. It is a potent stimulator of corticotropin synthesis of proopiomelanocortin and secretion of ACTH and other fragments of the precursor. Second, it is also now appreciated that vasopressin can be produced by neurones of the paraventricular nucleus and that this peptide also has an important function in regulating the secretory activity of the corticotrophs. Vasopressin has been colocalized with corticotropin-releasing factor in the neurons of the parvicellular division of the paraventricular nucleus.

In some animals, it appears that vasopressin is a more important secretagogue for ACTH than corticotropin-releasing factor and that the relative importance of these peptides in humans is not yet clear. In all animals studied, however, corticotropin-releasing factor and vasopressin potentiate one another's actions. Vasopressin actions are mediated by receptors on the corticotroph coupled to phosphatidylinositol second messenger systems and a protein kinase C while corticotropin-releasing factor exerts its action through classical cyclic adenosine monophosphate (AMP) second messenger systems and protein kinase A (Thompson and Smith 1989). One recently described mechanism for their potentiation is an action of vasopressin that increases the expression on the corticotroph cell surfaces of corticotropin-releasing factor receptors making the corticotroph more responsive to small amounts of corticotropin-releasing factor (Childs and Unabia 1989). It has been postulated that vasopressin and corticotropin-releasing hormone mediate the stress response to different types of stressors, but this idea awaits confirmation.

From the psychiatric perspective, this new understanding is important because it allows for a new link between limbic and hypothalamic dysfunction and dysfunction of the hypothalamic-pituitary-adrenal axis. Now, alterations in the neuroregulation of vasopressin and corticotropin-releasing factor must be considered in the explanation for the alterations that occur in this axis in depressive states. A further complexity is the recent appreciation that immune system disturbances can also affect the hypothalamic-pituitary-adrenal axis through the effects of lymphokines such as interleukin-1.

The dexamethasone suppression test has a noticeable effect on the hypothalamic-pituitary-adrenal axis in depression. Failure of the potent synthetic glucocorticoid dexamethasone to produce normal suppression of cortisol has been proposed as a diagnostic test for endogenous depression. While argument continues as to the sensitivity and specificity of this test and its clinical usefulness, it remains clear that in many patients with endogenous depression alterations have occurred in the normal functioning of the hypothalamic-pituitary-adrenal axis. Cortisol levels are frequently higher than normal, although they retain the usual diurnal rhythmicity. The adrenal response to injected ACTH is greater than in normal subjects suggesting a hypertrophied gland that has experienced increased stimulation by ACTH and possibly other fragments of the proopiomelanocortin peptide. ACTH levels have not been shown to be consistently elevated, and the ACTH response to injected corticotropin-releasing factor is diminished. The diminished response of the corticotrophs to corticotropin-releasing factor suggests that the pituitary gland is desensitised to it, as occurs with prolonged exposure of corticotrophs to the corticotropin-releasing factor and also in the presence of high levels of cortisol. In these circumstances, it is likely that vasopressin assumes a more important role in the regulation of cortisol levels compared with corticotropin-releasing factor. These disturbances remain an exciting key to understanding the disturbances occurring in the brain in endogenous depression.

Alterations in the Hypothalamic-Pituitary-Adrenal Axis in Pregnancy

That the hypothalamic-pituitary-adrenal axis is altered in pregnancy has been known since the 1960s when elevations in urine cortisol were described in pregnant women (Espiner 1966). More recently, it was noted that plasma cortisol levels rise as pregnancy advances; however, a substantial proportion of this elevation in cortisol consist of cortisol bound to transcortin, which is regulated by oestradiol in the pregnant woman's blood. Nevertheless, free (biologically active) cortisol has also been shown to progressively rise as pregnancy advances (Demey-Ponsart et al. 1982, Nolten and Rueckert 1981). Cortisol levels in the pregnant woman's blood continue to show the usual diurnal variation found in nonpregnant subjects and are also responsive to stressors (such as surgery) and demonstrate a pronounced rise at the time of labour (Namba et al. 1980, Nolten and Rueckert 1980, Cousins et al. 1983, Patrick et al. 1980). Interestingly, epidural anesthetics substantially decrease the cortisol response to labour and to ceasarian section. It remained a puzzle, however, that cortisol levels could progressively rise during pregnancy without producing Cushing's syndrome and without suppressing ACTH production from the pituitary and leading to the usual negative feedback suppression of cortisol release. It was postulated that increased levels of progesterone in the blood of pregnant women were displacing cortisol from its binding protein and that this was the reason the axis was disturbed in pregnancy. However, Genazzani and coworkers (1975) demonstrated the presence of ACTH in the placenta and provided an alternative explanation: that the placenta was influencing the maternal hypothalamic-pituitary-adrenal axis.

Proopiomelanocortin in the Placenta

Genazzani's identification of ACTH in the placenta and its prompt confirmation by Rees and associates (1975) provoked speculation that the elevation in cortisol levels found during pregnancy was due to the secretion of ACTH by the human placenta. Rees also demonstrated that dexamethasone did not normally suppress cortisol during pregnancy, a finding confirmed by several other groups. This nonsuppressibility of plasma cortisol by dexamethasone during pregnancy was easy to understand if ACTH was also being produced by the placenta which was not responsive to the normal control mechanisms regulating ACTH production by the pituitary. Interest subsequently turned to whether the placenta would produce fragments of the precursor molecule proopiomelanocortin.

Dorothy Krieger and coworkers (Liotta and Krieger 1980) demonstrated that indeed proopiomelanocortin was synthesised by the human placenta and the beta-endorphin was also synthesised within the placenta. Many workers have now demonstrated rising levels of beta-endorphin as pregnancy advances (Brinsmead et al. 1985, Goland et al. 1981, Newnham et al. 1984). This is of particular interest from the psychiatric perspective because of the possibility that beta-endorphins (which are structurally similar to morphine) might have behavioural effects. Indeed, intraventricular injections of beta-endorphin have been demonstrated to exert profound behavioural effects in laboratory animals, and some reports demonstrate analgesia following injections into the cerebrospinal fluid.

However, a major stumbling block in this argument is the ability of the beta-endorphin in the peripheral plasma to penetrate the blood-brain barrier. Indeed studies in laboratory animals, especially sheep, have demonstrated that during stressful situations such as hypoglycaemia, although plasma levels of beta-endorphin rise dramatically, no parallel change occurs in the cerebrospinal fluid (Owens and Smith 1987, Smith et al. 1986). In human studies during pregnancy, a dissociation has been demonstrated between plasma levels of beta-endorphin and the levels found in cerebrospinal fluid (Steinbrook et al. 1982). However, this does not mean that peripheral plasma beta-endorphin cannot affect brain function because the blood-brain barrier is altered in the area of the hypothalamus, where a fenestrated membrane forms, and penetration by peptides is possible. Thus the extent to which peripheral plasma beta-endorphin can penetrate the brain substance is still uncertain. This is particularly relevant when analyzing beta-endorphins during pregnancy where the elevations of peptide concentrations occur not for minutes or hours but for months. The possibility of neurones in this region becoming tolerant to the effects of the endogenous opiates during this prolonged exposure may have important implications for mood alterations associated with pregnancy.

Corticotropin-Releasing Factor During Pregnancy

Following the isolation of hypothalamic corticotropin-releasing factor and its characterisation by Vale and colleagues (1981), this peptide was soon identified in the human placenta and blood of pregnant women. Indeed, its plasma concentrations were quite remarkable and in the order of 10 ng/ml (Sasaki et al. 1987, Campbell et al. 1987). Subsequently, it has been demonstrated that the placenta is capable of synthesising corticotropin-releasing factor and secreting it (Smith et al. 1985).

The dramatic rises that occur in corticotropin-releasing factor concentrations in the blood as pregnancy advances has been confirmed by many groups. This has added a further level of complexity to understanding the hypothalamic-pituitary-adrenal axis in pregnancy. What part does placentally derived corticotropin-releasing factor play in the regulation of this axis? What role does corticotropin-releasing factor produced by the placenta have? The levels found in the blood as term approaches are certainly capable of exerting biological actions on corticotrophs of the pituitary, although some controversy remains in this area because of the presence in plasma of a specific binding protein for corticotropin-releasing factor, which to some extent diminishes its biological activity. However, concentrations of this binding protein do not increase during pregnancy, and therefore, the pituitary of pregnant women is exposed to increased concentrations of biologically active corticotropin-releasing factor (Orth and Mount 1987). Some of this releasing hormone is also present in larger molecular weight forms, some due to a combination of the binding protein with corticotropin-releasing factor and others due to the presence of the precursor peptide of corticotropin-releasing factor circulating in plasma (Chan et al. 1988).

In studies with laboratory animals and humans, prolonged exposure to corticotropin-releasing factor leads to desensitization of the corticotrophs to further stimulation (Thompson and Smith 1989). Congruent with this idea, it has been shown that women in the third trimester of pregnancy are relatively insensitive to the biological actions of corticotropin-releasing factor, i.e., little if any increase in cortisol secretion occurs following an injection of corticotropin-releasing hormone. However, as has been indicated in reference to nonpregnant women, it is likely that maintenance of the diurnal variation and stress responsivity of cortisol and the corticotrophs is dependent more on hypothalamic release of vasopressin than corticotropin-releasing factor. Corticotropin-releasing factor has been shown to have behavioural effects when injected into the cerebrospinal fluid, but once again, the ability of corticotropin-releasing factor to cross the blood-brain barrier is restricted, and therefore, its ability to influence behaviour by effects on the brain remains uncertain.

Postpartum Changes in the Hypothalamic-Pituitary-Adrenal Axis

Following delivery of the baby and expulsion of the placenta, the hormonal disturbances characteristic of pregnancy disappear. However, the timing of disappearance varies considerably with different hormones. Corticotropin-releasing factor and beta-endorphin levels in plasma return to normal within hours after a precipitous fall from the levels seen during labour, while plasma cortisol takes days if not weeks to return to normal. Evidence of a persisting disturbance in the hypothalamic-pituitary-adrenal axis in the postnatal period can be detected with dynamic tests. The blunted cortisol and ACTH response to injected corticotropin-releasing factor found in late pregnancy is also found in the early postnatal period and then gradually returns to normal. The dexamethasone suppression test is also abnormal in the postnatal period with many women showing a failure to suppress normally, but this too returns to normal over a period of several weeks (Smith et al. 1987, Owens and Smith 1987). Interest in the potential effects of breast-feeding has prompted studies into the effects of breast-feeding on plasma beta-endorphin concentrations, but no significant effects have been demonstrated in carefully controlled studies (Tulenheimo et al. 1985).

Alterations in the Hypothalamic-Pituitary-Adrenal Axis and Mood Disturbances in Antepartum, Parturient, and Postpartum Women

The dramatic hormonal changes characteristic of pregnancy and the association of pregnancy with significant mood changes before and after delivery have prompted researchers to investigate the potential relationship between the alterations in hormones and the mood disturbances. The placenta secretes a multitude of both steroid and peptide hormones, and the problems of researchers have been not so much to document the very readily determined changes in hormones but to decide which hormones to examine. Because the hypothalamic-pituitary-adrenal axis has an important role in the stress response and pregnancy (especially delivery) is clearly a significant stress, several workers have explored the relationship between changes in cortisol and mood alterations. With the realisation that significant changes also occur in the concentrations of beta-endorphin and corticotropin-releasing factor during pregnancy and the knowledge that both of these peptides can potentially have behavioural effects, interest in the relationship between changes in the hypothalamic-pituitary-adrenal axis in pregnancy and mood change has increased. Strengthening the rationale for this interest is the knowledge that several characteristics of endogenous depression—elevated plasma cortisol but preserved diurnal rhythm, blunted cortisol response to intravenous corticotropin-releasing hormone, and diminished cortisol suppression by dexamethasone—also occur in pregnancy.

Cortisol and Maternal Mood

One of the most interesting studies relating maternal mood to plasma cortisol is by Handley and coworkers (1977) who found that the development of postpartum blues was significantly related to plasma cortisol measured at thirty-eight weeks of pregnancy. Smith and associates (in press) have also studied the relationship between plasma cortisol during pregnancy and postpartum blues and found a weak association between postnatal mood disturbance and the change between cortisol measured at thirty-eight weeks and on Day 2 postpartum. The weaker association observed by Smith and associates may be related to the less-intensive studies they performed in the first postnatal week compared with the studies of Handley and coworkers, who obtained mood rating scores on most of their subjects during the first week. However, Smith and associates also examined the relationship between abnormalities in the dexamethasone suppression test done postnatally and the development of mood as another approach to examining the potential links between hypothalamic-pituitary-adrenal axis disturbance and alterations in affect. However, in this extensive study, no relationship could be demonstrated.

Beta-Endorphin and Postnatal Mood

Newnham and colleagues (1984) performed an extensive study examining the relationship between beta-endorphin and postnatal mood but were unable to clearly identify a relationship except that beta-endorphin levels at thirty-eight weeks of pregnancy correlated with the development of postpartum blues. A study by Smith and associates (in press) also examined beta-endorphin and a significant relationship was observed between the fall in beta-endorphin between thirty-eight weeks and Day 2 postpartum and the degree of mood disturbance developed during the first week. Further, those subjects showing most mood disturbance in the first week also had a high chance of developing depressed mood later in the postnatal period.

The hypothesis proposed by Smith and associates as a rationale for the study was that progressively rising plasma beta-endorphin levels during pregnancy caused an increase in beta-endorphin in the hypothalamic and limbic regions accessible through fenestrated blood barriers to circulating concentrations of beta-endorphin. The neurones in these regions, therefore became tolerant to elevated concentrations of beta-endorphin, and when these concentrations fell dramatically postnatally, increase of spontaneous neuronal firing occurred in a manner analogous to narcotic withdrawal. However, the relationships demonstrated in this study between altered levels of concentrations of beta-endorphin and mood disturbance were relatively weak with poor predictive power. Confirmation of this work will be required by studies at other centers before they can become a basis for identification of at-risk patients for clinical interventions. Smith and associates also sought a relationship between mood disturbance and plasma concentrations of corticotropin-releasing factor immunoreactivity, but no such associations were detected in this study of almost 100 subjects.

Current Views on the Relationship Between Mood Disturbance During Pregnancy and the Hypothalamic-Pituitary-Adrenal Axis

At this stage, while considerable endocrine similarities have been demonstrated between the changes in the hypothalamic-pituitary-adrenal axis observed in pregnancy and that found in endogenous depression and some statistical associations between plasma cortisol and beta-endorphin concentrations and changes in their levels and the development of mood disturbance, no proof has yet been obtained that there is a cause-and-effect relationship between these observed associations. It is possible that other changes found in pregnancy, such as alterations in the concentrations of brain amines and aminergic neuronal activity, may produce alterations both in mood status and in the hypothalamic-pituitary-adrenal axis resulting in the statistically observed associations among cortisol, beta-endorphin, and mood change. However, a causative role for beta-endorphin in mood changes cannot be excluded. The possibility that the placenta through the production of beta-endorphin–related peptides and corticotropin-releasing factor or other products of the placenta can affect maternal mood is an exciting idea for current and future study. Unfortunately, such studies will need considerable epidemiological, psychiatric, obstetric, and endocrine input if our understanding is to be advanced rather than retarded by inconclusive studies or spurious results produced by carelessly controlling for the many social, obstetric, and endocrine variables associated with pregnancy.

References

Brinsmead, M., Smith, R., Singh, B., Lewin, T., and Owens, P. (1985). Peripartum concentrations of beta-endorphin and cortisol and maternal mood states. *Aust. N.Z. J. Obstet. Gynaecol.*, 12:194–97.

Campbell, E. A, Linton, E., Wolfe, C., et al. (1987). Plasma corticotrophin-releasing hormone concentrations during pregnancy and parturition. *J. Clin. Endocrinol. Metab.* 64:1054–59.

Chan, E-C., Thomson, M., Madsen, G., Falconer, J., and Smith, R. (1988). Differential processing of corticotrophin-releasing hormone by the human placenta and hypothalamus. *Biochem. Biophys. Res. Comm.*, 153:1229–35.

Childs, G. V., and Unabia, G. (1989). Activation of protein kinase C and L calcium channels enhances binding of biotinylated corticotrophin-releasing hormone by anterior pituitary corticotropes. *Mol. Endocrinol.*, 3:117–26.

Cousins, L., Rigg, L., et al. (1983). Qualitative and quantitative assessment of the circadian rhythm of cortisol in pregnancy. *Am. J. Obstet. Gynecol.*, 145:411–16.

Demey-Ponsart, E., Foidart, J. M., Sulon, J., et al. (1982). Serum CBG, free and total cortisol and circadian patterns of adrenal function in normal pregnancy. *J. Steroid Biochem.*, 16:165–69.

Espiner, E. A. (1966). Urinary cortisol excretion in stress situations and in patients with Cushing's syndrome. *J. Endocrinol.*, 35:29.

Fowler, R. J. (1986). The mediators of steroid action. *Nature*, 320:20.

Genazzani, A. R., Fraidi, F., Hurliman, J., et al. (1975). Immunoreactive ACTH and cortisol plasma levels during pregnancy. *Clin. Endocrinol.*, 4:1–14.

Goland, R. S., Wardlaw, S. L., Stark, R. I., et al. (1981). Human plasma beta-endorphin during pregnancy, labour and delivery. *J. Clin. Endocrinol. Metab.*, 52:74–79.

Handley, S. L., et al. (1977). Mood changes in the puerperium and plasma tryptophan and cortisol concentrations. *Brit. Med. J.*, 2:18–22.

Liotta, A. S., and Krieger, D. T. (1980). In vitro biosynthesis and comparative postranslational processing of immunoreactive precursor corticotropin/beta-endorphin by human placental and pituitary cells. *Endocrinology*, 105:1504–11.

Namba, Y., Smith, J. B., et al. (1980). Plasma cortisol concentrations during caesarian sections. *Br. J. Anaesthesiol.*, 52:1027–31.

Newnham, J. P., Dennett, P. M., et al. (1984). A study of the relationship between circulating beta-endorphin–like immunoreactivity and postpartum "blues." *Clin. Endocrinol. Metab.*, 51:466–72.

Nolten, W. E., and Rueckert, P. A. (1980). Diurnal patterns and regulation of cortisol secretion in pregnancy. *J. Clin. Endocrinol. Metab.*, 51:466–72.

———. (1981). Elevated free cortisol index in pregnancy: Possible regulatory mechanisms. *Am. J. Obstet. Gynecol.*, 139:492–98.

Orth, D. N., and Mount, C. D. (1987). Specific high-affinity binding protein for human corticotropin-releasing hormone in normal human plasma. *Biochem. Biophys. Res. Comm.*, 143:411–17.

Owens, P. C., Smith, R., Brinsmead, M. W., et al. (1987). Postnatal disappearance of the pregnancy-associated reduced sensitivity of plasma cortisol to feedback inhibition. *Life Sci.*, 41:1745–50.

Owens, P. C., and Smith, R. (1987). Opioid peptides in blood and cerebrospinal fluid during acute stress. *Clin. Endocrinol. Metab.* 1:415–37.

Patrick, J., Challis, J., et al. (1980). Circadian rhythms in maternal plasma cortisol and estriol concentrations. *Am. J. Obstet. Gynecol.* 136:325–34.

Rees, L. H., Burke, C. W., et al. (1975). Possible placental origin of ACTH in normal human pregnancy. *Nature,* 254:620–22.

Sasaki, A., Shinkawa, O., et al. (1987). Immunoreactive corticotropin-releasing hormone in human plasma during pregnancy, labor and delivery. *J. Clin. Endocrinol. Metab.,* 64:224–29.

Smith, R., Gaillard, R. C., Bishof, P., Schoenberg, P., and Owens, P. C. (1985). Secretion of corticotropin-releasing factor and N-terminal pro-opiomelano-cortin by the isolated human placenta. *Proc. Endocrine Soc. of Australia,* 28: Abst. 42.

Smith, R., Owens, P. C., Lovelock, M., Chan, E-C., and Falconer, J. (1986). Acute hemorrhagic stress in conscious sheep elevates immunoreactive α-endorphin in plasma but not in cerebrospinal fluid. *Endocrinology,* 118: 2572–76.

Smith, R., Owens, P. C., Brinsmead, M. W., Singh, B., and Hall, C. (1987). The nonsuppressibility of plasma cortisol persists after pregnancy. *Horm. Metabol. Res.,* 19:41–42.

Smith, R., Grossman, A., Gaillard, R. C., et al. (1989). Circulating met-enkephalin and beta-endorphin: Studies in normal subjects and patients with renal and adrenal disease. *Clin. Endocrinol.,* 15:291–300.

Smith, R., Cubis, J., Brinsmead, M., Lewin, T., Singh, B., Owens, P., Chan, E-C., Hall, C., Adler, R., Lovelock, M., Hurt, D., Rowley, M., and Nolan, M. (in press). Mood changes, obstetrical experience and alterations in plasma cortisol, beta-endorphin and corticotrophin releasing hormone during pregnancy and the puerperium. *J. Psychosom. Res.*

Steinbrook, R. A., Carr, D. B., Datta, S., et al. (1982). Disassociation of plasma and cerebrospinal fluid β-endorphin–like immunoreactive levels during pregnancy and parturition. *Anaesth. Analg.* 61:893–97.

Thompson, M., and Smith, R. (1989). The action of hypothalamic and placental corticotropin-releasing factor on the corticotrope. *Mol. Cell. Endocrinol.,* 62:1–12.

Tulenheimo, A. R., Raisanen, I. J., Salminen, K. R., and Laatikainen, T. J. (1985). Plasma immunoreactive beta endorphin in the early puerperium and during suckling. *J. Obstet. Gynaecol.,* 6:47–50.

Vale, W., Speiss, J., Rivier, C., and Rivier, J. (1981). Characterization of a 41-residue ovien hypothalamic peptide that stimulates secretion of cortico-tropin and beta-endorphin. *Science,* 213:1394–97.

Chapter 14
Endocrine Function and Hormonal Treatment of Postpartum Psychosis

Junichi Nomura and Tadaharu Okano

Introduction

Many studies have been done on postpartum psychosis since Marcé described its characteristic feature as *délire triste,* or depressive confusion, in 1858 (Hamilton 1962, Pauleikhoff 1964, Brockington and Kumar 1982, Hatotani et al. 1983b, Nomura et al. 1986). However, the nosology and the etiology of postpartum psychosis are not yet clear, and we have difficulty in finding its proper place in the modern classification of mental diseases. The biological and psychological events surrounding childbirth are complex, but it appears indisputable that disorders in psychoneuroendocrine equilibria which result from parturition are related to postpartum psychosis. This chapter consists of clinical surveys, endocrine studies, and hormonal treatment of cases of postpartum psychosis. The relationship with maternity blues is also briefly discussed.

Clinical Survey of Postpartum Psychosis

Subjects

Among female patients who visited our psychiatric department of Mie University Hospital in Japan between 1968 and 1981, eighty-five patients (thirty-six inpatients and forty-nine outpatients) were chosen as subjects of this study. They had their first onset of mental disturbance within three months after delivery and were followed for more than one year after the onset. The patients with a previous psychiatric history were excluded from the survey. The percentage of postpartum psychosis in the entire female patient population was 1.8 percent and remained fairly constant during these years.

Clinical Pictures

According to Hatotani and coworkers (1983b), the clinical pictures of postpartum psychosis are described as depressed, acute paranoid-hallucinatory, confusional-delirious, languid-perplexed, and neurasthenic-hypochondriac. There is a tendency to shift from one set of symptoms to another. The fundamental varieties of postpartum illness are depression and/or acute psychosis. Depression encompasses mild or neurotic depression, major depression, and psychotic depression or depression with mood-congruent or mood-incongruent psychotic features. Acute psychoses mean *bouffée délirante*, an acute paranoid-hallucinatory state or confusional-delirious state, but they often overlap with psychotic depression. According to circumstances, patients with psychotic features may be diagnosed as having schizoaffective disorder.

In this study, subjects were limited to those who had their first episode after delivery. Depending upon their main symptoms, they were classified into three groups. Group I consisted of patients with major depression and comprised 34 percent of all subjects. Group II were patients with psychotic depression and/or acute psychoses and comprised 34 percent of the subjects. Their most common feature was a confusional-delirious state. Group III consisted of patients with neurotic depression and comprised 20 percent of the subjects. Their main clinical feature was a neurasthenic-hypochondriac state, sometimes accompanied by vegetative symptoms. Pure schizophrenia or mania was not observed in this study; if these syndromes are seen, they are likely to be relapses of illnesses that developed before delivery.

Onset of Illness

There is no general agreement regarding the time between delivery and onset of symptoms that defines postpartum psychosis. Brockington and Kumar (1982) suggested that the term should be limited to cases beginning within two weeks of delivery. In our study, as shown in Figure 14.1, 58 percent of patients had their onset within three weeks of delivery (early onset). However, in 42 percent of the patients, the illness began between one and three months after delivery (late onset). From these data, it might be reasonable to define the term "postpartum" as occurring within three months after delivery.

Clinical pictures were somewhat different, depending upon the time

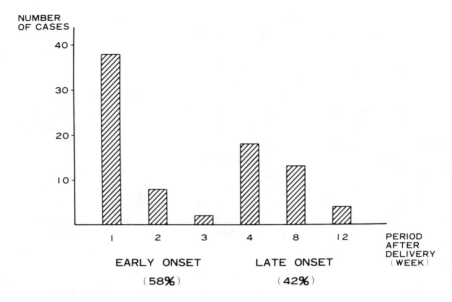

Figure 14.1. Onset of postpartum psychosis.

of onset. Among the patients with early onset, those with psychotic features (Group II) were more frequent than those with purely depressive symptoms (Group I). These patients with psychotic features and with early onset may correspond to postpartum psychosis in a narrow sense. In patients with late onset, patients with depressive symptoms (Group I) were more frequent than those with psychotic features (Group II). Patients with neurotic clinical pictures (Group III) did not show any correlation with the time of onset.

Course of Illness

In seventy-four cases, the long-term course was followed for about six years. Forty-five percent of the patients recovered without relapse; 39 percent had a relapse or recurrence; 16 percent experienced a chronic course for more than one year. Patients with a confusional-delirious state showed a higher tendency to relapse (53 percent) as compared with patients with major depression (25 percent). Among those who relapsed, 38 percent suffered further postpartum episodes. According to our previous study, 5 to 15 percent of postpartum psychoses developed into periodically recurring psychosis, a case of which will be presented later (Hatotani et al. 1983a).

Relationship with Maternity Blues

In another study on maternity blues, 122 healthy women were examined prospectively from early pregnancy until one month before delivery to obtain endocrine and psychological data (Okano 1988). Among them, twenty-two women (17.2 percent) were diagnosed by interview and self-rating scale as having maternity blues. The same interviewer examined the subjects again at one month after delivery. At this point, four subjects were diagnosed with postpartum depression. It thus appears that 2 percent of healthy pregnant women suffered from postpartum depression one month after delivery, and 9.5 percent of cases with maternity blues develop into postpartum depression. Cases with maternity blues also showed high scores of anxiety at one month after delivery. It may be important to follow carefully those with maternity blues for at least one month after delivery.

Endocrine Studies of Postpartum Psychosis

Thyroid Function in Postpartum Psychosis

Among eighty-five patients with postpartum psychosis, the levels of serum thyroxine (T_4), triiodothyronine (T_3), and thyroid-stimulating hormone (TSH) were measured in 10 patients with major depression (Group I) and in fifteen patients with psychotic depression and/or acute psychoses (Group II). The control values were obtained from the normal postpartum women one month after delivery. The results are shown in Table 14.1. Serum T_3 levels were significantly lowered in postpartum psychosis, especially in Group II. In addition, serum T_4 levels were significantly decreased and serum TSH levels were signifi-

TABLE 14.1. Thyroid function in postpartum psychosis.

	T_3 (ng/dl)	T_4 (μg/dl)	TSH (μU/ml)
Control [10]	143.2	8.4	2.7
	($\pm$13.3)	($\pm$1.0)	($\pm$0.8)
Postpartum Psychosis			
Group I [10]	108.3**	7.7	2.7
(Major depression)	($\pm$17.1)	($\pm$1.7)	($\pm$1.0)
Group II [15]	92.5**	6.6*	3.9*
(Psychotic depression)	($\pm$23.6)	($\pm$2.3)	($\pm$1.5)

Figures in brackets indicate number of subjects; figures in parentheses indicate mean $\pm$ standard deviation; *p $<$ 0.05; **p $<$ 0.001.

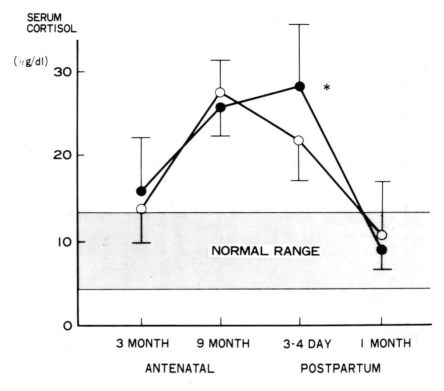

Figure 14.2. Serum-bound cortisol levels in antenatal and postpartum periods: ○ = normal subjects (34 cases); ● = subjects with maternity blues (8 cases); ⊥ = standard deviation; * = p 0.01.

cantly increased in Group II. These values were within normal ranges, and there were no physical symptoms of hypothyroidism. However, such diminished thyroid levels, even at a subclinical level, may have an unfavorable influence on symptoms and the course of postpartum psychosis and may give a clue to suggest thyroid therapy, as discussed later in greater detail.

Endocrine Findings in Maternity Blues

Among 122 subjects for the clinical survey of maternity blues, endocrine examinations were carried out in forty-two women. The serum levels of T_4, T_3, TSH, and bound cortisol were measured at 10:00 A.M. on four occasions: early pregnancy (12 weeks), late pregnancy (36 weeks), third- or fourth-day postpartum, and one month after delivery.

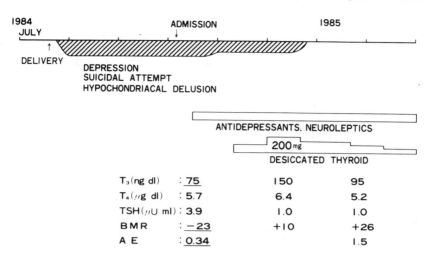

Figure 14.3. Clinical course of Case 1.

The levels of T_4 were decreased at one month after delivery. The levels of TSH showed a transient increase on the third- or fourth-day postpartum and returned to their previous levels by one month. However, the levels of thyroid hormones and their changes during the course of the study did not show any significant difference between the normal group and the group with maternity blues.

The serum levels of bound cortisol remained at high levels, especially toward the end of pregnancy. On the third- or fourth-day postpartum, cortisol levels began to decrease in the normal group. However, in the group with maternity blues, serum cortisol continued to increase on those days and were significantly higher than those in the normal group. The results are shown in Figure 14.2. At one month after delivery, serum cortisol returned to the normal range, and there was no difference between the two groups. We are now confirming the result in a second series of cases.

Hormonal Treatment of Postpartum Psychosis

Case 1: Age 34, Postpartum Psychotic Depression (Figure 14.3).

The patient delivered her third child at the age of thirty-four. From the tenth day after delivery, she complained of insomnia, anxiety, agitation, feelings of guilt, and depressive mood. She made

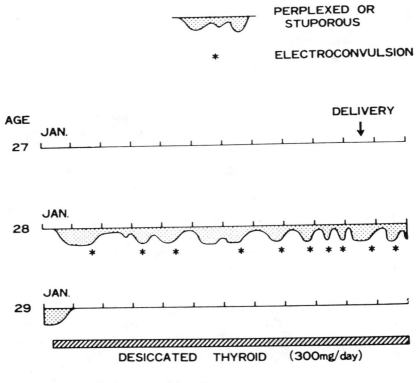

Figure 14.4. Clinical course of Case 2.

repeated suicidal attempts. She had cenesthopathy and a delusion of guilt. At the time of admission, serum T_3 was 75 ng/dl and basal metabolic rate was −23. Serum levels of T_4 and TSH were normal. Thyroglobulin antibodies and thyroid microsomal antibodies were not detected. The thyrotropin-releasing hormone (TRH) test was normal. These findings suggested slight hypofunction of the thyroid gland. Treatment with amitriptyline and fluphenazine was insufficient to bring about recovery. After the addition of desiccated thyroid, up to 200 mg per day, her psychic state improved rapidly.

In cases with an acute psychotic state, we often determine the ratio of androsterone to etiocholanolone (A/E ratio or androgen index) in 17-ketosteroids (17-KS) (Nomura et al. 1979 and 1983). The ratio is usually lowered during the acute psychotic state because of a decrease of the androgen fraction, probably reflecting the decrease of hepatic 5α-reductase which metabolizes testosterone to androsterone. The activity of this enzyme is increased by the thyroid hormone

and decreased by stress or stimulation of the ventromedial hypothalamic (VMH) nucleus. In our experience, the A/E ratio can be a
good indicator for thyroid therapy, and the hormone should be
administered so that the ratio increases to a level of more than 1.0. In
this case, the ratio was 0.34 while the patient was ill and increased to
1.50 after treatment with desiccated thyroid and recovery.

Case 2: Age 28, Postpartum Persistent Depression (Figure 14.4).

The patient became confused during the second month after her
first delivery at the age of 27. The perplexed or stuporous state
persisted for about one year. Neuroleptics were ineffective and electroconvulsive therapy (ECT) alleviated her symptoms for only a
short time. One year after the onset of illness, 300 mg per day of
desiccated thyroid was administered. This therapy caused the symptoms to disappear completely. She has had neither a relapse nor
residual symptoms since that time. In this patient, the A/E ratio was
0.78 during the psychotic period and increased to 2.12 after recovery under thyroid hormone treatment.

Case 3: Age 41, Recurrent Type of Postpartum Psychosis (Figure 14.5).

At the age of 29, this patient delivered a child prematurely because
of placenta previa and lost her baby soon after birth. She was irritable and sleepless for two weeks and then became languid, inert, and
sleepy. For about twelve years after the delivery, she suffered a
manic-depressive state concurrent with menstruation. Neuroleptics,
antidepressants, and lithium could not prevent recurrences. Review
of the endocrine status revealed hypothyroidism and luteal insufficiency. Basal metabolic rate (BMR) and serum levels of T_3 and T_4
were low. Serum TSH and its response to TRH were high. Basal
body temperature (BBT) did not show a biphasic pattern, and the
elevations of serum estrogen and progesterone during the luteal
phase were low. The A/E ratio was 0.42 to 0.53. It was believed that
these endocrine conditions had been induced by parturition and that
they probably played a part in the recurrence of the psychotic episodes. The administration of desiccated thyroid (150 mg per day)
and medroxyprogesterone acetate (10 mg per day) for ten days
during the luteal period alleviated the recurrent psychotic state.
When these hormones were discontinued, a delirious excitement
recurred. At present, the administration of these hormones and
lithium carbonate (200 mg per day) enables her to maintain emotional stability.

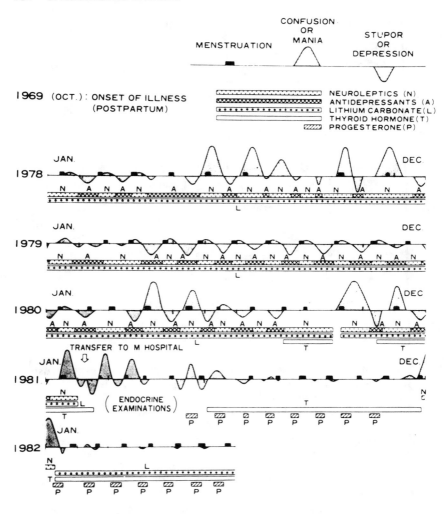

Figure 14.5. Clinical course of Case 3.

Case 4: Age 31, Postpartum Depression with Hashimoto's Disease (Figure 14.6).

This patient had two manic episodes in her early twenties and became depressed after her first delivery at the age of 25. At that time, the A/E ratio was low and the administration of desiccated thyroid (100 mg per day) was effective. After the second delivery, thyroid hormone was used prophylactically with success. At the age

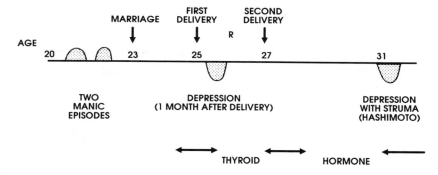

Figure 14.6. Clinical course of Case 4.

of 32, she became depressed without any apparent cause. A soft, diffuse struma was found at this time. Serum T_4 was 3.8 μg/dl, and the serum was positive for thyroid microsomal antibodies. She was diagnosed as almost certainly having Hashimoto's disease and benefited again from thyroid hormone therapy. It was likely that the subclinical hypothyroidism caused by Hashimoto's disease had long existed and played a part in her psychiatric illness. It has been reported that autoimmune diseases such as Hashimoto's disease may be aggravated as a postpartum autoimmune endocrine syndrome (Amino et al. 1982).

Case 5: Age 53, Sheehan's Syndrome (Figure 14.7).

This patient had her sixth delivery at the age of 33. She bled excessively because of premature separation of the placenta, and fell into a coma for thirty minutes. She had to be kept in bed for one month. For fifteen years after the delivery, she received no treatment and had various symptoms including general weakness, loss of pubic and axillary hair, loss of teeth, atrophy of the breast, dry skin, hypotension, headache, and low resistance to infection. At the age of 47, after physical exhaustion and sleeplessness, she suddenly fell into a confusional and agitated state. She recovered after a blood transfusion and was maintained by thyroid therapy (desiccated thyroid, 25 mg per day). When this was discontinued, she lost consciousness and became amnesic for two months. She was easily tired and inactive, and affect was blunted. Her intellectual ability was somewhat reduced.

As shown in Figure 14.8, the empty sella turcica was demonstrated by metrizamide CT-cisternography. Endocrine examination revealed the following: cortisol 1.0 μg/dl, ACTH 10 pg/ml, BMR -27,

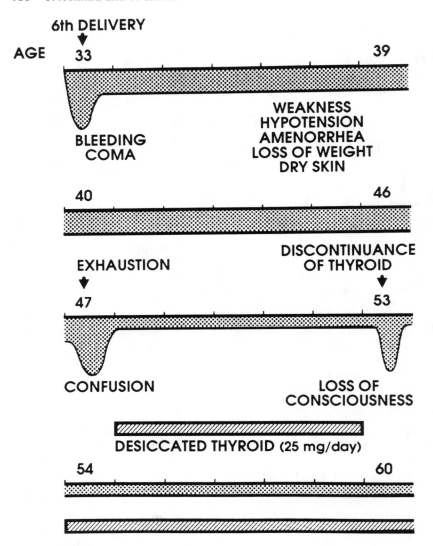

Figure 14.7. Clinical course of Case 5.

TSH 1.0 μU/ml, T$_4$ 3.9 μg/dl, T$_3$ 85 ng/dl, luteinizing hormone (LH) 3.9 mIU/ml, follicle stimulating hormone (FSH) 1.9 mIU/ml, and urinary estrogen 3.2 μg/day. There was no response of serum LH and FSH to luteinizing hormone–releasing hormone (LHRH) or of serum TSH to TRH. The electroencephalogram (EEG) showed general slowing and slight asymmetry in the frontotemporal area. In

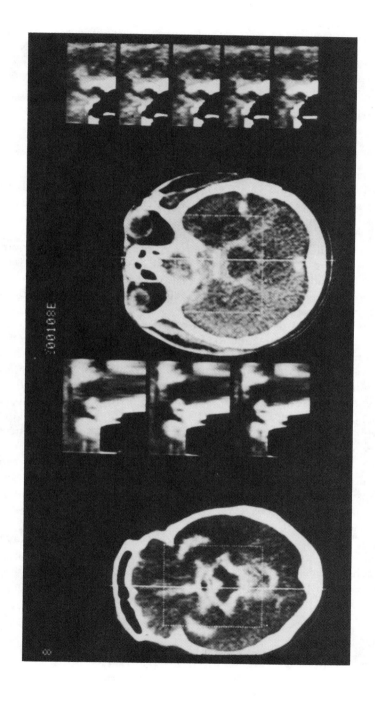

Figure 14.8. Metrizamide CT-cisternography of Case 5. Empty sella turcica in Case 5 (left) and control (right).

this case, it was obvious that the hypopituitarism after delivery (Sheehan's syndrome) had lasted for many years and had become a biological background for the psychotic breakdown (Sheehan and Davis 1982). Thyroid hormone was effective as a substitution therapy.

Discussion

Clinical Study

Our clinical and statistical results on postpartum psychosis agree in general with previous reports (Brockington and Kumar 1982, Paffenbarger 1982). If the term "postpartum psychosis" is limited to patients whose first episode of mental disorder occurred within three months after delivery, the most common clinical picture of postpartum psychosis broadly resembles an affective disorder. The cases encompass mild or neurotic depression, major depression, and psychotic depression. The patients with psychotic depression often show acute paranoid-hallucinatory or confusional-delusional states that may be mistakenly diagnosed as schizoaffective disorder.

It is interesting to note that the onset of postpartum psychosis has two peaks: one within three weeks after delivery and another between one and three months after delivery. There is no indication of the late onset in the report by Brockington and coworkers (1982). However, Hamilton (1982) pointed out that postpartum psychosis with early onset tends to show agitation and confusion, while psychosis with late onset tends to show depression. This tendency is also confirmed in our study. The difference in clinical pictures may be from differences of hormonal as well as situational background.

The prognosis of postpartum psychosis is generally believed to be excellent. In our results, however, about half of the patients had a relapse or recurrence or took a chronic course for more than one year. It seems important to follow carefully the course of each patient for a fairly long period.

It is important to know if the syndrome of maternity blues may be a predictor or prodrome of postpartum depression. Our data suggest that the possibility of suffering postpartum depression is several times greater in postpartum women who have had maternity blues. The data should be confirmed on a larger scale.

Endocrine Study

In the group with postpartum major depression, serum T_3 levels were significantly decreased. Hypofunction of the thyroid gland was more obvious in the group with postpartum psychotic depression. As was pointed out by Hamilton (1962) and Hatotani and associates (1983b), function of the hypothalamic-pituitary-thyroid axis may be lowered for several months after delivery, and this may be one of the biological factors responsible for aggravation, protraction, or recurrence of postpartum psychosis. In postpartum cases with slight hypothyroidism, it should also be determined if there is hypopituitarism as an abortive case of Sheehan's syndrome or Hashimoto's disease as a postpartum autoimmune disorder.

We observed that serum-bound cortisol level was raised in subjects with maternity blues when compared with normal subjects without maternity blues. The meaning of this finding should be further studied, but it is interesting to mention that Stein (1986) pointed out some clinical resemblance between the symptoms of maternity blues and Cushing's disease. It is also important to know if a disturbance of the hypothalamic-pituitary-adrenal axis may be related to the early postpartum cases with agitation, as suggested by Hamilton's model (1982).

Hormonal Treatment

Thyroid hormone has been used mainly for two purposes in psychiatry. One is to stop the recurrence of psychosis (Gjessing 1983), and the other is to enhance the effect of antidepressants (Prange et al. 1987). Both indications for thyroid hormone are applicable to certain patients with postpartum psychosis. In this report, thyroid hormone was used in the first way in Cases 2 and 3, and in the second way in Cases 1, 4, and 5.

In using thyroid for these cases, the usual thyroid tests are often too insensitive to be a useful indicator. As shown in the individual cases, the ratio of androsterone to etiocholanolone in urinary 17-KS is convenient for this purpose. The thyroid hormone is administered clinically in order to increase this ratio to at least more than 1.0. If postpartum psychosis develops into periodic psychosis concurrent with menstruation, as shown in Case 3, use of gonadal hormones may be considered. Hormonal treatments of periodic psychosis were described in detail by Hatotani and colleagues (1983a). Finally, an important caution is that excessive use of neuroleptics or antidepressants in patients with postpartum psychiatric illness may at times aggravate or protract clinical symptoms.

References

Amino, N., Mori, H., Iwatani, Y., et al. (1982). High prevalence of transient post-partum thyrotoxicosis and hypothyroidism. *N. Engl. Med. J.*, 306:849–52.

Brockington, I. F., and Kumar, R. (Eds.) (1982). *Motherhood and Mental Illness.* London: Academic Press.

Brockington, I. F., Winokur, G., and Dean, C. (1982). Puerperal psychosis. In I. F. Brockington and R. Kumar (Eds.), *Motherhood and Mental Illness,* pp. 37–69. London: Academic Press.

Gjessing, L. R. (1983). An essay on the syndrome of catatonia periodica. In N. Hatotani and J. Nomura (Eds.), *Neurobiology of Periodic Psychoses,* pp. 15–45. Tokyo: Igaku Shoin.

Hamilton, J. A. (1962). *Postpartum Psychiatric Problems.* St. Louis: C. V. Mosby.

———. (1982). Model utility in postpartum psychosis. *Psychopharmacol. Bull.* 18(3):184–87.

Hatotani, N., Kitayama, I., Inoue, K., et al. (1983a). Psychoendocrine studies of recurrent psychoses. In N. Hatotani and J. Nomura (Eds.), *Neurobiology of Periodic Psychoses,* pp. 77–92. Tokyo: Igaku Shoin.

Hatotani, N., Nomura, J., Yamaguchi, T., et al. (1983b). Clinicoendocrine studies of postpartum psychoses. In N. Hatotani and J. Nomura (Eds.), *Neurobiology of Periodic Psychoses,* pp. 93–104. Tokyo: Igaku Shoin.

Nomura, J., Hisamatsu, K., Hatotani, N., et al. (1979). Role of the central nervous system in hepatic steroid and ammonia metabolism. *Psychoneuroendocrinology,* 4:47–56.

Nomura, J., Hatotani, N., Hisamatsu, K., et al. (1983). Studies on the cerebrohepatic relationship with reference to the pathogenesis of acute psychoses. In N. Hatotani and J. Nomura (Eds.), *Neurobiology of Periodic Psychoses,* pp. 201–14. Tokyo: Igaku Shoin.

Nomura, J., Okano, T., Komori, T., et al. (1986). Clinico-endocrine studies of postpartum psychoses. In C. Shagass et al. (Eds.), *Biological Psychiatry 1985,* pp. 228–30. New York: Elsevier.

Okano, T. (1988). Clinicoendocrine study of maternity blues. *Mie Medical Journal.*

Paffenbarger, R. S., Jr. (1982). Epidemiological aspects of mental illness associated with childbearing. In I. F. Brockington and R. Kumar (Eds.), *Motherhood and Mental Illness,* pp. 19–36. London: Academic Press.

Pauleikhoff, B. (1964). *Seelische Störungen in der Schwangerschaft und nach der Geburt.* Stuttgart: Ferdinand Enke.

Prange, A. J., Jr., Garbutt, J. C., and Loosen, P. T. (1987). The hypothalamic-pituitary-thyroid axis in affective disorders. In H. Y. Meltzer (Ed.), *Psychopharmacology: The Third Generation of Progress,* pp. 629–36. New York: Raven Press.

Sheehan, H. L., and Davis, J. C. (1982). *Post-Partum Hypopituitarism.* Springfield, IL: C. C. Thomas.

Stein, G. (1986). Psychobiological changes associated with maternity blues. In C. Shagass et al. (Eds.), *Biological Psychiatry 1985,* pp. 222–24. New York: Elsevier.

Chapter 15
Psychiatric Manifestations in Patients with Postpartum Hypopituitarism

J. C. Davis and M. T. Abou-Saleh

During the last weeks of pregnancy the endocrine system is in a unique state. The blood levels of progesterone, 17α-hydroxyprogesterone, and the estrogens have been rising steadily and have now achieved much higher values than the highest peaks reached in the menstrual cycle. Prolactin levels are raised to about 10 or 12 times the nonpregnant levels, and placental lactogen, a hormone not found in nonpregnant women, is present in large amounts in the blood. Pituitary gonadotrophin secretion is suppressed, these hormones being replaced by placental chorionic gonadotrophin. Other less obvious changes are present, a possibly relevant one being a slight rise in the mean levels of circulating free or nonprotein-bound cortisol, which is the biologically active fraction (Demy-Ponsart et al. 1982).

At childbirth most of these changes are very suddenly reversed. The levels of the sex steroids and placental hormones fall rapidly. The secretion of prolactin by the pituitary does indeed continue at a high level after delivery and is partly maintained if the mother breast-feeds the baby, but even here there is a physiological change in the action of the hormone. In pregnancy the high level of estrogens blocks the action of prolactin in the breast tissue, but when estrogen levels fall abruptly, the prolactin causes lactation in the primed mammary gland.

It is a fairly general principle that a rapid change in the blood level of a hormone often produces psychological upsets in the transition period, even when the hormonal change is toward normal values. Thus estradiol implants for the management of menopause can cause grossly supra-physiological blood levels persisting for many weeks; when the level begins to fall, irritability and depression often occur, even though the plasma estradiol is still at a higher level than in normal women of reproductive age. Similarly, when long-continued or over-treatment by thyroxine in hypothyroidism or by cortisol in Addison's disease is corrected by adjusting the dose and the blood profile is converted to normal, the patients often complain of depression and tiredness for a few weeks. Therefore, when we consider the rapid and gross changes in hormones after labour and the concomitant changes in blood volume, together with anxieties and physical stresses of labour, the wonder is rather at the perfection of the mechanisms of adaptation resulting in about 90 percent of women having only trivial or no psychological disturbances rather than at the comparatively few unfortunates who do develop postpartum psychiatric illness.

In postpartum hypopituitarism the hormonal changes at labour are even more evident than those with normal delivery, for in this disease destruction of the anterior lobe of the pituitary occurs by infarction, i.e., tissue death from interruption of the blood supply. Although the fully developed form of this disease is now rare, it throws much light on the etiology of the mental disturbances in the postpartum period and is worth describing in some detail.

Postpartum Hypopituitarism, or Sheehan's Syndrome

The report of this condition by Simmonds in 1914 led to the term "Simmonds' disease," which is still used on the Continent, but there were some serious errors in the description that led to a confusion of true hypopituitarism with anorexia. These inaccuracies are corrected by Sheehan in a series of papers, especially Sheehan and Summers (1949), and the condition is now often called "Sheehan's syndrome."

Hypopituitarism arises in the following way. The vascular system in late pregnancy is in a sensitive state, and if for any reason the patient goes into a state of shock, infarction of various organs can occur. The commonest cause of shock is massive ante- or postpartum hemorrhage; retained placenta and abruptio placentae are the next commonest. The anterior lobe of the pituitary is a vulnerable organ at this time, perhaps because it is considerably enlarged (Erdheim and Stumme, 1909).

The mechanism of infarction is controversial: one theory ascribes it to disseminated intravascular coagulation, but we have argued elsewhere (Sheehan and Davis, 1988) that the primary cause is arterial spasm. In this theory, shock causes a spasm of the sensitive arteries to the hypophyseal portal system which supplies all, or very nearly all, of the blood flow to the anterior lobe. This spasm lasts two to three hours; at the end of this time the parenchymal cells of the affected areas of the lobe are all dead, except for a very thin outer rim which derives its oxygen supply from surrounding structures. As the endocrine cells in the anterior lobe do not, in humans, regenerate from the live remnants, the patient shows permanent hypopituitarism from this time, the severity depending on the extent of the necrosis. In general, tests of pituitary reserve begin to show deficiencies when about 85 percent of the lobe has been destroyed, and when 95 percent has been necrosed, a total loss of function ensues. The posterior lobe (neurohypophysis) only very rarely undergoes necrosis; however, following severe damage to the anterior lobe a very slow shrinkage of the posterior lobe follows over several years.

When trophic hormone secretion stops, the target endocrine glands show a loss of function and develop atrophy. The thyroid shrinks and the blood levels of thyroxine and triiodothyronine fall. The inner two zones of the adrenal cortex atrophy, and the production of cortisol ceases (the outer layer, the zona glomerulosa, is essentially independent of ACTH control and so continues to secrete aldosterone). The ovaries show no gross atrophy, but follicle development is aborted at a very early stage, and estrogen and progesterone secretion stops. In addition to the loss of trophic hormones, there is no secretion of growth hormone or, in severe cases, of prolactin.

As a result of this lack of endocrine function, a series of profound somatic and mental changes ensue. The most striking immediate event is that lactation ceases and the sensation of fullness disappears.* The patient becomes sensitive to cold and may sit huddled in extra layers of clothing or adjusts the heating to a level most people find uncomfortable. Over the next few weeks any suntan the patient may have begins to fade, and fresh exposure to the sun merely causes reddening without any resultant pigmentation. The pubic and axillary hair begin to thin and ultimately disappear; if the pubic hair has been shaved for the delivery it does not regrow. The body weight shows no great alteration. The general resistance to physical stresses is reduced, and a quite trivial infection may cause hypotension and a lapse into stupor or coma, sometimes ending fatally.

The mental changes in a severe typical case are highly significant. The general picture is that a profound apathy and mental slowdown set in. At first this may be ascribed to a hemorrhage, but it persists after

---

*A frequent complaint of new mothers in support groups is that they *are having* difficulty breast-feeding, or *had* difficulty breast-feeding and had to switch to bottle-feeding. Giving up breast-feeding is often mentioned as a source of personal disappointment. Also, a history of bleeding is not infrequently found in the informal communications (see also Sneddon, Chapter 8, on lactation problems in patients with postpartum emotional disorders).—EDS.

the hemoglobin levels are restored to normal. The patient is lethargic and sleeps for long periods. She shows much less interest in the baby than is normal, even if the birth has been eagerly awaited. She does not adequately regain her previous interests or social activities; little interest is taken in current affairs or reading or in her previous professional or business activities. She often becomes rather slovenly in dress, and spontaneous conversation is reduced though she replies when questioned. Her memory is impaired and she may reply to questions about previous events with a vague account that turns out on subsequent checking to be quite inaccurate. An outstanding feature is an almost total loss of libido and its associated emotions; thus in one case the discovery that the patient's husband was having an affair with another woman was received with an apathetic indifference. It will readily be seen that a previously well-adjusted household can soon deteriorate into a problem family.

Although this dull state of mental and physical inertia, if untreated, may persist for many years, it may be interrupted by crises affecting the general health or mental state. It has been mentioned that episodes of coma, often with hypothermia, may occur; these sometimes set in without any very obvious cause, but are often precipitated by infections, trauma, exposure to cold, or excessive fluid intake. Spontaneous recovery may occur, but sooner or later death may occur in an attack of coma. Independently of these, the general loss of drive may be punctuated by episodes of severe acute psychiatric disturbance. She may become paranoid, with delusions of reference or make accusations that the doctor is trying to poison her, for example. Auditory hallucination can be prominent, with voices giving meaningless information. In another form aggressive episodes occur in which she shouts abuse against anyone with whom she comes into contact, or she may become withdrawn and unresponsive, muttering incoherently. Even without hormone treatment, these acute episodes may clear up spontaneously, with reversion to the previous apathetic state, but sometimes severe psychotic disturbances may last for months. A precipitating factor for these crises is not usually discovered.

The electroencephalogram (EEG) in chronic hypopituitarism usually shows a generalized theta activity replacing the alpha activity, the change being most marked in the occipital region.

The above account is based on patients studied before corticosteroids were generally available for treatment or in cases where the diagnosis had been missed. Treatment of chronic cases with replacement doses of cortisone (25 mg in the morning, 12.5 mg in the evening, or equivalent doses of hydrocortisone or artificial steroids) usually produces a most dramatic improvement. Indeed, it is one of the quickest instances of restoration to health in medicine. The general level of mental and physical spontaneous activity rises to normal within a day or two, with the restoration of the patient's social, family, and intellectual interests before her illness.

Cortisone therapy usually leads to a brisk diuresis as the water retained slowly over a long period is excreted quickly; indeed, this diuresis can be so brisk that a false diagnosis is made of diabetes insipidus which has been "unmasked" by the steroid therapy, but unlike true diabetes insipidus the diuresis only lasts for two or three days.

Cortisone therapy rapidly restores the EEG to normal. Libido may be restored to some extent by cortisone, but usually estrogens are needed as well as cortisone to restore it fully. Estrogens without cortisone have little effect.

The role played by thyroid replacement is not too easy to assess. There is a resemblance between the hypopituitary mental state and the condition of primary hypothyroidism and "myxedema madness." However, before steroids were available, thyroid therapy by itself produced little benefit in hypopituitarism. Today, cortisol therapy is usually started together with thyroxine, so it is difficult to separate the part played by thyroxine in the combined therapy.

Advances in obstetrics and blood transfusions have now made postpartum necrosis a rare disease in the Western world, and the few cases that do occur are usually treated promptly. Nevertheless, the condition has been described here in some detail to serve as a model of the profound effects of severe hormone alterations on the mental state. There is, however, some evidence suggesting that a transitory period of partial hypopituitarism may occur in the puerperium after a normal labour. Thus at this time, there is a fall in growth hormone response to arginine stimulation (Katz et al. 1969), and about 50 percent of diabetics show a sudden fall in insulin requirements, which might be a minor form of the Houssay phenomena (Hepp and Roth 1967). The failure of some women to achieve adequate lactation may also be a manifestation of impaired pituitary function. As mentioned above, the anterior lobe is enlarged at term and shrinks rapidly after delivery, and possibly a slight degree of arterial spasm, insufficient to produce cell death but enough to diminish function temporarily, might occur.

To summarise then, a series of sudden and profound endocrine changes occur at about the time of labour, and the coexisting occurrence of pituitary necrosis certainly leads to several mental disturbances. There are some similarities and differences between these and the typical picture of postpartum psychiatric illness.

Implications for the Etiology of Postpartum Psychiatric Illness

The weeks and months following childbirth are a period of high vulnerability for psychiatric disturbance. At least half of the mothers develop "blues," one in five experience postnatal depression, and one in a thousand suffers from a psychotic condition. Although the causes of these conditions remain uncertain, hypotheses have been proposed involving psychological, social, and biological factors.

Most mothers experience distress and insomnia four to five days following childbirth. These symptoms are short-lived, usually lasting for a few hours, but in a minority they are a harbinger of postnatal depression or the more rare and sinister development of postpartum psychosis (postpartum psychotic depression). These "blues" have been associated with hormonal changes, and studies have shown an association with lower concentrations of circulating estrogens, progesterone, cortisol, and prolactin. In these studies, individual hormones were measured often using older and less sensitive assay techniques. Moreover, the total bound hormones were measured. There are no investigations yet of a multiple hormone profile and measurement of concentrations of free circulating hormones.

The determinants of postnatal depression have been extensively investigated, and studies have indicated an important contribution of psychological, social, and biological factors. There is, however, some controversy as to whether women are at greater risk for depression in the postpartum period than at other times. It has been suggested that the increased risk could be accounted for by the aggregation of nonspecific causative factors. Women who develop postnatal depression have often had a previous experience with the illness, show personality traits that dispose them to depression (excessive anxiety, lack of self-confidence, and low self-esteem), lack of family, particularly marital support, and experience of stressful life events prior to their illness.

Biological factors have been classified into nonspecific factors, which contribute to depression occurring at other times, and specific factors, which are particularly associated with pregnancy, childbirth, and the postpartum period. Studies by Handley and coworkers (1977) report an association between depressive symptoms developing within two weeks from childbirth and low plasma tryptophan concentrations which is consistent with findings in depression occurring at other times. Studies of the hypothalamic-pituitary-adrenal axis have been less rewarding. There is no association between postpartum depressive symptoms and circulating cortisol concentration either at baseline or following dexamethasone administration despite the high circulating levels of cortisol and the increased rate of nonsuppression to dexamethasone observed in the postpartum period, changes that have been strongly associated with depressive illness (Abou-Saleh 1988). Of interest is the report by Railton (1961) who obtained good results in treating and preventing postpartum depression using prednisolone.

Hamilton (1962) postulated the involvement of thyroid dysfunction in the causation of postpartum psychiatric illness. This was based on the well-documented occurrence of psychiatric disturbance in thyroid disorders, particularly hypothyroidism, and of the transient hypothyroidism during the puerperium. Total plasma thyroxine levels fall in all women from the third postpartum week. His hypothesis was tested in a study by Grimmell and Larsen (1965) who found lower serum protein-bound iodine (PBI) in women with postpartum depression compared with normal controls. A recent study, however, found no significant differences in thyroid function or the presence of thyroid antibodies between thirty hospitalized psychotic postpartum women and thirty control subjects matched for age and time since delivery (Stewart et al. 1988). The fall in total plasma thyroxine and PBI is mainly due to a fall in thyroxine-binding globulin and probably does not indicate any significant change in the level of free (biologically active) thyroid hormones. The condition of postpartum thyroiditis, while surprisingly common if looked for, does not appear to be associated with postpartum depression (Mekki et al. 1989).

The specific involvement of hormones in the etiology of postpartum depression has been postulated by a number of investigators. This is based on the observation of dramatic changes in concentrations of estrogen, progesterone, and prolactin in the two weeks from childbirth and the common occurrence of mood disturbance in the premenstrual period in association with similar changes in concentration of these hormones. Postpartum depression has been related to higher levels of prolactin concurrent with low levels of estrogen and progesterone (Steiner 1979). Dalton (1980) has specifically linked postpartum and premenstrual depressive symptoms to lower levels of progesterone which she confirmed in the study of its efficacy in preventing postpartum depression. Twenty-seven women were treated with 100 mg progesterone administered intramuscularly for seven days followed by 400 mg progesterone suppositories twice a day for sixty days. She reported no episodes of postpartum depression within six months from childbirth. This was, however, an uncontrolled study, and its findings are therefore inconclusive. Alder and Cox (1983) interestingly found that women who took oral contraceptives during the postpartum period were more likely to be depressed in the months following childbirth than those not taking oral contraceptives and who breast-fed their babies.

Postpartum and Premenstrual Psychoses

Of all the psychiatric conditions occurring in this period, psychoses have attracted most attention. Postpartum psychosis has been recognised as a distinct entity from the nineteenth century, antedating the introduction of the main distinction between schizophrenia and manic-depressive psychosis and was linked to childbirth. Studies of the profile of symptoms and diagnoses of women with postpartum psychoses have shown that the majority of these patients have bipolar (manic-depressive) psychosis, and the temporal link with childbirth has been carefully examined. It was shown that at least two-thirds of the illnesses start within two weeks of childbirth, inviting speculation on the biological determinants of this condition.

The development of postpartum psychosis has been specifically related to dramatic changes in circulating hormones within the first two weeks after childbirth, e.g., prolactin (Abou-Saleh 1982) and estrogen (Cookson 1981). One speculation is that the reduction in these hormones is mediated by changes in monoamine function: both estrogen (Hruska and Silbergeld 1980) and prolactin (Hruska et al. 1982) have antidopamine effects. It has been hypothesised that the sudden and rapid drop in levels of these hormones exposes supersensitive post-synaptic receptors, providing a trigger mechanism for the illness in those who are disposed to develop bipolar disorders.

It is conceivable that other hormones such as cortisol and thyroxine might also be implicated and that the transient hypopituitarism in the postpartum period might be conducive to this trigger mechanism. A corollary of this hypothesis is obtained in the recognised entity of premenstrual relapse of postpartum psychosis which has a similar symptom profile and is associated with similar dramatic changes in circulating estrogen, progesterone, and prolactin. Brockington and coworkers (1988) reported eight patients with postpartum psychosis who rapidly recovered then relapsed shortly before the onset of their first menstrual period after delivery. Five of them had repeated premenstrual relapses. There have been no studies to test these hypotheses, including the exploration of the therapeutic usefulness of hormone therapy in these conditions or as a preventive measure.

There are certain similarities between psychiatric manifestations of postpartum hypopituitarism and postpartum psychiatric conditions with respect to their symptoms and the temporal relationship to the dramatic hormonal changes. It is conceivable that some women with postpartum hypopituitarism who become psychotic are disposed to develop this condition. However, the dramatic therapeutic response of these conditions to hormone replacement would support the notion that they are organic psychoses which are probably wholly caused by this biological insult.

References

Abou-Saleh, M. T. (1982). Mania associated with weaning: A hypothesis. *Br. J. Psychiatry,* 140:547–48.

———. (1988). How useful is a dexamethasone suppression test? *Current Opinion in Psychiatry,* 1:60–65.

Alder, E. M., and Cox, J. L. (1983). Breast-feeding and post-natal depression. *J. Psychosom. Res.,* 27:139–44.

Brockington, I. F., Kelly, A., Hall, P., and Deakin, W. (1988). Premenstrual relapse of puerperal psychosis. *J. Affective Disord.,* 14:287–92.

Cookson, J. C. (1981). Estrogens, dopamine and mood. *Br. J. Psychiatry,* 139: 365–66.

Dalton, K. (1980). *Depression after Childbirth.* Oxford: Oxford University Press.

Demey-Ponsart, E., Foidort, J. M., Sulon, J., and Sodoyez, J. C. (1982). Serum CBG, free and total cortisol and circadian patterns of adrenal function in normal pregnancy. *J. Steroid Biochem.,* 16:165–69.

Erdheim, J., and Stumme, E. (1909). Über die Schwangerschaftsveränderung der Hypophyse. *Z. Beitr. Path. Anat.,* 46:1–132.

Grimmell, K., and Larsen, V. L. (1965). Post-partum and depressive psychiatric symptoms and thyroid activity. *J. Am. Med. Women's Assoc.,* 20:542–46.

Hamilton, J. A. (1962). *Postpartum Psychiatric Problems.* St. Louis: C. V. Mosby.

Handley, S. L., Dunn, T., Baker, J. M., Cockshott, C., and Gould, S. (1977). Mood changes in the puerperium and plasma tryptophan and cortisol concentrations. *Br. Med. J.,* 2:18–22.

Hepp, H., and Roth, U. (1967). Post-partum metabolite status in diabetes mellitus. *Geburtshilfe Frauenheilkund,* 27:368–75.

Hruska, R. E., Pitman, K. T., Silbergeld, E. K., and Ludmer, L. M. (1982). Prolactin increases the density of striatal dopamine receptors in normal and hypophysectomized male rats. *Life Sci.,* 30:547–53.

Hruska, R. E., and Silbergeld, E. K. (1980). Estrogen treatment enhances dopamine receptor sensitivity in the rat striatum. *Eur. J. Pharmacol.* 61:367–400.

Katz, H. P., Grumbach, M. M., and Kaplan, S. L. (1969). Diminished growth hormone response to arginine in the puerperium. *J. Clin. Endocrinol.,* 29: 1414–19.

Mekki, M. C., Lazarus, G. H., and Hall, R. (1989). Post-partum thyroiditis. *Saudi Med. J.,* 10:21–24.

Railton, I. E. (1961). The use of corticoids in postpartum depression. *J. Am. Med. Women's Assoc.,* 16:450–52.

Sheehan, H. L., and Davis, J. C. (1982). *Post-Partum Hypopituitarism.* Springfield, IL: C. C. Thomas.

Sheehan, H. L, and Summers, V. K. (1949). The syndrome of hypopituitarism. *Q. J. Med.,* 18:319–78.

Steiner, M. (1979). Psychobiology of mental disorders associated with childbearing. *Acta Psychiatr. Scand.,* 60:449–64.

Stewart, D. E., Addison, A. M., Robinson, E., Joffe, R., Burrow, G. N., and Olmsted, M. P. (1988). Thyroid function in psychosis following childbirth. *Am. J. Psychiatry,* 145:1579–81.

Chapter 16
Reproductive-Related Depressions in Women: Phenomena of Hormonal Kindling?

Barbara L. Parry

Introduction

Women have a higher incidence of depression than men (Weissman and Klerman 1977). The most likely time for a woman to become depressed is during the postpartum period; the least likely time is during pregnancy (Paffenbarger 1982). In fact, many women experience euphoria during pregnancy. As Paffenbarger writes, "It leads us to ask whether the low attack rate during pregnancy is the result of some protective physiological, psychological, or social process and whether the sudden increase immediately following delivery is due to release of that defense."

This chapter examines the role of reproductive hormones on the course of postpartum affective illness by viewing it in the context of other psychiatric syndromes related to reproductive function in women.

Pregnancy is associated with increased levels of reproductive hormones and improved mood; the postpartum period is associated with decreased levels of reproductive hormones and depressed mood. Similarly, euphoria is most likely to occur during the late follicular (periovulatory) phase of the menstrual cycle when estradiol levels are increasing, and depression often occurs during the late luteal (premenstrual) phase of the cycle when these hormone levels are declining. Thus, both during pregnancy and the late follicular phase of the menstrual cycle, hormone levels are increasing and mood is generally high. Alternatively, during the postpartum period and the premenstrual phase of the menstrual cycle, hormones are declining, and this is a vulnerable time period for depression to occur. Thus, during both the puerperium and the menstrual cycle, different emotional states are associated with different phases of the reproductive hormonal cycle.

In patients with seasonal affective disorder (SAD), another disorder that predominates among women (Rosenthal et al. 1984), euphoria tends to occur during one particular phase of the annual cycle (summer) and depression during another phase (winter). The underlying hormonal influences of this disorder are unknown. However, the cyclicity of SAD symptoms with alleviating or mitigating influences on mood has parallels in both puerperal and menstrually related mood disorders. Thus, whether it be the puerperal, menstrual, or seasonal cycle, euphoria tends to occur at one particular phase (i.e., during pregnancy, midcycle, or summer) and depression at another particular phase (postpartum, premenstrual, or winter). Rapid-cycling mood disorders, defined as four or more affective episodes a year (Dunner et al. 1977), likewise show cyclic mood changes that may be precipitated (particularly in women) by changes in hormonal state.

The phenomenology of these mood disorders suggests that different cycle phases may have differential protective and predisposing effects on the course of affective illness. The fact that at least in puerperal and menstrually related mood disorders, different hormonal influences are present at each cycle phase suggests that reproductive hormones may help mediate the course of affective illness during different cycle phases.

Further evidence for this hypothesis is suggested by other clinical examples where changes in the reproductive hormonal milieu may precipitate mood changes. Examples include oral contraceptives, hormonal replacement therapies, and menopause. In contrast to puerperal, seasonal, and menstrual influences that enhance cyclicity, the influence of oral contraceptives and menopause serve to dampen the cyclicity of ovarian function. The fact that both cyclic-enhancing and cyclic-dampening influences can result in depression again underlines the need to examine the independent effect of reproductive hormone levels on mood. Perhaps there is a therapeutic window for the amplitude of reproductive hormonal change at different stages of the life cycle: too much deviation from the optimal level or timing of cyclicity in either direction may make predisposed individuals more vulnerable to mood disorders.

In order to examine the interaction between affective illness in women and reproductive hormonal states, the types of affective illness in which women predominate will be reviewed first, and then the phenomenology of different reproductive hormone levels that are linked with depressive mood changes (oral contraceptives, premenstrual phase of the menstrual cycle, the postpartum period, and meno-pause) will be examined.

Depression in Women

Depression is a major mental health problem in women. Women, com-pared with men, have a greater lifetime risk for depression, and this risk appears to be increasing with time (Gershon et al. 1987, Weissman et al. 1984). Women predominate with respect to unipolar depression (Weissman and Klerman 1977), the depressive subtype of bipolar ill-ness (Angst 1978), and cyclical forms of affective illness such as rapid-cycling manic-depressive illness (Dunner et al. 1977) and seasonal affective disorder (Rosenthal et al. 1984). In addition, events associated with the reproductive cycle are capable of provoking affective changes in predisposed individuals. Examples include depression associated with oral contraceptives (Parry and Rush 1979), the luteal phase of the menstrual cycle (Dalton 1964), the postpartum period (Hamilton 1962), and possibly menopause (Angst 1978, Winokur 1973, Weissman 1979). Sex differences in the rates of depression began to appear in adolescence (Weissman et al. 1987), a time of major change in the neuroendocrine reproductive axis. Thus, the fluctuation of ovarian steroids during specific phases of the reproductive cycle may bear some relationship to the particular vulnerability of women for affective dis-orders.

The reproductive hormones could exert their effects on mood di-rectly or indirectly by their effect on the neurotransmitter (McEwen and Parsons 1982), neuroendocrine (Meites et al. 1979), or circadian systems (Albers et al. 1981, Wehr 1984), all of which have been impli-cated in the pathogenesis of affective illness.

One clinical model for studying the relationship of ovarian hor-mones and affective illness is the affective changes associated with the postpartum period. One scientific advantage of studying postpartum psychiatric illness is that patients at risk can be identified. High-risk patients include those with previous affective illness or previous post-partum psychiatric illness (Kendell et al. 1987). Of those women with a previous postpartum depression, 50 percent are likely to develop a subsequent postpartum depression (Reich and Winokur 1970). Of those women with a prior history of postpartum psychosis, one in three are likely to develop a subsequent postpartum psychosis (Brockington and Kumar 1982).

Episodes of postpartum psychiatric illness warrant treatment, not only because they may become progressively more severe, but also because they may worsen the course of affective illness. Several studies (cf. Brockington et al. 1981) suggest that 30 percent of women with a postpartum affective illness may later develop nonpuerperal-related affective illnesses. This pattern of illness parallels the longitudinal course of affective illness in which episodes tend to become more severe, more frequent, and more spontaneous (independent of life events) not only with age but as a function of the number of prior episodes (Kraeplin 1921, Zis and Goodwin 1979, Post et al. 1984).

The recurrent and progressive course of behavioral dysfunction in postpartum psychiatric illness and affective illness is consistent with a model of conditioning, behavioral sensitization, and electrophysiological kindling—phenomena found to be more robust in females (Post et al. 1984). A prediction of this model would be that experiencing repeated episodes of untreated postpartum affective illness would lead to greater degrees of behavioral pathology and to recurrences that were less treatment-responsive than the initial episode. Another prediction of this model is that untreated episodes would sensitize women in particular to the development or exacerbation of other affective illness.

Some evidence for this clinical phenomena comes from observations that the postpartum state (or the termination of pregnancy) may worsen the course of rapid-cycling bipolar disorder (Protheroe 1969, Herzog and Detre 1974, Wehr et al. unpublished observations), premenstrual syndrome (Brockington et al. 1988), and menopause (Bratfos and Haug, 1966).

Reproductive-Related Depressions

Phenomenology of Affective Syndromes
Associated with the Reproductive Cycle

Based on an extensive, albeit not necessarily exhaustive, review of each major reproductive-related depression, the strength and consistency of findings for the relationship between reproductive events and mood as well as cognitive and behavioral symptoms will be summarized. Whenever possible, an attempt is made to distinguish affective symptoms from affective syndromes (a persistent elevation in several symptoms or a disorder).

Menstrual Cycle–Related Symptoms and Menarche

At least 20 percent and as many as 80 percent of women report mild to minimal mood or somatic changes premenstrually (Davis 1985). The percentage of women who experience severe premenstrual symptoms is unknown but has been estimated to be 5 percent. Our understanding of possible menstrual cycle-related changes has been limited by retrospective assessments, which are known to correlate poorly with prospective measures. In addition, research has been limited by a lack of consensus on what constitutes a significant change in symptoms or in a syndrome. The most commonly reported symptoms occurring premenstrually include depression; irritability; hostility; anxiety; changes in sleep, appetite, energy, and libido; and somatic symptoms. Obvious parallels exist between some of the symptoms reported premenstrually and some of the symptoms of several subtypes or possible variants of affective disorders, including atypical depression (e.g., hypersomnia, hyperphagia, lethargy). The bulk of evidence suggests that premenstrual symptoms are age-linked, with the onset sometimes occurring during adolescence and the highest prevalence occurring in the late twenties to early thirties (Golub 1988, Logue and Moos 1985).

Despite the apparent link in timing of symptoms to the menstrual cycle in some women, a causal relationship has not been proved. Whereas certain complaints may coincide with the premenstrual phase, a cyclic mood disorder may at times continue independent of the menstrual cycle. For example, cycles of both menstruation and affective symptoms may overlap for months or years and then dissociate, or symptoms occurring monthly may continue even after the cessation of ovarian functioning (Morton 1950, Craig 1953, Dalton 1964). This means that interrupting the endogenous menstrual cycle—whether by oral contraceptives (Morris and Uhdry 1972, Lewis and Hoghughi 1969) or by menopause (Craig 1953, Dalton 1964, Muse et al. 1984) does not necessarily ensure an absence of cyclic symptoms. In terms of a diagnostic strategy, for example, symptoms that appear to be premenstrual are less likely to be strictly controlled by the menstrual cycle itself if they worsen with the use of oral contraceptives; symptoms are more likely to be truly related to the menstrual cycle if they improve with the use of oral contraceptives. Thus premenstrual symptoms may sometimes represent an independent mood cycle that periodically is associated with the timing of the menstrual cycle (i.e., technically, the mood cycle is said to be "entrained" to the menstrual cycle).

If the menstrual cycle is related to mood or behavior changes in some women, then we might expect the onset of changes to occur at menarche. There is evidence that the sex difference in depression first arises with the onset of puberty (Kandel and Davis 1982). In a careful study of hormonal and psychological shifts during early adolescence (Nottelmann et al. 1984), there were gender differences in the pattern of correlations for pubertal stage; gonadotropin secretion; gonadal and adrenal steroid hormone secretion; and changes in the self-perception of cognitive, social, and physical characteristics. In adolescent women, shifts in gonadotropin and gonadal steroid hormone levels parallel changes in measures of competence. However, the clinical significance of such hormone and cognitive or behavioral changes is unknown.

Oral Contraceptive Use

Depression, as a side effect of oral contraceptive (OC) use, has been reported in 30 to 50 percent of women, although most of the data come from studies using higher doses than are now commonly used (Lewis and Hoghughi 1969, Kane et al. 1969). Most studies found an increase in OC-related depressed mood, affective lability, irritability, decreased energy, and pessimism. There is disagreement about OC-related changes in libido and sleep, with reports of both increases and decreases. Appetite and psychomotor function are minimally affected. The possibility of diurnal mood variations with OC use has not been adequately addressed. However, features of melancholia, such as diurnal variation in mood and suicidal preoccupation, are not thought to be prominent (Hamilton and Murphy 1983; Mueller, unpublished manuscript, Contraceptive Evaluation Branch, Center for Population Research, National Institute of Child Health and Human Development, Bethesda, MD, March 1984).

The onset of OC-induced biological changes occurs within approximately two to three months. Psychiatric side effects account for approximately 40 percent of OC discontinuations and most often occur within the first three to six months of use. An absolute pyridoxine (vitamin B_6) deficiency occurs in 20 percent of women taking OCs, with a relative deficiency occurring in 80 percent. Pyridoxine therapy reverses the deficiency in approximately two months, with an improvement in depression at approximately four to six weeks (Adams et al. 1973, Parry and Rush 1979, Glick and Bennett 1981).

Pregnancy

The gonadal steroid changes during pregnancy are much greater in magnitude than are gonadal steroid changes that occur during the menstrual cycle (or those resulting from the suppression of these hormones with OC use) (Hamilton et al. 1988). Mood changes may occur during pregnancy but most often occur in individuals predisposed to affective disorders. Women with panic disorder may show an improvement in panic symptoms during pregnancy (George et al. 1987). Pregnancy is generally associated with a relatively low incidence of psychiatric disorders. In fact, the incidence of mental illness is substantially lower during pregnancy (7.1 per 10,000 woman-years) compared with the incidence during nonchildbearing periods (35.1 per 10,000 woman-years) (Paffenbarger, 1982).

Postpartum Psychiatric Illness

Postpartum illness may manifest in a variety of symptoms and syndromes. The clinical picture that develops may resemble any one of the major categories of psychiatric illness (i.e., depression, mania, delirium, organic syndromes, or schizophrenia). As with menstrual cycle–linked changes, the most common syndrome of severe postpartum illness is depression. Severe postpartum affective syndromes should be distinguished from maternity or baby blues in terms of the severity and frequency of symptoms, the time course of the illness, and its epidemiology (Hamilton 1989).

Maternity blues, characterized by mild depression, crying, irritability, anxiety, and fatigue, generally occur on the third or fourth day after delivery. Elation may also occur at this time. Symptoms are usually transitory, lasting from one to two days to one to two weeks. Perhaps because of the lack of a consensus definition, the reported incidence of mild postpartum (recent deliveries) dysphoria varies but appear to be between 50 and 80 percent (Stein 1979, Buesching et al. 1986).

In contrast, more serious mental illness following childbirth, such as postpartum depression, which is characterized by symptoms of a major affective disorder, occurs in 10 percent of women and may have a delayed onset of six weeks to three to four months after delivery and a course of six months to one year (Hamilton 1989). Some evidence suggests that prenatal depression predicts postpartum depression (Buesching et al. 1986, Stein 1979). First episodes of bipolar illness in women often have their onset in the postpartum period (Bratfos and Haug 1966, Reich and Winokur 1970).

Puerperal psychosis (defined as severe mental illness requiring hospitalization) occurs after approximately one delivery in 1,000 (Brockington and Kumar 1982). If a patient previously has had a postpartum psychosis, the probability of having another episode is one in three. Puerperal psychosis usually has an acute onset, occurring within two weeks of delivery. Patients with puerperal psychosis experience more confusion and mania compared with nonpuerperal psychotic patients who have more schizophrenic symptoms (Brockington et al. 1981), and postpartum mood changes are generally associated with confusion, disorientation, and other cognitive changes compared with other conditions associated with mood change. Sleep disturbance appears to be a common prodromal symptom.

Menopause

Another predictable time of hormonal change occurs in most women's lives at approximately age 50, with the gradual cessation of ovarian function. A report by a scientific group from the World Health Organization (1981) defined menopause as the "permanent cessation of menstruation resulting from the loss of ovarian follicular activity." Strictly speaking, menopause refers to the last episode of menstrual bleeding, and women are commonly referred to as being postmenopausal if they have not experienced menstrual bleeding for one year (Carr and MacDonald 1983).

Menopausal symptoms may include various features of depression such as sleep disturbance (often related to hot flashes), fatigue, irritability, and other mood changes. The report of the World Health Organization (1981) concluded that there is an increase in psychological symptoms (as opposed to an affective syndrome) occurring one to two years before the cessation of menses and a decrease in symptoms one to two years after menopause (Jaszmann et al. 1969, Hallstrom 1973, Ballinger 1975). There appears to be an associated increase in consultations for emotional problems among women in the perimenopausal and early postmenopausal age groups (Shepherd et al. 1966). Moreover, this age group receives more prescriptions for psychotropic drugs compared with women from other age groups as well as men of similar ages (Skegg et al. 1977).

Using a cross-sectional approach to assess symptoms in women across segments of the life cycle (as grouped by the following age ranges: 13 to 19 years, 20 to 29 years, 30 to 44 years, 45 to 54 years, and 55 to 64 years), Neugarten and Kraines (1965) reported on several depression-related items (e.g., "tired feelings," "irritable and nervous," and "feel blue and depressed"). These researchers noted two peaks of depressive symptoms occurring between ages 20 and 29 and again perimenopausally (i.e., in the age group of 45 to 54 years for those subjects who were not clearly premenopausal or postmenopausal in that they experienced irregular cycles). However, the authors did not clarify whether their findings are specific for women, are related to reproductive events such as menopause, or are simply age-related in either sex.

A study by Bungay and colleagues (1980) demonstrated that women at about the time of menopause (defined as age 50) showed age-related peaks in the following symptoms compared with men: difficulty in making decisions, loss of confidence, night sweats (which are related to sleep difficulty), anxiety, forgetfulness, difficulty in concentration, tiredness, and feelings of worthlessness. These gender differences persisted even when the researchers controlled for age-related life events, such as children leaving home. However, other depression-related symptoms changes were not significantly affected in women during the menopausal time period (e.g., difficulty sleeping, loss of interest in sexual relations, loss of appetite).

Though both a follow-up (Winokur 1973) and a cross-sectional study (Weissman and Klerman 1977) did not find an increase in severe psychiatric illness (i.e., a syndrome) in these age groups, work by Angst (1978) demonstrates a bimodal onset of depressive illness in women, with peaks occurring in the early twenties and in the age range of 40 to 50 years. Also, Reich and Winokur (1970) demonstrated an increase in affective illness occurring at the time of menopause. Descriptions by Kraepelin (1921) also suggest an increased onset of depression after the cessation of reproductive functioning. There may be a change in the course of affective illness at the time of menopause. Kukopulos and coworkers (1980) in a longitudinal study of patients with bipolar illness found that menopause coincided with the induction of rapid cycles of mood (three or more episodes a year).

Many postmenopausal women use estrogen replacement. There are reports of improved sleeping patterns for postmenopausal women during estrogen treatment (Schiff et al. 1979, Thomson and Oswald 1977), although this improvement may partly result from alterations in the number of waking episodes associated with hot flashes (Carr and MacDonald 1983). Estrogen therapy may improve well-being in some patients with treatment-resistant depressions (Gerner 1983), including women who are depressed around the onset of menopause (Furuhjelm et al. 1976). The use of estrogen in combination with tricyclic antidepressants has also been investigated. In a double-blind, placebo-controlled study (Shapiro et al. 1985), both premenopausal and postmenopausal women who had failed to respond to adequate trials of at least two antidepressants were treated with conjugated estrogen in combination with imipramine (Tofranil). Two of the eight postmenopausal women showed a marked decrease in depressive symptoms. One of the three premenopausal women was bipolar, however, and became manic. The extreme antidepressant responses tended to occur within one to two weeks of treatment. Aside from two transient episodes of uterine bleeding, there were no marked side effects. The blood levels of imipramine were not changed by the addition of estrogen. Although there was no overall improvement in depression, treatment may be enhanced if we can begin to identify subgroups of women who are likely to be responsive to this type of adjunctive therapy. Estrogen treatment also may induce rapid-cycling (Oppenheim 1984).

Relationships Among Reproductive-Related Depressions

We do not have enough research evidence to determine whether there are definitive predictive relationships between various reproductive-related events. We suggest that cyclic or possibly recurrent affective changes (i.e., changes occurring either premenstrually or in the post-partum period, especially with repeated pregnancies) may have more phenomenological or other similarities compared with acyclic (or less recurrent) affective changes (i.e., changes occurring with menopause apart from cyclicity in use of synthetic hormones).

Recurrence and cyclicity versus acyclicity may be one factor in producing symptoms. Additionally, the time course of hormonal changes (acute versus chronic) may influence the presentation of symptoms. For example, there is an unusually low incidence of psychiatric disorders in pregnancy (except for women who are predisposed to affective disorders), suggesting that the change or variability in reproductive hormones rather than their absolute level may increase some women's risk for symptoms (Hamilton 1984). The relative lack of psychiatric correlates during pregnancy, when there are chronically elevated levels of steroid hormones, contrasts sharply with the symptomatic changes sometimes occurring with more acute hormonal elevations; these differences may reflect adaptive alterations in gonadal steroid receptor functioning.

In view of shared symptoms as well as certain shared aspects of hormonal change, we wondered whether positive or negative experiences associated with one reproductive event would predict experiences with others. Several reports have suggested that pregnancy-related symptoms predict vulnerability to OC-related psychiatric side effects such as depression (Nilsson et al. 1967, Kane 1977). Women who experience difficulty in tolerating OCs have been observed to report a greater number of moderate to severe premenstrual cramps, as assessed retrospectively (Graham and Sherwin 1987).

Premenstrual changes may predispose to the development of severe maternity blues (Ballinger et al. 1979, Nott et al. 1976), and premenstrual mood changes may be exacerbated following a postpartum depression (Dalton 1964, Brockington et al. 1988). In a study by Dennerstein and coworkers (1988), a group of thirty-eight women with moderate to severe premenstrual syndrome were selected by rigorous criteria. A premenstrual rise in symptoms was confirmed by prospective symptom ratings. Of the thirty-eight women, twenty-six (68 percent) reported a history of postpartum depression (compared with approximately 10 percent of the general female population). Thirty-five had taken oral contraceptives at some time, with thirty-two (92 percent) reporting some degree of side effects in general (type unspecified) compared with approximately 30 percent of the general population of OC users in this country who discontinue OCs because of depressive side effects and approximately 40 percent who experience some degree of side effects in general. Although we know very little about the possible relationship between premenstrual and perimenopausal changes, a history of OC-induced side effects may be a relative contraindication to the use of estrogens postmenopausally (Craig 1983).

Regarding possible links between reproductive events and affective disorders (Kolakowska 1975), we now know that a lifetime history of major depression is associated with retrospectively and prospectively assessed reports of severe premenstrual changes (Endicott et al. 1981, Halbriech and Endicott 1985), and that this relationship is probably, to some extent, reciprocal. Women suffering from an affective disorder—diagnosed independently of the postpartum period—risk a 10 to 40 percent chance of having an episode of affective disorder during the postpartum period (Bratfos and Haug, 1966). Moreover, women with bipolar affective disorder who have previously experienced an affective postpartum psychosis are at a 50 percent risk for subsequent puerperal psychotic episodes (Reich and Winokur 1970).

In general, high levels of prenatal depression are associated with increased evidence of depressive symptoms at six weeks postpartum (Buesching et al. 1986).

Depression occurring in association with the reproductive cycle may sensitize a woman to future depressions. Alternatively, a major affective disorder may be exacerbated or precipitated during, for example, a premenstrual period (Halbriech and Endicott 1985). There are anecdotal reports that after treatment cycles of bipolar illness with lithium, premenstrual and seasonal mood cycles persist or become more prominent. Price and Dimarzio (1986) report patients with rapid-cycling disorders have an increased tendency to have more severe forms of premenstrual syndrome, though Wehr and colleagues (1988) found no convincing relationship between manic-depressive cycles and menstrual cycles in their patients with rapid-cycling disorders.

Thus, the cyclicity of affective disorders in the form of rapid-cycling bipolar illness or seasonal affective disorder may be compounded by periodic affective change occurring in association with the premenstruum, with pregnancy and the postpartum period, and with altered reproductive hormonal milieu induced by oral contraceptives or gonadal hormone treatments.

Mechanisms of Reproductive-Related Depressions

With the kindling model of depression in mind (Post et al. 1984), one wonders whether such periodic reproductive-related depressions may sensitize women to future affective episodes (Zis and Goodwin 1979).

Rapid-cycling bipolar illness and seasonal affective disorder are examples of cyclic forms of mood disorders that predominate in women. The interaction of reproductive hormones, particularly with thyroid hormones in rapid-cycling affective disorder and with melatonin in seasonal affective disorder, may provide clues to the pathogenesis of reproductive-related depressions. The increased incidence of hypothyroidism occurring postpartum (Amino et al. 1982) or in winter may in part account for rapid-cycling mood disorders and depression, which may occur at these times, respectively. Another cyclic mood disorder, which can be viewed as a form of rapid-cycling, is recurrent premenstrual depression in which thyroid (Brayshaw and Brayshaw 1986) and melatonin (Parry et al. 1987) disturbances also have been implicated. Melatonin may play a role not only in the pathogenesis of seasonal premenstrual syndrome (Parry et al. 1987) but in nonseasonal forms of this disorder as well. Recent studies demonstrate that patients with premenstrual depression have circadian disturbances of melatonin secretion compared with normal controls and may respond to bright light treatment (Parry et al. 1987). Similar studies of melatonin in postpartum mood disturbances would seem worthwhile and are currently underway.

How cyclic depressions related to reproductive events may affect other forms of cyclic affective disorders is unknown, but a relationship does seem to exist. Work with animals may provide models and possibly shed light on the mechanisms involved. For example, the predisposition of women with thyroid impairment to cyclic forms of depression has a parallel in an animal model. Richter and coworkers (1959) produced abnormal cycles of motor activity experimentally in female animals, but not male animals, by partial thyroidectomy. As in rapid-cycling patients, treatment with thyroid extract abolished the abnormal behavioral cycles, which returned after cessation of treatment. Richter hypothesized that the abnormal, regular cycles of activity were produced by the effect of thyroid deficiency on homeostatic mechanisms controlling luteotropin (prolactin) release (possibly related to the effect of TRH on prolactin). He installed similar cycles by daily subcutaneous injections of prolactin.

Similar cycles were also produced by inducing pseudopregnancy, a condition that stimulates pituitary secretion of prolactin which acts on the ovary to produce persistent corpora lutea and the secretion of progesterone. Ovariectomy abolished the running activity; estrogens increased it. Longer abnormal activity cycles were produced by giving the rats anhydrohydroxyprogesterone. These findings parallel certain clinical findings. As occurs in affective illness, the abnormal activity cycles became shorter with time. Also, both the hypothyroid state and estrogen in human females are associated with the induction of rapid-cycling mood disorders (cf. Parry 1989, Wehr et al. 1988).

Reproductive hormones also modulate hormonal, neurotransmitter, and biologic clock mechanisms that have each been the focus of hypotheses about the pathophysiology of affective disorders. Estrogen and progesterone can alter the biosynthesis, release, uptake, degradation, and receptor density of norepinephrine, dopamine, serotonin, and acetylcholine (Oppenheim 1983, McEwen et al. 1982). The gonadal steroids also modulate other hormonal mechanisms (thyroid, cortisol, prolactin, and opiates) that affect neurotransmitter systems (Rausch and Parry 1987, Meites et al. 1979, Buckman et al. 1980, Ojeda et al. 1977).

Gonadal hormones may alter biologic clock mechanisms, which also have been implicated in the pathophysiology of affective disorders (Wehr 1984). Estrogen shortens the period of circadian activity in ovariectomized hamsters and rats (Morin et al. 1977, Albers et al. 1981). The onset of activity occurs earlier on days of the estrous cycle when endogenous titers of estradiol are high in intact hamsters. Progesterone delays the onset of activity in intact rats by antagonizing the effect of estrogen (Axelson et al. 1981). Estrogen, in addition to shortening the free-running period and altering the phase relationship of the activity rhythm to the light-dark cycle, increases the total amount of activity, and decreases the variability of day-to-day onsets of activity. These findings parallel clinical work by Wever (1984) who found that the mean free-running sleep-wake cycle period is significantly shorter in women than in men (28 minutes). The wake episode is shorter (1 hour 49 minutes), and the sleep episode is longer (1 hour 21 minutes) in women compared with men. Thus, the fraction of sleep is longer for females than males. The circadian temperature rhythm was similar in both sexes. According to Wirz-Justice and associates (1984), women sleep longer than men, at all times of the year. When in free-running conditions, women tend to become internally desynchronized, particularly in the summer by shortening the period of their sleep-wake cycle.

Thus, the inherent cyclicity of the female reproductive hormones, by destabilizing or sensitizing neurotransmitter, neuroendocrine, and biologic clock mechanisms, may set the stage for the development of cyclic affective disorders.

While the cyclicity of the endocrine milieu may increase the vulnerability to episodic depressions in women, it may protect against the development of the many chronic illnesses more characteristic in men. The investigation of hormonal contributions to affective illness in women and the examination of the way in which the course of these illnesses is affected by reproductive events of the life cycle may increase our understanding of affective illness and potentially provide alternative treatment strategies.

Summary

Women are at higher risk than men to develop depressive episodes during the reproductive years. Furthermore, women are vulnerable to depressions associated with oral contraceptives, abortion, the premenstrual period, the puerperium, and menopause. The phenomenology and biologic mechanisms involved in these illnesses perhaps should be viewed in the context of other manifestations of the link between depression and female reproductive functions. For example, women are especially vulnerable to a rapid-cycling form of affective illness and to hypothyroidism, an associated factor for this form of affective disorder. The postpartum period is also associated with impaired thyroid function, and there are reports of the induction of rapid cycles of mood following the termination of pregnancy. Thus, alterations in thyroid hormones may be a feature of both postpartum and rapid-cycling forms of affective disorder in women.

A previous history of a postpartum depression places a woman at a high risk for the development of a subsequent puerperal episode. Also, difficulties during pregnancy may predispose a woman to the development of other reproductive-related depressions. The role reproductive hormones play in this possible sensitization phenomenon needs to be examined in order to understand the relationship of depression to the female reproductive cycle.

References

Adams, P. W., Rose, D. P., Folkard, J., et al. (1973). Effect of pyridoxine hydrochloride (vitamin B_6) upon depression associated with oral contraception. *Lancet*, 1:897–904.

Albers, E. H., Gerall, A. A., Axelson, J. F. (1981). Effect of reproductive state on circadian periodicity in the rat. *Physiol. Behav.*, 26:21.

Amino, N., More, H., Iwatani, Y., et al. (1982). High prevalence of transient postpartum thyrotoxicosis and hypothyroidism. *N. Engl. J. Med.*, 306:849.

Angst, J. (1978). The course of affective disorders. II. Typology of bipolar manic depressive illness. *Arch. Gen. Psychiatry,* Nervankr 226:65.

Axelson, J. F., Gerall, A. A., and Albers, E. (1981). Effect of progesterone on the estrous activity cycle of the rat. *Physiol. Behav.*, 26:631.

Ballinger, C. B. (1975). Psychiatric morbidity and the menopause: Screening of a general population sample. *Br. Med. J.*, 3:344–46.

Ballinger, C. B., Buckley, D. E., Naylor, G. J., et al. (1979). Emotional disturbance following childbirth and the excretion of Cyclic AMP. *Psychol. Med.*, 9:293–300.

Bratfos, D., and Haug, J. O. (1966). Puerperal mental disorders in manic-depressive females. *Acta Psychiatr. Scand.*, 42:285–94.

Brayshaw, N. D., and Brayshaw, D. D. (1986). Thyroid hypofunction in premenstrual syndrome. *N. Engl. J. Med.* 315:1486.

Brockington, I. F., Cernik, K. F., Schofield, E. M., et al. (1981). Puerperal psychosis. Phenomena and diagnosis. *Arch. Gen. Psychiatry*, 38:829–33.

Brockington, I. F., Kelly, A., and Deakin, W. (1988). Premenstrual relapse of puerperal psychosis. *J. Affective Disord.*, 14:287–92.

Brockington, I. F., and Kumar, R. (Eds.) (1982). *Motherhood and Mental Illness.* London: Academic Press.

Brockington, I. F., Winokur, G., and Dean, C. (1982). Puerperal Psychosis. In I. F. Brockington and R. Kumar (Eds.), *Motherhood and Mental Illness*, pp. 37–70. London: Academic Press.

Buckman, M. T., Srivasteva, L. S., and Peake, G. T. (1980). Regulation of prolactin secretion by endogenous sex steroids in man. *Prog. Reprod. Biol.*, 6:66.

Buesching, D. P., Glasser, M. L., and Frate, D. A. (1986). Progression of depression in the prenatal and postpartum periods. *Women Health*, 11:61–78.

Bungay, G. T., Vessey, M. P., and McPherson, C. K. (1980). Study of symptoms in middle life with special reference to menopause. *Br. Med. J.*, 281:181–83.

Carr, B. R., and MacDonald, P. C. (1983). Estrogen treatment of postmenopausal women. *Adv. Intern. Med.*, 28:491.

Craig, G. M. (1983). Guidelines for community menopausal clinics. *Br. Med. J.*, 286:2033–36.

Craig, P. E. (1953). Premenstrual tension and the menopause. *Med. Times*, 81:485.

Dalton, K. (1964). *The Premenstrual Syndrome.* London: Heineman Medical.

———. (1977). *The Premenstrual Syndrome and Progesterone Therapy*, pp. 17, 72, 118. Chicago: William Heineman.

Davis, M. (1985). Premenstrual syndrome. In *Report of the Public Health Service Task Force on Women's Health*, Vol. 2, pp. 11–85. Washington, DC: Government Printing Office.

Dennerstein, L., Morse, C., and Gotts, G. (1988). Perspective from a PMS clinic. In L. H. Gise, N. G. Kase, and R. L. Berkowitz, (Eds.), *The Premenstrual Syndromes*, pp. 109–18. New York: Churchill Livingstone.

Dunner, D. L., Patrick, V., and Fieve, R. (1977). Rapid cycling manic depressive patients. *Compr. Psychiatry*, 18:561.

Endicott, J., Halbreich, U., Schact, S., et al. (1981). Premenstrual changes and affective disorders. *Psychosom. Med.*, 43:519–30.

Furuhjelm, M., and Fedor-Freybergh, P. (1976). The influence of estrogens on the psyche in climacteric and postmenopausal women. In P. A. VanKeep, P. A. Greenblat, and M. Albeaux-Fernet (Eds.), *Consensus in Menopause Research*. Baltimore: University Park Press.

George, D. T., Ladenheim, J. A., and Nutt, D. J. (1987). Effect of pregnancy on panic attacks. *Am. J. Psychiatry,* 144:1078–79.

Gerner, R. H. (1983). Systemic treatment approach to depression and treatment-resistant depression. *Ann. Psychiat.,* 13:37–49.

Gershon, E. S., Hamovet, J. H., Guroff, J. J., and Nurenberger, J. I. (1987). Birth-cohort changes in manic and depressive disorders in relatives of bipolar and schizoaffective patients. *Arch. Gen. Psychiatry,* 44:314.

Glick, I. D., and Bennett, S. E. (1981). Psychiatric complications of progesterone and oral contraceptives. *J. Clin. Psychopharmacol.,* 1:350–67.

Golub, S. (1988). A developmental perspective. In L. H. Gise, N. G. Kase, and R. L. Berkowitz (Eds.), *The Premenstrual Syndromes,* pp. 7–19. New York: Churchill Livingstone.

Graham, C. A., and Sherwin, B. B. (1987). The relationship between retrospective premenstrual syndrome reporting and present oral contraceptive use. *J. Psychosom. Res.,* 31:45–53.

Halbriech, U., and Endicott, J. (1985). Relationship of dysphoric premenstrual changes to depressive disorders. *Acta Psychiatr. Scand.,* 71:331.

Hallstrom, T. (1973). *Mental Disorder and Sexuality in the Climacteric.* Stockholm: Scandinavian University Books, Esselte Studium.

Hamilton, J. A. (1962). *Postpartum Psychiatric Problems.* St. Louis: C. V. Mosby.

———. (1984). Psychobiology in context: Reproductive-related events in men's and women's lives. *Contemp. Psychiatry,* 3:12–16.

———. (1989). Postpartum psychiatric syndromes. In B. L. Parry (Ed.), *Women's Disorders. The Psychiatric Clinics of North America.* Philadelphia: W. B. Saunders.

Hamilton, Jean, and Murphy, D. L. (1983). Characteristics of depression induced by oral contraceptives. Presented at the Conference on Depression and Mood Changes Among Oral Contraceptive Users, Contraceptive Evaluation Branch, Center for Population Research, National Institute of Child Health and Human Development, Bethesda, MD, February 1983.

Hamilton, Jean, Parry, B. L., and Blumenthal, S. J. (1988). The menstrual cycle in context, II: Human gonadal steroid hormone variations. *J. Clin. Psychiatry,* 49:480–84.

Herzog, A., and Detre, T. (1974). Postpartum Psychoses. *Dis. Nerv. Syst.,* 35: 556–59.

Jaszmann, L., VanLith, N. D., and Zaat, J.C.A. (1969). The perimenopausal symptoms. *Med. Gynaecol. Sociol.,* 4:268–77.

Kandel, D. B., and Davis, M. (1982). Epidemiology of depressive mood in adolescents. *Arch. Gen. Psychiatry,* 39:1205–12.

Kane, F. J. (1977). Iatrogenic depression in women. In W. E. Fann (Ed.), *Phenomenology and Treatment of Depression.* New York: Spectrum.

Kane, F. J., Treadway, R., and Ewing, F. (1969). Emotional change associated with oral contraceptives in female psychiatric patients. *Compr. Psychiatry,* 10:16–30.

Kendell, R. E., Chalmers, J. C., and Platz, C. (1987). Epidemiology of puerperal psychoses. *Br. J. Psychiatry,* 150:662–73.

Kolakowska, T. (1975). The clinical cause of primary recurrent depression in pharmacologically treated females. *Br. J. Psychiatry,* 126:336–45.

Kraeplin, E. (1921). *Manic Depressive Insanity and Paranoia.* Edinburgh: E. and S. Livingstone, Ltd.

Krailo, M. D., and Pike, M. C. (1983). Estimation of the distribution of age at natural menopause from prevalence data. *Am. J. Epidemiol.*, 117:356.

Kukopulos, A., Reginaldi, P., Laddomada, G. F., Serra, G., and Tondo, L. (1980). Course of the manic depressive cycle and changes caused by treatments. *Pharmakopsychiatrie*, 13:156.

Lewis, A., Hoghughi, M. (1969). An evaluation of depression as a side effect of oral contraceptives. *Br. J. Psychiatry*, 115:697–70.

Logue, C. M., and Moos, R. H. (1985). Perimenstrual symptoms: Prevalence and risk factors. *Psychosom. Med.*, 48:388–414.

McEwen, B. S., and Parsons, B. (1982). General steroid action on the brain: Neurochemistry and neuropharmacology. *Ann. Rev. Pharmacol. Toxicol.* 22: 555.

Meites, J., Bruni, J. F., Van Vugt, P. A., et al. (1979). Relation of endogenous opioid peptides and morphine to neuroendocrine functions. *Life Sci.*, 24: 1325.

Morin, L. P., Fitzgerald, K. M., and Zucker, I. (1977). Estradiol shortens the period of hamster circadian rhythms. *Science*, 196:305.

Morris, N. M., and Uhdry, J. R. (1972). Contraception pills and day-by-day feelings of well-being. *Am. J. Obstet. Gynecol.*, 113:763–65.

Morton, J. H. (1950). Premenstrual tension. *Am. J. Obstet. Gynecol.*, 60:343.

Muse, K. N., Cetel, N. S., Futterman, L. A., et al. (1984). The premenstrual syndrome: Effects of "medical ovariectomy." *N. Engl. J. Med.*, 311:1345–49.

Neugarten, B. L., and Kraines, R. J. (1965). Menopausal symptoms in women of various ages. *Psychosom. Med.*, 27:266–73.

Nilsson, A., Jacobson, L., and Ingemanson, C. A. (1967). Side-effects of an oral contraceptive with particular attention to mental symptoms and sexual adaptation. *Acta Obstet. Gynecol. Scand.*, 46:537–56.

Nott, P. N., Franklin, M., Armitage, C., et al. (1976). Hormonal changes and mood in the puerperium. *Br. J. Psychiatry*, 128:379–83.

Nottelmann, E. D., Susman, E. J., Blue, J. H., et al. (1984). Gonadal and adrenal hormone correlates of self concept in early adolescence. Presented at the Annual Meeting of the Society for Pediatric Research, San Francisco, May 1984.

Ojeda, S. R., Castro-Vazques, A., and Jameson, H. E. (1977). Prolactin release in response to blockade of dopaminergic receptor and to TRH injection in developing and adult rats. Role of estrogen in determining sex differences. *Endocrinology*, 100:427.

Oppenheim, G. (1983). Estrogen in the treatment of depression: Neuropharmacological mechanisms. *Biol. Psychiatry*, 18:721.

———. (1984). A case of rapid mood cycling with estrogen: Implications for therapy. *J. Clin. Psychiatry*, 45:34.

Paffenbarger, R. S., Jr. (1982). Epidemiological aspects of mental illness associated with childbearing. In I. F. Brockington and R. Kumar (Eds.), *Motherhood and Mental Illness*, pp. 19–36. London: Academic Press.

Parry, B. L. (1989). Reproductive factors affecting the course of affective illness in women. In B. L. Parry (Ed.), *Women's Disorders. The Psychiatric Clinics of North America*, pp. 207–20. Philadelphia: W. B. Saunders.

Parry, B. L., Berga, S. L., Kripke, D. F., and Gillin, J. C. (1988). Melatonin in Premenstrual Syndrome. American College of Neuropsychopharmacology, San Juan, Puerto Rico, December 1988.

Parry, B. L., Rosenthal, N. E., Tamachin, L., and Wehr, T. (1987). Treatment of a patient with seasonal premenstrual syndrome. *Am. J. Psychiatry,* 144:762.

Parry, B. L., and Rush, A. J. (1979). Oral contraceptives and depressive symptomatology: Biologic mechanisms. *Compr. Psychiatry,* 20:347.

Post, R. M., Rubinow, D. R., and Ballenger, J. C. (1984). Conditioning, sensitization and kindling: Implications for the course of affective illness. In R. M. Post and J. C. Ballenger (Eds.), *Neurobiology of Mood Disorders.* Baltimore: Williams and Wilkins.

Price, W. A., and Dimarzio, L. (1986). Premenstrual tension syndrome in rapid-cycling bipolar affective disorder. *J. Clin. Psychiatry,* 47:415.

Protheroe, C. (1969). Puerperal psychoses: A long-term study 1927–1961. *Br. J. Psychiatry,* 115:9–30.

Rausch, J. L., and Parry, B. L. (1987). The effect of gonadal steroids on affective symptomatology. In O. G. Cameron (Ed.), *Presentations of Depression.* New York: John Wiley and Sons.

Reich, T., and Winokur, G. (1970). Postpartum psychoses in patients with manic depressive disorder. *J. Nerv. Ment. Dis.,* 151:60.

Richter, C. P., Jones, G. S., and Biswanger, L. (1959). Periodic phenomena and the thyroid. *Arch. Neurol. Psychiatry,* 81:117.

Rosenthal, N. E., Sack, D. A., Gillin, J. C., et al. (1984). Seasonal affective disorder: A description of the syndrome and preliminary findings with light therapy. *Arch. Gen. Psych.,* 41:72.

Schiff, I., Regestein, Q., Tulchinsky, D., et al. (1979). Effects of estrogen on sleep and psychological state of hypogonadal women. *J.A.M.A.* 242:2405–7.

Shapiro, B., Oppenheim, Q., and Zohar, J., et al. (1985). Lack of efficacy of estrogen supplementation to imipramine in resistant female depressives. *Biological Psychiatry* 20:576–78.

Shepherd, M., Cooper, B., Brown, A. C., et al. (1966). *Psychiatric Illness in General Practice.* London: Oxford University Press.

Skegg, D. C., Doll, R., and Perry, J. (1977). Use of medicines in general practice. *Br. Med. J.,* 1:1561–63.

Stein, M. (1979). Psychobiology of mental disorders associated with childbearing. *Acta Psychiatr. Scand.,* 60:449–64.

Thomson, J., and Oswald, I. (1977). Effect of œstrogen on the sleep, mood, and anxiety of menopausal women. *Br. Med. J.,* 2:1317.

Wehr, T. A. (1984). Biological rhythms and manic depressive illness. In R. M. Post and J. C. Ballenger (Eds.), *Neurobiology of Mood Disorders.* Baltimore: Williams and Wilkins.

Wehr, T. A., Sack, D. A., and Rosenthal, N. E. (1988). Rapid cycling affective disorder. Contributing factors and treatment responses of 51 patients. *Am. J. Psychiatry,* 145:179.

Weissman, M. M. (1979). The myth of involutional melancholia. *J.A.M.A.* 242:742.

Weisman, M. M., and Klerman, J. L. (1977). Sex differences and the epidemiology of depression. *Arch. Gen. Psychiatry* 34:98–111.

Weissman, M. M., Leaf, P. J., Holzer, C. E., et al. (1984). The epidemiology of depression: An update on sex differences in rates. *J. Affective Dis.,* 7:179.

Weissman, M. M., Gammon, D., John, K., et al. (1987). Children of depressed parents: Increased psychopathology and early onset of major depression. *Arch. Gen. Psychiatry,* 44:847.

Wever, R. A. (1984). Properties of human sleep-wake cycles: Parameters of internally synchronized free running rhythms. *Sleep* 7:27.

Winokur, G. (1973). Depression in the menopause. *Am. J. Psychiatry,* 130:92.

Wirz-Justice, A., Wever, R. A., and Aschoff, J. (1984). Seasonality in free running rhythms in man. *Naturwissenschaften* 71:316, 1984.

World Health Organization. (1981). Report of a World Health Organization Scientific Group, Research on the Menopause. World Health Organization Technical Report Series 670. Geneva.

Zis, A. P., and Goodwin, F. K. (1979). Major affective disorder as a recurrent illness. A critical review. *Arch. Gen. Psychiatry,* 36:835.

Chapter 17
Prophylactic Measures

James Alexander Hamilton
and Deborah A. Sichel

Psychiatric illness after childbirth is fraught with many unique hazards. When the hazards are ignored, tragic consequences may ensue. If the hazards are understood and attended to they become much less threatening. The word "prophylactic" is derived from a Greek word which means "to stand guard before," or "to take precaution against."

This chapter examines some of the specific hazards associated with postpartum illness and suggests measures that may be taken to guard against them. In Chapter 5, Elizabeth Herz describes preventive measures related to general care and management of postpartum patients. The first part of this chapter presents a variety of pharmacological measures, some of which are in transition and/or rapid development. The second part of this chapter discusses the prevention of some special hazards that are related to various unique qualities of postpartum illness.

The likelihood of severe psychiatric illness in an unselected obstetrical population is at least one per 1,000 deliveries. In most of these cases, women require treatment on a hospital psychiatric unit. These cases, designated as "severe," do not include women with mild to moderate depressive symptoms, where the incidence estimate runs from 5 to 12 percent of all women delivering. If a patient has previously had a severe postpartum illness with onset within the first two weeks after delivery and is pregnant again, the likelihood of recurrence is one in three (Bratfos and Haug 1966, Reich and Winokur 1970, Garvey et al. 1983). This is an increase of over 300 times, not 300 percent. Women with major depressions of late onset are also high-risk patients. The exploration of pharmacological agents to prevent recurrence has been confined mainly to high-risk patients. The risk of recurrence of postpartum symptoms of lesser severity is also high, but the hazard has less numerical documentation.

The pharmacological approaches and other prophylactic measures described in this chapter are based on investigative approaches that fall short of ideal experimental conditions. Except for a few retrospective studies, there is little information in the postpartum field which is confirmed by first-class experimental work. Postpartum illness is an area of medicine that has been overlooked for most of the twentieth century. If irrefutable experimental evidence for prophylactic measures is demanded, one will have to wait for many years.

Pharmacological Prophylaxis in High-Risk Patients

Several approaches to pharmacological prophylaxis are described; all depend on the administration of prophylactic medication *beginning very soon after delivery,* optimally, in the delivery room. The hormonal prophylactic regimens are not regimens which are intended for *treatment.* This rule is absolute in the case of estrogen and pyridoxine. The hormonal approaches discussed in this chapter must be regarded as preliminary and still experimental. Alternative strategies that use psychotropic medications will also be discussed in this chapter; these represent tested interventions. However, if pituitary ischemia initiates the pathophysiological sequence, there is no evidence that psychotropic medications will prevent this.

The Estrogen Approach

In 1957, one of the authors (J.H.) had a patient who experienced a severe postpartum psychosis. She was hospitalized for several weeks and eventually recovered. Two years later she became pregnant again. In cases such as these, termination of pregnancy is one possible solution. If this is rejected, the psychiatrist is confronted with a serious problem. This was the situation when the author met Dr. Emory Page, an investigator of the effect of administered estrogen on lactation. Dr. Page made the observation that in his experimental group, patients were remarkably free of maternity blues (Page 1959).

The early symptoms and the timing of a serious postpartum psychotic depression often resemble those of maternity blues. Beyond this, the possibility of an association between the two had not been suggested. However, grasping for a straw, the psychiatrist administered long-acting estrogen at delivery to the high-risk patient. She developed no postpartum psychiatric symptoms (Hamilton 1962). Other patients at high risk for a recurrence of severe postpartum illness were treated similarly. By 1977, 35 cases of estrogen prophylaxis in high-risk patients could be reported; none had a recurrence (Hamilton 1977). Eventually, a total of 50 patients with prior postpartum illness, moderate to severe, received estrogen prophylaxis; none had a recurrence.

Early use of estrogen prophylaxis depended on a single injection of a long-acting estrogen, administered immediately after delivery. This was later extended with oral estrogen over two weeks and reduced gradually. Most of the cases reported by the author (J.H.) made use of estrone (Theelin) 10 mg in oil at delivery, followed by conjugated estrogens (Premarin) 2.5 mg twice daily for Days 1 to 7 then 2.5 mg daily for Days 8 to 14.

More recent cases treated by the other author (D.S.) acknowledge the reasonable and widely held concern for thromboembolic phenomena which have occurred occasionally in connection with estrogen administration. Should a thromboembolic event occur, the first appropriate step is to discontinue the estrogen. If a bolus of long-acting estrogen was present from an intramuscular injection, estrogen might continue to be released over a period of several days. Various approaches are being explored, including substitution of intravenous estrogen for the first dose and the supplementation of this with subcutaneous heparin, or by transdermal estrogen patches.

In the matter of timing, it is to be noted that with loss of the placenta, serum estradiol falls to one-fifth of its pregnancy level in five hours, and to one-fifth of this level, or lower, in the succeeding twenty-four hours (Tulchinsky 1980). A reasonable inference is that the slope of the estrogen fall may be a primary factor in activating the mechanism which leads to psychiatric symptoms and illness.

No instances of thromboembolic phenomena have been reported with estrogen prophylaxis. Nevertheless, both authors believe that the concern regarding long-acting estrogen administered postpartum is valid, and that prophylactic use of estrogen should be considered as a research activity rather than as a recommended procedure at this time.

The Progesterone Approach

Many nineteenth-century observers, including Marcé, reported that psychiatric reactions early in the puerperium often showed improvement or apparent recovery, only to recur just prior to the first menstrual period (Marcé 1862). One of the authors (D.S.) has observed that premenstrual recurrence over a period of several months may be a common phenomenon in the recovery from postpartum psychiatric illness. Early in the twentieth century it became known that the progesterone level of the serum dropped prior to menstruation. Billig and Bradley (1946) reported on twelve patients who were treated successfully with progesterone administered to cushion their recurring premenstrual fall. Others tried progesterone for other conditions with varying reports of success or failure.

The London physician Katharina Dalton (1985) reported a diminished incidence of postpartum psychiatric reactions when progesterone is administered at delivery and continued until after the first menstrual period. Her population was identified as women who have had at least one medical consultation for "depression" following childbirth. This population includes cases of mild and moderate severity and also cases that required psychiatric hospitalization. After the women in this population had another child, they were questioned by letter regarding whether they had had a recurrence. Affirmative answers were received from 68 percent. This figure was used as a baseline to compare with observed recurrences from a similarly defined population who were given progesterone at delivery and for several weeks thereafter. Groups with this prophylactic regimen were reported to have had recurrence rates ranging from 6 to 10 percent. Dalton's regimen was 100 mg of progesterone intramuscularly at delivery and for seven days, followed by progesterone suppositories, 400 mg twice daily for two months or until the onset of menstruation.

The authors are seriously concerned about a number of recurrences of severe postpartum illness following "progesterone prophylaxis" which have come to their attention during the past two years. When Dalton's own reports are studied, the criteria for identification of "recurrence" appears to be different for the control and experimental groups. The double-blind requirement was not fulfilled. A recent study with double-blind controls yielded results that question the prophylactic action of progesterone suppositories (Freeman et al. 1990).

The Pyridoxine Approach

A third approach to chemical prophylaxis has been reported by the British psychiatrist Diana Riley (1982 and 1984). Working with high-risk patients, she administered orally 100 mg of pyridoxine *after* delivery and daily for twenty-eight days to an experimental group. Placebos were given to a matched control group. The recurrence rate was several times higher in the control group than in patients who received pyridoxine. The experimental circumstances were good but not perfect. No rationale was given by Riley, but it may be noted that pyridoxine is a metabolic precursor of serotonin.

The authors have insufficient information to assess the efficacy of the pyridoxine method. One of us (J.H.) has used it in conjunction with the estrogen method, and there appear to be no contraindications or hazards. With the emergence of problems with the two hormonal approaches, pyridoxine deserves careful study.

Psychotropic Drug Prophylaxis

Three chemical interventions for prophylaxis have been described. The authors acknowledge that in most circumstances, clinicians are faced with high-risk situations and need to make solid practical decisions for their patients. While preliminary study of estrogen prophylaxis appears promising, no double-blind study has been undertaken and no distinct diagnostic groups selected. Thus, it remains highly experimental and we cannot recommend its safe use outside a strictly controlled study design. We do not recommend progesterone since its efficacy is now in question for prophylaxis in high-risk patients.

An alternative is to review carefully which psychotropic medications were effective in achieving remission of symptoms in the prior postpartum illness. In most cases these will include lithium, antidepressants, and antipsychotic drugs.

In most situations of potential recurrence, reinstitution of lithium immediately after delivery, with rapid achievement of therapeutic blood levels, is recommended. It may also be prudent to add a low dose of antipsychotic drug for the first few weeks, preferably one of the potent, less sedating agents like haloperidol, perphenazine, or trifluperazine. Lithium levels should be monitored in the first week, as water and electrolyte changes may modify excretion and produce toxicity. After the first week postpartum this should normalize. As always, thyroid function must be monitored, particularly with treatment with lithium.

In situations of potential recurrence of nonpsychotic major depression, attention should be paid to the time of onset in relation to delivery. Antidepressant medication may be begun somewhat before the prior time of onset. The medication of choice would be that to which the patient previously responded favorably. The aggressive pharmacological approach will usually preclude breast-feeding, particularly when lithium is administered. The appropriateness of breast-feeding while taking other psychoactive drugs is discussed by Erickson et al. (1979), Sovener and Oisulak (1979), and Brixen-Rasmussen et al. (1982). These matters require extensive planning and collaboration between physicians and other health care specialists. Alternatives should ·be discussed with the patient. Close monitoring in the weeks following delivery is necessary. Given that recurrent postpartum illnesses tend to be progressively more severe, we feel that to preempt relapse affords the best care for a woman, with significant reduction of psychological morbidity and its sequelae.

The term "prophylaxis" has other broad connotations. There are special hazards other than recurrence that need to be guarded against. Protection against some of these hazards is discussed below.

Prevention of Psychological Trauma

Postpartum psychiatric illness often brings anxiety, confusion, insomnia, and aberrations of consciousness which have never been experienced before. The anxiety is often reported to be more severe than any prior anxiety. Patients often use graphic terms to describe the anxiety: "My veins were on fire," or "My chest seemed as if it would explode," or "I could feel pounding everywhere in my body."

As the sensations of anxiety develop, many patients are very concerned about the absence of a reasonable cause. They say, "If a burglar were pointing a gun at me, I might consider such a reaction appropriate. But there is no burglar." Anxiety is equated with fear, and one expects fear to reflect a dangerous situation. In the anxiety of postpartum illness, the absence of a fearful object is likely to increase the anxiety inherent in the illness.

The human mind is curious, and in the absence of an apparent cause, the patient tends to seek a cause. Guilt-laden events from the past may be revived and associated with the symptoms. Where religious indoctrination has encouraged rigid notions of right and wrong, some patients may believe that possession by the devil or punishment for sins may explain their disturbing experiences.

The slow and insidious development of major postpartum depression generates other self-deprecatory ideas. Lacking energy and being depressed in mood, the patient is likely to feel that she is not competent to care for her infant, or that she has failed at motherhood.

The patient's search for a cause of the anxiety, confusion, depression, and other symptoms hits usually upon a wrong answer, an answer that is truly threatening to the patient, to her self-image, and to her feeling of competence in the role of motherhood. This wrong answer is enormously anxiety-producing. The inferno of anxiety is now fired from two directions: the agitation and apprehension, which is inherent in postpartum illness, and the fear generated by the implications of the answer, which the patient has fabricated: failure, incompetence, insanity, or punishment for sin. The key to reducing psychological stress and trauma is to convince the patient that she has a real and acute illness, that the illness has a physiological cause, that the cause is likely a chemical or hormonal imbalance incidental to the readjustment back to the nonpregnant state. In other words, the patient has a medical illness with psychiatric symptoms.

The role of the physician in providing this strategic explanation of symptoms is not always an easy one. It may be assumed that most patients have already come to some self-deprecatory explanation of their symptoms before medical attention is sought. In the first examination, the physician should be as thorough as possible in eliciting the details of current symptoms. Past history of medical illnesses and prior pregnancies is obtained. Prior depressive reactions are inquired about, but the examiner should not dwell upon psychological pressures, interpersonal conflicts, or sexual stresses. Inquiry about energy level, sleep patterns, and disturbing dreams may yield useful information.

At the end of the examination, the diagnosis should be stated without evasiveness or ambiguity: postpartum depression, postpartum psychosis, or postpartum panic disorder. The severity should be stated as accurately as it can be estimated. It is important to state that the cause of the condition is related to adjustments of body chemistry after delivery and that the process of readjustment may take several weeks, but the eventual outcome is expected to be total recovery. All therapeutic actions are explained as efforts to facilitate the body's return to the equilibrium that existed before pregnancy.

Every person who comes in contact with the patient is educated thoroughly regarding the policy of diagnosis and interpretation. Hospital staff members who communicate with the patient are trained to treat her as if she has an acute, not a chronic, illness. The association of present symptoms with past events or stresses, a commonplace topic of discussion among patients and sometimes staff in psychiatric facilities, is discouraged. Family members are educated along similar lines (Hamilton 1985).

Prevention of Suicide

Suicide is a real and present hazard in postpartum psychiatric illness. In the early agitated psychosis, the mercurial quality of symptoms makes it impossible to predict the course of thinking from one hour to the next. The impulsiveness of these early cases, the drive to put ideas into action, requires constant surveillance. With a major postpartum depression of later onset, a secretly held obsession of futility and failure may lead to a planned suicide attempt. This is the reason why the psychosis and the severe depression should be cared for in a facility with excellent staff and psychiatric controls.

Suicide outside the area of control should be considered from the beginning of treatment. Patients will go home on leave and will be discharged from the hospital eventually. It is an awkward time to first warn the family of suicidal hazards when the patient is ready to leave the hospital. A preferred alternative is to conduct a conference with one or more family members before seeing the patient for the first time, or as a second choice, immediately after seeing the patient. This provides an opportunity to learn about the patient and about the present illness. Relatives are told about the special qualities and hazards of postpartum illness, and the excellent prognosis *if* the case is managed wisely. The need for quiet surveillance and faithful reporting is stressed. This is particularly important when the patient is on leave, and after release from hospital care. An additional benefit of the conference is that the family can learn that the treatment program is based on special characteristics of postpartum illness. With this information, they are likely to remain committed to the program.

Prevention of Infanticide

Some cases of infanticide occur during the early weeks after delivery. These are usually cases of postpartum psychotic depression (postpartum psychosis). In most cases, the psychosis has been identified before the infanticide occurs. Behavior that is obviously irrational and disturbed leads prudent and knowledgeable people to introduce control measures.

Infanticide may occur when patients are not obviously psychotic or irrational most of the time. At least half of the infanticides take place eight, ten, or many more weeks after delivery, when the early agitation and hyperactivity of the postpartum psychotic depression has *apparently* subsided. The history is usually that of a woman who had indications of, or the diagnosis of, psychosis, who may or may not have been hospitalized, and who is at home attempting to take care of her responsibilities. She is confused, depressed, and tired most of the time, and she has occasional episodes of vivid hallucinations, often "voices," and delusions. Usually her memory for these experiences is vague. The episodes may be accompanied by unexplained, irrational statements. Family members are often aware of these apparent lapses into odd behavior, but they overlook them because it is apparent that the patient is trying to fulfill her responsibilities and get well.

The episodes of vivid hallucinations and delusions, sometimes accompanied by violence, are particularly characteristic of psychoses after childbirth. Early in the course of illness, similar episodes may move into other psychotic presentations, so that they are a part of the total picture of psychosis. Several weeks later, when the usual appearance of the patient may be of a mild to moderate depression, abrupt episodes of grossly psychotic behavior tends to be regarded as residuals from an illness that has generally improved. The patient's diagnosis may have been changed from psychosis to depression.

The old German psychiatric literature described this unique postpartum syndrome as a persisting cloud of confusion, wherein patients occasionally slipped into episodes of violent agitation and vivid hallucinations, then slipped away from the acute episodes, usually without clear recollection or understanding of what had happened, or with but fragmentary recollection of the experiences during the agitated or acute phase. The term "amentia" from the Latin "without mind," was applied to the syndrome. Nineteenth-century observers held that the confusion or delirium of postpartum cases was *different* from that which occurred in other psychiatric syndromes. It was compared to the confusion of the sleepwalker. The designation "amentia" has given way to terms like "mania" in the modern German nomenclature. Professor Bernhard Pauleikhoff of Münster reviewed the syndrome for the Marcé Society (1984) and describes it again in Chapter 18.

Retrospective analysis of patients who commit infanticide is almost nonexistent in the psychiatric literature. One of the authors (J.H.) has interviewed a number of these women and has reviewed detailed records of seventeen cases. In most of them, it was apparent that the patients, six or more weeks after childbirth, were suffering from confusion plus symptoms which were regarded as moderate depression. They were subject to occasional attacks of grossly psychotic thinking, sometimes with psychotic behavior as well. Usually the origins of such episodes could be traced to the early weeks after delivery. Patients typically tried to conceal the disturbed ideation, tried to control it by "willpower." (The possibility has not escaped us that many cases of suicide by new mothers, which may occur many weeks or months after delivery, may be the result of episodes of amentia, but we have no data or experience with postpartum suicide to support this idea.)

What can the physician do to anticipate and counter the hazard of amentia, particularly when it appears only occasionally, and many weeks after delivery? A very important step, early in the treatment of postpartum psychotic depression, is the establishment of a degree of rapport that will insure the reporting of continued episodes of amentia. Knowledge of the continuation or cessation of episodes of amentia will aid in the determination of an appropriate date for hospital discharge and the relaxation of surveillance after discharge. The early and open discussion of these episodes tends to desensitize patients to them, and this may contribute to their cessation.

Beyond identification and desensitization, are there special kinds of treatment that could expedite the elimination of these episodes? Two fragile clues may be recorded. In Pauleikhoff's study of 350 hospitalized postpartum patients, fifty were said to have had persistent episodes of amentia (Pauleikhoff 1984). The average time until complete remission of the episodes was three months after delivery. With three months as an average, quite a few patients waited longer for complete remission.

The experience of one author (J.H.) was different. Among over four hundred patients hospitalized for the spectrum of postpartum illness, not more than four or five had psychotic thinking beyond the tenth week postpartum. There were two idiosyncracies of case management. The first was that patients with any appreciable degree of depression, slowed mentation, excessive fatiguability, or continuing diminished sexual responsiveness, found themselves on a maintenance dose of thyroxine. Very few of these symptoms persisted.

The second idiosyncracy had to do with a careful psychiatric evaluation of hospitalized and discharged patients which took place six or seven weeks after delivery. The purpose of this evaluation was to search for any indication of distorted ideation, aberrations of consciousness, or mood disturbances. The rationale was that if such conditions were continuing, this suggested an acute condition could be turning into a chronic one. If the evaluation disclosed that thinking was impaired or distorted, even episodically, patients were given a short series of electroconvulsive treatments (ECT), rarely more than four or five treatments. Over all, approximately 5 percent of our patients received ECT.

As indicated earlier, the two idiosyncracies of treatment are no more than clues. However, one of the other, or both, could explain the virtual absence of late amentia as a subacute residual from the acute psychosis. There were no suicides or infanticides.

Ensuring a Complete Diagnosis

Since the exhaustive clinical descriptions of the nineteenth century, it has been noted that some postpartum cases, ranging downward from 30 percent to 5 percent or less, fail to recover and remain chronic. The older studies of chronic cases described a mental state which was indistinguishable from dementia. In 1858, L. V. Marcé noted that cases which became chronic had a variety of physical disabilities and stigmata.

Almost 100 years later, the Swiss psychiatrist V. S. Bürgi (1954) studied chronic postpartum cases, confirmed Marcé's observations, found additional physical symptoms and signs, and said that the patients resembled textbook pictures of various kinds of hormonal disorders. The Japanese psychiatrists Noboru Hatotani and Junichi Nomura (1983) studied such chronic cases, treated them aggressively with a variety of hormones, and reported favorable results in many cases (see Chapter 14).

From 1937 through 1982, the endocrine pathologist H. L. Sheehan of the University of Liverpool reported on cases of postpartum hypopituitarism associated with excessive blood loss at delivery. Sometimes most of the pituitary is destroyed by ischemic necrosis. While Professor Sheehan was attending to the physical aspects of these patients, he noted two psychiatric syndromes, an agitated psychosis and a depression. In 1961, one of us (J.H.) consulted Professor Sheehan, who suggested that we might be looking at cases of similar etiology, but from different perspectives. Professor Sheehan was developing a simple treatment for his patients which they took for the rest of their lives, with marked and rapid relief from psychiatric symptoms and considerable relief from most of their physical symptoms. The treatment consists of thyroxine plus cortisone acetate. The author (J.H.) was using thyroxine extensively for depressive symptoms beginning three weeks or more after delivery. It was the mistake of my life that I did not follow Sheehan's suggestion and use a corticoid for early postpartum psychosis (Sheehan 1961, quoted by Hamilton 1962; Sheehan and Davis 1982).

The discussion here concerns four hypothetical conditions:

1. The usual situation is one in which the blood supply to the pituitary diminishes after childbirth, the secretion of pituitary tropic hormones, thyrotropic hormone, and ACTH returns to the prepregnancy level, and the thyroid, adrenals, and other glands controlled by the pituitary settle back to their prepregnancy levels.
2. The "sluggish pituitary" is a situation in which the pituitary tropic hormones decrease to levels that are temporarily quite low, the activity of one or more target glands decreases correspondingly to levels well below the prepregnancy level, and then over a period of months, the pituitary and the target glands return gradually to a functional level that comes close to the prepregnancy level.
3. The "different equilibrium" is a situation in which, after the readjustment from the pregnancy equilibrium, the various hormonal levels settle into a new equilibrium in which one or more of these substances is maintained at a level lower than optimal. An example of this occurs when the thyroid is damaged by autoimmune thyroiditis and cannot produce an adequate amount of

thyroxine, despite constant stimulation from an excess of thyroid-stimulating hormone (TSH).

4. The "damaged pituitary" is a situation in which the downward postpartum readjustment of the pituitary and other endocrine systems is complicated by a marked loss of blood. The blood supply to the pituitary may be compromised further by vascular spasm in the small arteries which supply the pituitary. Blood coagulates in these vessels, and this is followed by necrosis of most of the pituitary secretory cells. This condition, postpartum hypopituitarism or Sheehan's syndrome, is a permanent affliction which has many life-threatening physical complications, together with psychiatric presentations of psychosis and depression. When Sheehan's syndrome is treated with cortisone and thyroxine, the psychiatric symptoms disappear very rapidly. Many of the physical complications are improved, but more slowly.

The hypothesis is advanced that the four hypothetical conditions described above may form a continuum, from the ideal situation (No. 1) through the "sluggish pituitary" and/or the "different equilibrium" (Nos. 2 and 3) to the "damaged pituitary" (No. 4). If this were true, intermediate conditions might be expected.

Recent experience reveals two kinds of intermediate conditions. The first condition involves the initial presentation of a patient with postpartum psychotic depression or a major postpartum depression. After several months, the patient fails to recover and settles into a chronic condition, usually with multiple physical complaints as well as chronic psychiatric symptoms. In cases of this kind, it is suggested that if continuing deficits in the pituitary are searched for, it is likely that they will be found. One of the authors has seen two such cases in the past three years. A case is reported from India (Khanna et al. 1988). Still another is described as Case 5 in Chapter 14.

A second type of intermediate condition is one in which a patient has recovered from a postpartum psychiatric illness and is found to have a sign which appears to reflect at least minor pituitary damage. The sign is an increased vulnerability to sunburn, a decreased capacity to tan when one is exposed to the sun. We now have seen two cases of this phenomenon. Susan Hickman (1989) has conducted an informal survey of recovered patients and confirms that this is not rare. The connection of the tanning phenomenon to the pituitary is worth reviewing.

Adaptive changes in skin color are important protective mechanisms for many amphibians. This phenomenon is accomplished by melanin-containing skin cells (melanocytes) which are under the control of pituitary melanocyte-stimulating hormone (MSH). Varieties of MSH have been found to perform a similar function in some mammals. However, MSH appeared to be absent from the serum of humans. Indeed, an "intermediate lobe" of the pituitary, within which MSH was formed, was absent in many mammals, including man. Within the last decade, a chain of amino acids corresponding to the sequence of MSH has been found to be present in human and also bovine adrenocortico-tropic hormone (ACTH). This chain of amino acids is believed to perform the function of stimulating melanocites in tanning (Sawyer et al. 1982, Hadley 1984). Thus the diminution in tanning capability may be the "fingerprint" which identifies some degree of residual damage to the pituitary after a postpartum psychiatric illness.

It would appear that the foregoing bits of information represent additions to observations of postpartum psychiatric illness made years ago by Marcé and Bürgi, cases of psychiatric illness which became chronic and developed stigmata that can now be related to hormonal deficits. Apparently, when cases of acute postpartum illness evolve into chronic disability, even mild disability, it would seem prudent to con-sider thorough physical evaluation. Such evaluation may require the tools and information that are limited usually to endocrinologists. The routine measurements of the clinical laboratory are sometimes mis-leading, as indicated in the following section.

Prevention of Laboratory Misdirection

The diagnosis and treatment of postpartum psychiatric illness begins, in most cases, during the first few weeks after delivery. It is within this time frame that serum levels of critical variables are not static. For the most part, they are moving down toward their prepregnancy levels. One of them, the serum level of thyroxine, may have an upward spike in the early puerperium, if the patient has autoimmune thyroiditis. The single determination of a serum variable resembles taking one shot at a moving target.

The decision against using supplementary thyroxine in postpartum depression is sometimes made on the basis of a single serum thyroxine determination. Serial determinations might point toward a downward trend. If a downward trend is established, and if symptoms of depres-sion are present, the authors believe that it may be appropriate to begin supplementary thyroxine after the third or fourth week postpartum. We are of the opinion that thyroxine should be started with a small dose (0.05 mg daily). The dose is titrated with monitoring of symp-toms, pulse, and further thyroxine determinations.

The foregoing position holds that the serum thyroxine does not need to be at an arbitrary low level before supplementation is started. This view is not revolutionary. Many thyroid specialists exercise some flexibility in their decisions to administer thyroxine. For example, writing in the fifteenth edition of *Cecil's Textbook of Medicine*, the distinguished thyroidologist Leslie J. DeGroot (1980) states that thyroid measures tend to be less severely depressed in patients with hypothyroidism of pituitary origin, and "in these subjects the values tend to overlap the normal range."

The position that a hypothyroid state can exist with a serum thyroxine level within "normal limits" is strengthened by the Harvard endocrinologist Daniel D. Federman in his section on the thyroid in *Scientific American Medicine*. Professor Federman (1988) notes that while T_4 is low in 85 percent of hypothyroid patients, it is within "normal limits" in 15 percent. The most frequent reason for this potentially misleading T_4 value, according to Federman, is an elevated thyroxine-binding globulin. The two principal reasons for the elevation of thyroxine-binding globulin are pregnancy and high estrogen. While the pregnancy levels of estrogen disappear soon after delivery, this provides no assurance that the pregnancy excess of the thyroxine-binding globulin goes away quickly. On the contrary, the data of Danowski (1953) indicate that a high level of globulin may remain for an average of three weeks, sometimes longer.

One further limitation of thyroid assessment measures may be mentioned. The determination of the serum level of the thyroid-stimulating hormone (TSH) is a valuable supplement to T_4 in many conditions. In primary thyroid disorder, the TSH level tends to be high, while this is not the case if a thyroid deficit is of pituitary or hypothalamic origin. In any given case of postpartum thyroid deficit, the cause may be primary (as in autoimmune thyroiditis) or secondary (reflecting a sluggish postpartum pituitary) or both. Thus, while TSH may be a useful index, it is not a simple solution to the problem of suspected postpartum thyroid deficit.

Measurement of cortisol in the puerperium presents a potential source of error. The symptoms of postpartum psychosis usually develop during the first fortnight after delivery. Total cortisol has risen to double its prepregnancy level by the third trimester, and two or three weeks are required for it to fall back to its previous level (Gibson and Tulchinsky 1980). Total serum cortisol sampled during the first two or three weeks is bound to be high or "normal." However, about 95 percent of this total cortisol is bound and physiologically inactive. If cortisol deficit is a factor in early postpartum illness, it must be the active, free fraction.

Measurement of free serum cortisol is a research laboratory function. It is a very changeable value, and a pulse of ACTH from the pituitary could elevate the serum level quickly, to a point compatible with improved function of the cerebral cortex. Perhaps a twenty-four-hour measurement of urinary free cortisol would be a useful test, but this has not been established.

There is a real need for specific laboratory tests for use in postpartum psychiatric illness. Until such tests are developed, the standard tests should be used with consideration of the changing quality of hormone levels in the early weeks after childbirth.

References

Billig, O., and Bradley, J. D. (1946). Combined shock and corpus luteum hormone therapy. *Am. J. Psychiatr.,* 102:783–87.

Bratfos, O., and Haug, J. (1966). Puerperal mental disorders in manic-depressive females. *Acta Psychiat. Scand.,* 42:285–94.

Brixen-Rasmussen, L., and Halgren, J., et al. (1982). Amitriptylene and nortriptylene excretion in human breast milk. *Psychopharmacology* (Berlin) 76: 94–95.

Bürgi, V. S. (1954). Puerperalpsychose oder Diencephalosis puerperalis? *Schweitz. Med. Wochensch.,* 84:1222–25.

Dalton, K. (1984, 1985). Progesterone prophylaxis. Paper presented to the Marcé Society, San Francisco, 1984. Progesterone prophylaxis used successfully in postnatal depression. *The Practitioner,* 229:507–8.

Danowski, T., et al. (1953). Is pregnancy followed by relative hypothyroidism? *Am. J. Obstet. Gynecol.,* 65:77–80.

DeGroot, L. J. (1979). The thyroid. In P. Beeson, W. McDermott, and J. Wyngaarden (Eds.), *Cecil's Textbook of Medicine.* 15th Edition, p. 2133. Philadelphia: W. B. Saunders.

Erickson, S., and Smith, G., et al. (1979). Tricyclics and breastfeeding. *Am. J. Psychiatr.,* 136:1483.

Federman, D. D. (1988). Endocrinology. In D. Federman (Ed.), *Scientific American Medicine.* New York: Scientific American Inc.

Freeman, E., and Rickels, K., et al. (1990). Ineffectiveness of progesterone suppositories in treatment for premenstrual syndrome. *J.A.M.A.* (July 18), 264(3):349–53.

Garvey, M., and Tuason, V., et al. (1983). Occurrence of depression in the postpartum state. *J. Affective Dis.,* 5:97–101.

Gibson, M., and Tulchinsky, D. (1980). The maternal adrenal. In D. Tulchinsky and K. Ryan (Eds.), *Maternal-Fetal Endocrinology.* Philadelphia: W. B. Saunders.

Hadley, M. E. (1984). *Endocrinology.* Englewood Cliffs, N.J.: Prentice-Hall.

Hamilton, J. A. (1962). *Postpartum Psychiatric Problems.* St. Louis: C. V. Mosby.

———. (1977). Puerperal psychoses. In J. Sciarra (Ed.), *Gynecology and Obstetrics.* New York: Harper & Row.

———. (1982). Model utility in postpartum psychosis. *Psychopharmacol. Bull.,* 18(3):184–87.

———. (1985). Guidelines for therapeutic management of postpartum disorders. In D. G. Inwood (Ed.), *Postpartum Psychiatric Disorders.* Washington, DC: American Psychiatric Press.

Hatotani, N., and Nomura, J., et al. (1983). Clinicoendocrine studies of post-partum psychoses. In N. Hatotani and J. Nomura (Eds.), *Neurobiology of Periodic Psychoses*. Tokyo: Igaku Shoin.

Hickman, S. (1989). Personal communication.

Khanna, S. A., and Ammini, S., et al. (1988). Hypopituitarism presenting as delirium. *Int. J. Psychiatr. Med.*, 18:89–92.

Marcé, L. V. (1858). *Traité de la folie des femmes enceintes, des nouvelles accouchées et des nourrices*. Paris: J. B. Baillière et Fils.

———. (1862). *Traité pratique des maladies mentales*. Paris: J. B. Baillière et Fils.

Page, E. (1959). Personal communication.

Pauleikhoff, B. (1984). *Amentia*. Address of the Distinguished Scholar. San Francisco: The Marcé Society.

Railton, I. E. (1961). The use of corticoids in postpartum depression. *J. Am. Med. Women's Assoc.*, 17:450–52.

———. (1984). The use of prednisolone for postpartum psychiatric problems. San Francisco: The Marcé Society.

Reich, T., and Winokur, G. (1970). Postpartum psychoses in patients with manic-depressive disease. *J. Nervous and Mental Disorders*, 151:60–68.

Riley, D. (1982, 1984). Pyridoxine prophylaxis. London and San Francisco: The Marcé Society.

Sawyer, T., and Hadley, M., et al. (1982). Design and comparative biological activities of highly potent analogues of alpha-melanotropin. *J. Med. Chem.*, 25:1022–27.

Sheehan, H. L. (1961). Personal communication, noted in Hamilton 1962.

Sheehan, H. L., and Davis, J. C. (1982). *Post-Partum Hypopituitarism*, Springfield, IL: C. C. Thomas.

Sovner, R., and Oisulak, P. (1979). Excretion of imipramine and desipramine in human breast milk. *Am. J. Psychiatr.*, 136:451–52.

Tulchinsky, D. (1980). The postpartum period. In D. Tulchinsky, and K. J. Ryan (Eds.), *Maternal-Fetal Endocrinology*. Philadelphia: W. B. Saunders.

Part IV
Unfinished Business

With only a few years of "enlightenment" regarding postpartum psychiatric illness, it is not surprising to find knowledge and practice incomplete, contradictory, at loose ends, or at best, in progress.

L. V. Marcé divided his cases into a disorder of early onset, usually psychosis, and a disorder of late onset, usually a depression. Lacking a meaningful official nomenclature, professionals have searched for terms that would permit them to communicate with each other regarding postpartum patients, i.e., to find a workable technical jargon. Chapters 18 and 19 look carefully at old and new information about symptom patterns, seeking the most useful and accurate terms for communication. Professor Bernhard Pauliekhoff of Münster, world authority on postpartum symptoms and their progression over time, describes the early mercurial psychotic disorder and notes that patients often have early severe depressive episodes. It may then evolve into a late depression, sometimes punctuated by psychotic episodes. "Postpartum psychotic depression" is defended as the most accurate designation in Chapter 18. The depression that begins two or more weeks after delivery, without psychotic symptoms, is reviewed in Chapter 19. The term "major postpartum depression" is advocated for this disorder.

Infanticide is a rare catastrophic outcome of postpartum illness. The American justice system, largely because of confusing and contradictory guidance from psychiatry, has been erratic in its judgments and penalties in cases of infanticide. In Chapter 20 R. Kumar and Maureen Marks review the long history of legal and medical collaboration in England which has resulted in a rational, consistent, and humane approach to these cases. In Chapter 21, Daniel Maier-Katkin examines criminological issues that constitute the background of this problem. Chapter 22 deals with the defense of infanticide cases. Susan Hickman and Donald LeVine describe the procurement and use of defense evidence.

Chapter 23 takes up health insurance problems of postpartum patients. The present official terminology provides a tempting opportunity for insurance companies to disallow claims for postpartum psychiatric illness. Mark DeBofsky indicates legal principles and precedents that support claims for the costs of postpartum patient care, and he suggests how disallowal of claims can be discouraged.

The patient's husband is a key figure in the care and rehabilitation of the postpartum patient. Robert Hickman is a pioneer in the often-neglected field of integrating the husband into the therapeutic process. His experiences and formulation are presented in Chapter 24.

Irrefutable evidence is a rarity in the study of postpartum psychiatric illness or any other illness, for that matter. While large research projects with long follow-up, large numbers of cases, and good statistical and experimental controls could provide valuable information, there are no signs that this level of research will be conducted in the near future. Ethical issues, economic constraints, and competing priorities all conspire against it. In the final chapter it is noted that when present knowledge is assembled, a few simple but critical studies might provide the confidence required to embark on promising therapeutic regimes.

Chapter 18
Toward the Diagnosis of Postpartum Psychotic Depression

Bernhard Pauliekhoff

Well over 100 years have elapsed since the impressive descriptions of the clinical pictures of postpartum psychiatric illness were written by J.E.D. Esquirol, L. V. Marcé, and others. The continuing difficulty of diagnosis is illustrated by the fact that in all of these years, no clear diagnostic terms or definitions for these conditions have been established. Diagnosis and effective treatment are inseparable. These difficult illnesses are a great burden and a distress to both patients and their entire family. This is made worse when, as a result of the psychosis, self-destructive or criminal acts occur.

My thoughts on this matter are based on a lifelong study of the symptoms of psychiatric illness and their progression over time. This has been called upon in the course of an 8-month correspondence with J. A. Hamilton. A principal topic of the dialogue was the choice of an accurate designation for the psychosis which is the subject of this chapter.

In his 1858 treatise on psychiatric illness related to childbearing, Marcé acknowledges the important contribution of Esquirol in his preface: "Many individual publications in France and elsewhere since Esquirol regarding the mental illnesses following pregnancy have attracted attention to this variety of illness. The outstanding monograph, however, remains the monograph in the first book of Esquirol's works, a learned paper which is a classic, as are all of the writings of this eminent master" (Marcé 1858).

In his major 1838 handbook, Esquirol, the esteemed leader of psychiatric reform in France, wrote an extensive chapter on the mental

---

This chapter was translated by James Hamilton.—EDS.

illnesses of "Newly Delivered and Nursing Mothers" (Esquirol 1838). Even at that time he complained and warned:

Although much is known and written about illnesses related to childbirth, very little has been said about mental illnesses which occur at this time of life. This is responsible for my determination to write this chapter, in the hope that in this way some light may be brought to this field, a field which is important because of the great number of women who are afflicted. The number of women who are mentally ill during or after nursing is a number which is much greater than one might believe. In Salpêtrière, we count about one-twelfth of the psychiatrically ill women who are victims of this kind of illness. There are years when this proportion increases to one-tenth; during the years 1811, 1812, 1813, and 1814 there were ninety-two cases admitted who became ill with or soon after the beginning of lactation. From these ninety-two women, sixty were admitted during the years 1812 and 1813, during which the total admissions were 600.

Despite this earnest reminder and the striking frequency of postpartum illness, there was little improvement in this unsatisfactory situation until the founding of The Marcé Society at the University of Manchester in 1980. Esquirol found among the ninety-two women in his study, eight cases of "confusion," thirty-five cases of "depression and monomania," and forty-five cases of "mania." In all three of these diagnostic groups, particularly those designated as confusion and mania, undoubtedly a large number of patients would fit the diagnosis of postpartum psychotic depression. However, a realistic comparison between the formerly and presently named diagnoses is not feasible, since we do not yet agree upon clear diagnostic categories.

Easier and more certain than this is a comparison between the ages of patients. Esquirol reported that twenty-two of his patients were ages 20 to 25, forty-one were 25 to 30, sixteen were 30 to 35, eleven were 35 to 40, and two were 43 years old. In our 1964 study the age distribution is shown in Table 18.1.

The age at the time of illness has remained the same, with the peak incidence in the 25 to 29 age group, as this is the age of highest incidence in the 1964 sample. Most of the patients were married. In Esquirol's group, sixty-three were married and twenty-nine were single. In our sample, one hundred sixty-eight were married, twenty were premarital and twelve were unmarried.

Esquirol stressed the importance of the consistency of the interval between delivery and the first appearance of psychiatric symptoms: "From our women, twenty-one became ill between the fifth and the fifteenth day postpartum, seventeen from the fifteenth to the sixtieth day, nineteen from the second to the twelfth month, during the nursing period, and nineteen became ill at the time of voluntary or involuntary weaning. From this one could conclude (1) that mental illness

TABLE 18.1. Age of onset of 200 Münster cases of postpartum psychosis.

Age in years	<20	20–24	25–29	30–34	35–39	40–45
Number of cases	3	24	62	61	39	11

occurs more frequently after delivery than during nursing and (2) that the danger of mental illness decreases with time, after delivery."

From our study, the following distribution (Figure 18.1) indicates the time intervals after delivery when the psychoses of 200 patients began.

The foregoing distribution was reviewed and checked, and has considerable reliability, in spite of the fact that in any single case it is not easy to determine, and the reports of the patients on the date of symptom onset are not as reliable as reports from members of the family.

Postpartum psychotic depression usually begins the third to the fifth day after delivery, so that there is usually expert observation at this time [in Germany but not in the United States, where earlier discharge from the hospital is the rule.—EDS.]. Around the tenth day a phase of melancholy sets in, as the young mother leaves the hospital. Also at this time, several symptoms related to various elements of the situation in which the young mother finds herself develop. In diagnosis and therapy, the type of clinical picture and time of onset may be very important for the optimal treatment of the patient.

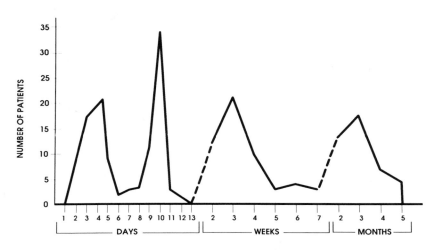

Figure 18.1. Post-delivery time intervals marking the onset of psychosis.

Up to the present time, postpartum psychotic depression has appeared in the literature under several names. Hamilton (1962) spoke of "postpartum delirium," and noted that this illness was more likely to develop out of a normal healthy state than from prior symptoms or illness such as febrile disease. In the German literature, more than 100 years ago, the concept of amentia (*a mente,* "without mind") was attached to the disorder, precisely because the patients behaved as if they had lost their minds. The clinical picture, as was often noted, usually included a dreamy confusion, which was characteristic for this psychosis, as distinct from the confusion found in a toxic delirium, for example, delirium tremens of chronic alcoholism. In the amentia of women who have recently delivered a baby, there is no decline or dissolution of consciousness as in ordinary delirium but rather an exit into a dream and psychotic world from which the patient quickly awakens, usually without remembering the content or events of her dreamy disordered mental status. As distinguished from affective states, where the details of the acute illness are remembered, patients with postpartum illness remember only fragments or have no recall.

To make clear the phenomena of the illness, the following case is presented.

A 21-year-old nurse, who was married during her pregnancy, felt somewhat better than usual during pregnancy. The birth of her child was on September 22, 1983. "Afterward I felt fine," reported this fully recovered woman at a review examination in August 1986. "Celebration was appropriate for the birth of the child. I was particularly happy that it was a girl. There was nothing unusual about my condition after delivery. I was in the hospital through the fifth postpartum day. Once during these days I cried, as often happens with young mothers. As to the possibility of other psychological changes during the time I was in the hospital, I can neither confirm nor deny that they occurred. I was so happy, and also I may have been quite talkative. The physician and the nurses were not aware that anything unusual was taking place. I do not know if we went from the hospital to home, or if we first went by the home of my mother-in-law. I do not remember getting home. I only recall that my husband picked me up at the hospital. Also, I have no recollection of my first day at home. Everything was in total chaos. I took care of and fed the child, but I was ready on the first day to run to town and make some purchases. I bought all kinds of things, sports clothes and many other articles.

"I was at home two or three days and then had an automobile accident at a street crossing. The other car had a bent fender, and I gave the driver my insurance number. In the evening I visited my sister and brought her children gifts. I can partly remember this day, but not everything. Oddly, I don't know if I returned home. Once I was with the infant in a pharmacy, and asked if I could leave the child there. I found everything easy, and the environment was perceived by me as unremarkable. I now ask myself, how the child went along with my behavior without crying, and why other people did not realize that something was wrong. Possibly the child thought that I was drunk.

"On October 1, I celebrated my birthday. I invited many people, but before the party I took off with the infant to visit a flea market about 40 to 50 miles distant. By the time I returned, most of the guests had left. I wanted to buy a home, and many other things. It was chaotic. It is a puzzle to me that nothing more happened. That became clear as the days passed. I quarreled with my husband, and during the week of my birthday in October 1983, I ended up in a psychiatric hospital. At that time I was hardly sleeping at all. I read and wrote a great deal. When I was taken in the ambulance to the hospital, I didn't know my destination. My husband and my brother-in-law went along. I thought that we would visit a house. While under medication in the hospital, I felt quiet and weary; I could hardly move. While on medication I had cramps. That was terrible; I was stiff and could hardly move."

After this statement, which was verified by other people, the psychosis continued as a manic-colored psychosis, "total chaos." The patient was treated for six weeks in a psychiatric hospital, where the erroneous diagnosis of schizophrenia was given. After discharge at her own demand, she made a serious suicide attempt. Then on January 17, 1984, she borrowed and signed a note for 30,000 German marks. Later on, by court action in 1986, the question was addressed as to whether, at the time of her signature, she was responsible. Although it was not apparent to the people with whom she was dealing that she was psychotic, it was decided that she was psychotic at the time with amentia and not responsible. Further, it was the opinion of the court that at that time she had no awareness of the nature of her crime, that her thinking was severely distorted and agitated.

Her mood in the months of December 1983 and January 1984 was described by the young mother, when interrogated later, as "depressive, indifferent, withdrawn, and suspicious." This coloring of the classic picture could be attributable to various medications, but these hardly influenced the deep psychotic disturbance. The medications were varied without improvement. This fact contributed to the indication of an erroneous diagnosis. In February, the patient suddenly recovered. On June 1 she went back to her work as a pediatric nurse.

In cases of this kind we are often asked by judges if during the illness of many months there are "lucid intervals" during which the patient may be clear and rational. This question should be answered in the negative, since the patient is in the midst of a psychosis, even if lay people and even physicians are not aware of this. In the case of the patient described here, her physician evaluated her correctly in court so that her "offense" was not penalized.

With her dreamy psychotic state, the patient lives in another world and is unable to control her behavior. She misinterprets her situation and environment fully, sees her husband as an enemy and does not recognize her own child. She may see herself as a movie actress or another person in public life, and not find this unusual. Occasionally, angels or devils appear in her psychotic episodes or dream life, and these lead to other hallucinations that influence her behavior. The paranoid and hallucinatory phenomena all fit together in the illness and are usually not understood as delusions. The patient is continuously restless with the mood happy, anxious, or full of despair. The psyche is very sensitive and changeable, as is often described in the literature. Manic and depressive states may almost overlap, and they often follow one another so that, depending on the condition which is predominant, various diagnoses are made, such as confused mania, an endogenous depression, or an atypical affective psychosis. Because of the hallucinations and delusions, a schizophrenia is often diagnosed.

This is not a mixture of psychoses, but rather a characteristic disorder, sui generis, which in its clinical course always returns to its own peculiar qualities.

Particularly characteristic, in distinction from other psychoses, is the onset and course of the illness. In our 1964 retrospective study, we saw as many women as possible who had become ill in the years from 1930 to 1960. Compared with twenty-three endogenous psychoses which began during pregnancy, the selected group consisted of 235 patients who had an amentia or other psychiatric diagnosis after childbirth. The findings of this study were later extended through further research, so that we have a large number of lifelong histories to consider. Again and again, we found that while postpartum psychotic depression is a strenuous and difficult psychosis, it is one with a very good prognosis for recovery. These women rarely become ill later in life. At the most, they may have a minor depressive reaction at menopause.

In spite of this good prognosis, the amentia postpartum or the postpartum psychotic depression, at least in its early symptoms, is hardly an easy disorder to treat. During the treatment of patients, it was always possible to see the validity of this rule: the traumatic psychosis after childbirth, with its changes between manic and depressive features, as well as its paranoid and hallucinatory phenomena, usually begins a few days after delivery, peaks quickly, and continues for months (on the average three months), and then suddenly a full recovery occurs. In the absence of a physical condition or cause that can be established, there is a tendency to make a discouraging and wrong diagnosis of schizophrenia. Frequently, many therapeutic approaches to the symptoms and the course of the psychosis have a negative effect on the illness, acting to increase as well as to prolong the illness. In the end, the psychosis goes into remission, as quickly as it began, frequently to the surprise of the physician. The patient, almost from one hour to the next, becomes well and awakened, as if from a stressful dream. Usually, there appears to be no reason for this sudden improvement, which does not seem to be associated with any obvious change in the physical status of the patient. In some cases there was a change in the situation that might be a cause of the remission. Patients who with a particularly bad prognoses were transferred to a hospital for chronic diseases and shortly after their arrival or a few days later were *fully recovered.*

As an example of this striking and sudden improvement of an acute psychosis is the history of a patient who so impressed the distinguished psychiatrist Robert Gaupp that he recounted her clinical history many years later. The occasion was a memorial to another distinguished psychiatrist, Karl Bonhoeffer, on his seventy-fifth birthday (Gaupp 1942–43). Gaupp recalled his year as an assistant to Karl Wernicke in Breslau fifty years earlier and remembered a patient who was of particular scientific interest. However, the patient was not a case of paranoia, which might have been expected because Gaupp devoted his life to the study of paranoia, but rather of a psychosis after childbirth.

"May I, from this time of our earlier work with Wernicke in Breslau," began Gaupp in his long case history from which is selected here a few passages, "recall a particular account of a problem we faced? A young Breslauer woman, a few days after delivery, was overcome with acute anxiety and a catatonic, negativistic stupor.

"She had removed her clothes and stood with a masklike face. Her nourishment and cleanliness were dubious. Our efforts to penetrate the negative stupor were futile. The stupor continued. When her husband visited later, she clung to him when it was time to go to her room. The husband decided against our advice to take her home. I felt that his plan was unworkable. He felt differently; his wife was dressed with the usual resistance and went mutely to his carriage. We felt that he would soon become aware of the need for professional help and bring her back to the hospital. That did not happen. I received a letter from the man a few days later that it had gone well with his wife to return home, that she began to speak again on the way home, and that she had greeted her children happily on arrival. Her self-assurance was immediately apparent, and they had all dined while she told them a great deal about the hospital. She continued well. I asked the husband to have her visit the clinic. She came within a few days and appeared as a cheerful, smart, lovely lady. She confirmed what her husband had written, she had *awakened* on the trip home, and had good recollections and amiable feelings for her time in the hospital."

With the aid of this impressive case history, Gaupp spoke against the one-sided "scientific" methods, with their stern physiological considerations, with which his teacher Wernicke had considered patients. He suggested the following facts were particularly significant: A rich inner life with a fully inactive motor system, recovery in a very short time with her return to her home and her children, recovery of a strong happy emotional capability, and recall of many experiences which those present would tend not believe that she perceived. Until today, it is not possible to say or prove or even decide why, over months, this acute clinical picture continued. Then on the way home she suddenly improved.

Many things are unexplained: What is the essential quality of the illness? What explains the rapid healing when she left the hospital? What explains recovery on the occasion of hospital transfers or other changes of environment? In the hospital, with unchanged care, one might expect that the illness would have continued for weeks or longer. Then there is the question of whether release several weeks earlier would have been equally therapeutic. These things, in our present state of knowledge, are difficult or impossible to answer.

This example is a case of a young mother with a postpartum psychotic depression with a good memory of events that took place in the hospital. However, this fact does not mean that her full memory was recovered. Memory acts in various ways with different patients.

Among the many unsolved problems with this illness is a basic understanding of the somatic relationships, and an equal understanding of the psychological relationships. Only a realistic look at these often misunderstood qualities of the psychosis can lead to optimal care, and only on this basis can patients and their relatives be wisely advised. The somatic and psychological causes and conditions do not work against each other, but they influence the changes of the psychosis together. The mental life does not react solely to the organic background. It is in consideration of this that the disease picture and its development in the course of the life history becomes meaningful, since the psychosis cannot be separated from the early mental life and personality. The psychosis is bound firmly to the biography, and it is through the analysis of the biography that it is possible to achieve the most accurate understanding of the psychological life. All acute psychoses demonstrate sharp changes in biography and personality. These changes point to connections between isolated phenomena and disease processes of the brain.

Of particular interest in postpartum psychotic depression is the time of its appearance, the few days after delivery. This is in contrast with the entire course of pregnancy, when very few psychoses appear. Compared with our twenty-three patients* with a psychiatric illness during pregnancy (Pauliekhoff 1964), Marcé found of his 310 cases, only twenty-seven cases that appeared during pregnancy. During the period after delivery, 180 cases developed (Marcé 1858). In spite of an interval of over 100 years, the studies agree that the proportion of cases during pregnancy to cases during the puerperium is 1 : 10. From this, it is noteworthy that in the three months after delivery, about ten times the number develop than in all nine months of pregnancy, so that the relationship, considering equal intervals of time, is much greater than 1 : 10. In the first months of pregnancy, some manifestations of depression occur. These are often a reaction to an unwanted pregnancy. In general, pregnancy may act as a protection against the emergence of a psychosis. This is also true for some neurological diseases, such as multiple sclerosis.

In general, pregnancy and postpartum psychoses are rarely distinguished from each other. They are, nevertheless, complete opposites, and their differences are important for diagnosis and therapy.

Women who are psychologically labile and who suffer vegetative disturbances often feel unusually well during pregnancy. If psychiatric illness begins during pregnancy, the prognosis is for a chronic course, and the illness requires very careful supervision.

Although psychiatric illness that develops soon after childbearing rarely occurs in later life, it does occur occasionally in both mother and daughter, and also in grandmother, mother, and daughter, as we have seen and as is described in the literature. Nevertheless, in these familial situations, this is not a clearly hereditary predisposition. Facts of this kind need to be put together in the interest of both mother and child. Above all, it is important to bear in mind the rarity of psychoses during pregnancy and its frequency after delivery, and the need to develop reasons for this.

Never, as some of the literature wrongly states, are these conditions solely traceable to the young mother who finds herself immobilized by child care, and because of this becomes upset and ill. Against this are endocrine and other physical and mental factors to consider. During pregnancy the woman is hopeful and may tend to minimize her new duties. After delivery, an entirely different situation is present, with

*Of about 200 cases.—Eds.

unusual demands that must be taken care of unconditionally and cannot be evaded.

It is very easy to distinguish postpartum psychotic depression from illness that begins later, at least ten days after childbirth. This corresponds to release from the hospital in my 1964 case study, and it produced a peak on the curve of when first symptoms occurred (see Figure 18.1). Women with depression after childbearing retain orderly and rational thinking, unlike the *amentia* observed in the psychoses (postpartum psychotic depression). They may leave the hospital without a feeling of health and courage; they may be unhappy, helpless, and disinterested. The young mother may not derive pleasure from her child. She may worry that she may inflict harm on her child, or she may make errors in its care. Sadness as a temperament illness in the German language meets this condition of depression and hopelessness. Melancholy phases may reappear after later pregnancies and may return in later life. As with the situation after childbirth, the depression may recur at the time of engagement or marriage of a child. Finally, these endogenous-depressive illnesses tend to reappear after a variety of situations, for example, moving to other living quarters, changing jobs, during a "rest cure," and after minor accidents. The situation after childbirth, with its special features may be a releasing factor not unlike that in other situations of change for these postpartum depressions. Each situation creates a disturbance of rhythm and, in its provocation, creates a new rhythm.

Puberty, pregnancy, birth, the puerperium, and menopause are important life cycle events for women. Psychological stresses and also psychoses may emerge without always demonstrating a clear causal relationship with physical factors. Particularly in puberty and at menopause, physical changes are blamed without paying attention to the psychological problems of these events in the life cycle. In no way are body and soul independent of physical activities in the brain. Even more, the course of mental activity follows time and sensory patterns, as well as its own development and individuality. Pregnancy, birth, and the puerperium with their significant readjustments of hormonal and metabolic balances also deeply influence psychological well-being. The whole human being with body, soul, and mind must be studied if we are to achieve a suitable diagnosis and an optimal treatment.

In the variety of postpartum psychiatric disorders and in their various courses, further studies will reveal a clearer differentiation and prognosis. Psychotherapeutic measures and social support are in all disorders at least as important as medical treatment. As is the case in any psychiatric problem, we are not dealing with an isolated symptom, but rather we must pay attention to the whole person as well as her family.

References

Esquirol, J.E.D. (1838). Die Geisteskrankheiten in Beziehung zur Medizin und Staatsarzneikunde. In's Deutsche übertr. v. W. Bernhard. 2 Bd. Berlin.

Gaupp, R. (1942–43). Rückblick und Ausblick. Offener Brief an Karl Bonhoeffer bei Vollendung seines 75. Lebensjahres. Z. Neurol., 175:325.

Hamilton, J. A. (1962). Postpartum Psychiatric Problems. St. Louis: C. V. Mosby.

Marcé, L. V. (1858). Traité de la folie des femmes enceintes, des nouvelles accouchées et des nourrices. Paris: J. B. Baillière et Fils.

Pauleikhoff, B. (1964). Seelische Störungen in der Schwangerschaft und nach der Geburt. Ihre häufigkeit, Entstehung, lebensgeschichtliche Problematik, Diagnose, Prognose und Therapie. Stuttgart: Ferdinand Enke Verlag.

———. (1986). Endogene Psychosen als Zeitstörungen. Zur Grundlegung einer personalen Psychiatrie unter Berücksichtigung ihrer historischen Entwicklung. Hürtgenwald: Pressler.

Chapter 19
Major Postpartum Depression

Galina M. Gorodetsky, Richard H. Trapnell, and James Alexander Hamilton

"Distressed perplexity" has been used to describe a mental state present in many patients with psychiatric illness after childbirth (Hoch and Kirby 1919). Patients are confused, perplexed, disturbed, and/or distressed. They are not functioning well and usually know it.

Readers of psychiatric literature and those who try to understand media coverage of postpartum illness are perplexed, perhaps also distressed, by words that have different meanings in different contexts. The most perplexing word of all is "depression." In ordinary usage, "depression" is a state of dejection or sadness, sometimes with reasonable cause, sometimes without apparent cause. In psychiatric usage, "depression" may designate a serious mental disorder, a disorder that requires very careful psychiatric care, often hospitalization in a facility equipped and staffed for the treatment of such cases. The full psychiatric label for this disorder is "major depression."

The problems of definition become more confused when the area of interest is narrowed to psychiatric conditions that follow childbearing. At the level of lesser severity, the term "postpartum depression" is sometimes used to designate a condition of malaise, discontent, and dysphoria, the incidence of which is on the order of one new mother in ten, or over 300,000 in the United States each year. Most of the studies of these "one-in-ten" depressions have been made on defined cross sections of obstetrical populations. Diagnoses have been made by psychological testing and standardized interviews of all of the obstetrical patients in the defined population.

In many studies, the standardized test and interview items have been patterned after criteria such as those developed by R. L. Spitzer and associates (1978) for standardizing the assessment and diagnosis of psychiatric patients. Thus criteria designed to standardize the diagnosis of psychiatric patients have been translated into questionnaire items and standardized interview questions. An implicit assumption is made that affirmative answers to certain questions justify the designation of such persons as depressed. There is an additional assumption in much of the literature that individuals so diagnosed are comparable to clinical cases which present for psychiatric care through the process of patient's complaints, the observations and apprehensions of relatives, and physician referral.

There exists, therefore, a special usage of the word "depression," which for clarity, may be designated as "test-derived depression." In contrast, the concept of depression which is derived from experience with identified psychiatric patients may be called "clinically-derived depression." No experiment has established the equivalence or direct comparability of these two concepts. It is possible that the test-derived depressions, on the average, are quantitatively less severe than clinic-derived depressions. It is also possible that the circumstances related to the answering of formal questions in a test and measurement atmosphere, as contrasted with the psychiatric clinic or office, may lead to qualitative differences between the two groups. This chapter does not discuss test-derived depression in any detail. An excellent literature review of test-derived depression is that of M. W. O'Hara and E. Zekoske (1988).

This chapter is concerned with a clinical entity that is defined in terms of patients who have been referred or who are self-referred for psychiatric care and who are depressed to such a degree that responsible and informed professionals have felt the patients have a disorder which merits psychiatric care and treatment, sometimes in a facility especially equipped and staffed to treat them. This is referred to as a major postpartum depression.

Like the major depression of *DSM-III-R*, major postpartum depression has three degrees of severity, mild, moderate, and severe (American Psychiatric Assocation 1987). A severe depression usually has a real and present hazard of suicide and almost always should be treated with the special protection of a psychiatric facility. This same risk applies, in lesser degree, to moderate depressions, and skilled judgment is needed to decide who should be cared for on an outpatient basis. Depressions of mild severity are usually appropriate for treatment at home.

Among psychiatric conditions that follow childbearing, there are two main disorders, postpartum psychotic depression and major postpartum depression. Both disorders include the adjective "postpartum" in their recommended designation, since this term conveys very important implications regarding etiology, prophylaxis, symptoms and signs, course, treatment, prognosis, and special hazards. In Chapter 18 Bernhard Pauliekhoff describes the unique qualities of postpartum psychotic depression, its relation to parturition, the many psychotic presentations of the disorder, and the unpredictable mercurial manner in which different symptoms develop. Also, Pauliekhoff points out how the early, agitated mercurial disorder often has a depressed state as one of its early presentations, as well as a late phase of dull depression. Pauliekhoff notes that the late depressed phase may be interrupted by explosive psychotic episodes. The violence of some of these psychotic episodes is a compelling reason for identification of this disorder as postpartum psychotic depression.

Cases of postpartum psychotic depression and of major postpartum depression constitute the most serious postpartum illnesses. Along with a few chronic schizophrenics and a few cases of character and personality disorders, they make up the hospitalized cases of postpartum illness. Altogether, these hospitalized cases occur at a rate of about one per 1,000 births. Cases of postpartum psychotic depression outnumber hospitalized major postpartum depressions by roughly six or eight to one. This figure is based on a review of the case histories of seventy-nine patients who were Marcé's own hospital cases, where only six were depressions without indications of psychosis (Marcé 1858). This small percent of the hospitalized cases conforms to the experience of the authors of this chapter. The proportion of uncomplicated depressions is increased greatly when outpatient cases are included, since many cases of mild and moderate major postpartum depression do not require hospitalization. However, even when the outpatients are included, the number of clinically diagnosed postpartum depressions falls far short of the 10 percent of all new mothers designated depressed by tests and measurements.

Most cases of major postpartum depression begin insidiously after the third week postpartum. Initial symptoms are loss of energy and appetite. Insomnia is common. Hair loss may occur. Patients appear pale and weak, and they may have palpitations. Lactation is often difficult and insufficient. Constipation and peripheral edema may develop. The apparent physical symptoms often precede the symptoms that appear to be psychiatric. ("Les désordres de la santé physique précèdent presque toujours les désordres intellectuels," Marcé 1858, page 338).

Psychiatric symptoms are not slow to follow: memory becomes poor, ideas are not clear, patients make confused statements, they do not feel well. At first, the symptoms do not seem overpowering, but gradually, the activities and stimulations that ordinarily cheer and renew individuals fail to do so. Gradually, by insensible gradations, the patients arrive at a state of severe depression. Everything seems hopeless; suicide becomes a preoccupation. The patients often feel that they have failed as a mother. They feel sick, without any energy at all. In this confusion there is little left but to cry, the *délire mélancholique* or *délire triste* of Marcé.

Once established, most cases of major postpartum depression continue for many weeks or months. Physical signs such as peripheral edema, cold extremities, and increased sensitivity to cold may increase. Fatigue is omnipresent. Speech and mentation are noticeably slowed, but the content remains rational, if somewhat confused. If recovery takes place spontaneously, this is usually a slow process.

As major postpartum depression reaches its peak, symptoms and signs may be reminiscent of an hypothyroid or myxedematous state. Laboratory measurements may confirm this suspicion, or serum T_3 and T_4 levels may be within normal limits or low normal. These are patients that some have found to be responsive to thyroid or thyroxine (Stössner 1910, Hamilton 1962, Baker 1967). Current practice is to begin with a low dose, monitor carefully with pulse and repeated T_4 assays, and increase the thyroxine gradually. As thyroid replacement therapy begins to take effect, usually within a fortnight, physical signs and depression disappear concurrently.

For many years, even when thyroid deficit was suspected, the suspicion was often discarded after a finding of serum T_4 within normal limits. This decision, however, runs counter to the observations of many endocrinologists, such as Daniel D. Federman, who notes that, while 85 percent of hypothyroid patients have low T_4 levels, the remaining 15 percent test within the normal range (Federman 1988). This position is extended by Leslie J. DeGroot (1980, pages 2, 133), who writes in *Cecil's Textbook of Medicine,* "Both the T_4 and the RAIU (radioactive iodine units) tend to be less severely depressed in patients with hypothyroidism of pituitary origin, and in these subjects the values tend to overlap the normal range."

At the present time, the authors are of the opinion that no single laboratory test can be depended upon to provide a reliable diagnosis of hypothyroidism in postpartum patients. At least two mechanisms can decrease the effective thyroxine level. One is the decreased activity of the thyroid gland in response to the decrease in pituitary thyrotropic hormone from the sluggish postpartum pituitary gland (Tulchinsky 1980). Another is the phenomenon of autoimmune thyroiditis, which may cause a temporary elevation of serum thyroxine followed by a deficit (Amino et al. 1976). In the former, the thyroid deficit is secondary to a diminution of pituitary activity; in the latter, the thyroid deficit is primary. In any single individual, a symptom-producing postpartum thyroid deficit may be attributable to either of these mechanisms, or both mechanisms may operate concurrently.

Fortunately, there is a rapidly developing awareness of thyroid involvement in mental illness, especially among women, as seen in the illuminating review by Victor I. Reus (1989). It is likely that the study and measurement of thyroid function in the puerperium will advance rapidly. Meanwhile, a rule of thumb for all cases of postpartum psychiatric illness would be to begin with a serum thyroxine and thyroid-stimulating hormone levels and a measurement of autoimmune antibodies then to continue with serial T_4 determinations at weekly intervals. The repeated T_4 studies will determine a trend that will help in the decision to begin thyroid drugs, which are almost never indicated before three weeks postpartum.

Psychological management of all postpartum psychiatric illness requires attention to the dominant theme of such illness, a theme of failure, incompetence, and inadequacy, a theme of self-accusation and self-denigration. As physicians themselves come toward a recognition of physical mechanisms in postpartum illness, opportunities become apparent for displacing the patient's theme of failure. The approach and strategy may differ according to whether the patient is psychotic or depressed. In the former, the physician *acts* consistently as if a physical illness were being treated. In major postpartum depression, it is appropriate to state that the disorder is a serious one and that it requires very careful management, particularly of physiological mechanisms. Further, the physical problems are the result of a normal hormonal slowdown, one that has overshot its mark and needs to return to normal balance with the rest of the (now) unpregnant body. Then, as the effects of medication begin to manifest themselves, physician and patient engage in a process of assessing progress.

At the theoretical level, how is the effectiveness of thyroxine on late depressive syndromes of postpartum psychotic depression explained? It is apparent that the early psychotic manifestations of the early psychosis cannot be explained by a deficit in T_4 or T_3 since both are ample in the first fortnight. However, when the sluggish postpartum pituitary creates a deficit in free cortisol, it may create a deficit in thyroxine synthesis as well. The difference is that while the cortisol deficit may become clinically apparent after three days, it requires two to three weeks for thyroxine to become clinically apparent. In other words, the depression often apparent after the postpartum psychosis cools may have a thyroid deficit component. But the most important reason for distinguishing between the two disorders is that while a psychotic exacerbation is a fair possibility in the late postpartum psychotic depression, it is unlikely in the major postpartum depression. Suicide ruminations and attempts in cases of major postpartum depression under treatment reflect the physician's difficulty in conveying the organic nature and the curability of major postpartum depression.

Earlier in this chapter, an effort was made to distinguish between different usages of the word "depression." At the one pole is major postpartum depression, whose *severe* cases comprise about 10 percent of hospitalized postpartum cases, or only a few hundred in the United States each year. Cases of moderate or mild severity that come to clinical attention may total several thousand patients and probably do not exceed 10,000 per year. The frequency of these clinically attended patients does not begin to approach the frequency of test-derived depressions, roughly 10 percent of obstetrical cases, or over 300,000 per year in the United States.

Major postpartum depressions and the test-derived depressions have similarities and differences. Both have a similar timing: onset is often two to four weeks after delivery, and usually slow spontaneous recovery occurs after several months or a year. The physical complaints are similar, but they may be more disabling in major postpartum depression. Many cases of both conditions that persist for many months tend to improve with another pregnancy and regress or recur after the second pregnancy. There is a familial trend in both types, but it is not overwhelming.

One difference is that the intensive study of the test-derived depressions with psychological tests prior to pregnancy, during pregnancy, and after delivery suggest that the prepregnancy, predelivery symptoms tend to reappear in the postpartum period. This has not been established with major postpartum depression, although the experience of a prior depression, unrelated to childbearing, is a predisposing factor in some cases. Most cases of the first occurrence of a severe postpartum illness, psychosis, or depression seem to have no significant psychiatric precursors; they appear "out of the blue."

The resemblances between major postpartum depression and the less severe but very frequent test-derived depressions raise this question: Is it possible that these conditions may be related and that to some clinically useful degree they represent greater or lesser degrees of similar pathophysiologic mechanisms?

If the answer to this question is affirmative, a second question suggests itself: if thyroid deficit, an elevated symptom threshold to the postpartum thyroxine level, or any other organic mechanism is accepted as a factor in the etiology of major postpartum depression, could this mechanism play a significant role in an appreciable proportion of the depressions isolated by testing procedures?

With the vast resources of modern experimental science, it would seem feasible to obtain answers to these questions.

References

American Psychiatric Association (1987). *Diagnostic and Statistical Manual of Mental Disorders,* 3rd ed., revised. Washington, DC: American Psychiatric Press.

Amino, N., Miyai, K., et al. (1976). Transient hypothyroidism after delivery in autoimmune thyroiditis. *J. Clin. Endocrinol. Metab.* 42:296–301.

Baker, A. A. (1967). *Psychiatric Disorders in Obstetrics.* Oxford: Blackwell.

DeGroot, L. J. (1979). The thyroid. In P. Beeson, W. McDermott, and J. Wyngaarden (Eds.), *Cecil's Textbook of Medicine,* 15th Edition. Philadelphia: W. B. Saunders.

Federman, D. D. (1988). The thyroid. In D. Federman (Ed.), *Scientific American Medicine.* New York: Scientific American Inc.

Hamilton, J. A. (1962). *Postpartum Psychiatric Problems.* St. Louis: C. V. Mosby.

Hoch, A., and Kirby, G. (1919). A clinical study of psychoses characterized by distressed perplexity. *Arch. Neurol. Psychiatr.,* 1:415–58.

Marcé, L. V. (1858). *Traité de la folie des femmes enceintes, des nouvelles accouchées et des nourrices.* Paris: J. B. Baillière et Fils.

O'Hara, M. W., and Zekoski, E. M. (1988). Postpartum depression: A comprehensive review. In R. Kumar and I. F. Brockington (Eds.), *Motherhood and Mental Illness,* Vol. 2. London: Wright.

Reus, V. I. (1989). Behavioral aspects of thyroid disease in women. In B. L. Parry (Ed.), *Women's Disorders, Psych. Clin. North Am.* 12:153–66.

Spitzer, R. L., Endicott, J., and Robins, E. (1978). Research diagnostic criteria: Rationale and reliability. *Arch. Gen. Psychiatry,* 36:773–82.

Stössner, K. (1910). Ein Fall von Myxödem im Anschluss an Gravidität. *München Med. Wochenschr.* 57:2531–33.

Tulchinsky, D. (1980). The postpartum period. In D. Tulchinsky and K. J. Ryan (Eds.), *Maternal-Fetal Endocrinology.* Philadelphia: W. B. Saunders.

Chapter 20
Infanticide and the Law in England and Wales

R. Kumar and Maureen Marks

Introduction

There are some notable exceptions to the maxim that all individuals are equal in the eyes of the law. English law (Infanticide Act 1938) treats a mother who kills her infant differently from any other person, including the father, who commits a similar offence. The history of infanticide is as old as that of human society, but a history of sacrifice of the newborn to propitiate the gods, to strengthen the race, or to control the population (see reviews by Langer 1974, Eisenberg 1981, McKenna 1983, Darbyshire 1985) does not provide a rationale for exempting mothers, as opposed to others, from severe punishment for a particularly shocking offence. Nor does the fact that childbirth and infancy are times of maximum vulnerability, with infant mortality rates that are exacerbated by poverty, malnutrition, social customs, and primitive medicine, provide any *specific* mitigation for mothers who kill their children. The explanation for special treatment in law of child-bearing women lies in the recognition that, for reasons that are still poorly understood, they are "at risk" of becoming mentally ill following the birth, and that, while the balance of mind is disturbed, they may, on impulse or through neglect, kill their infants.

The treatment of infanticidal women in England has not always been lenient or consistent, and this review will attempt to trace the history of the development of the current legislation and to examine its basis. If there are special grounds for pleading diminished responsibility for mental illness related to childbearing, then it must first be established that there is a definite causal link between the process of reproduction and the occurrence of mental illness. If such a link does exist, what are the limits of the association? Are there some kinds of mental illnesses that qualify for special leniency while others do not? Can the current application of the law in England shed any light on these questions? Finally, if there is a sound medical basis for a plea of diminished responsibility in the special circumstances that surround childbirth, is there not a case for seeking consistency across different countries in the way that their laws deal with infanticide?

Historical Background

In Ancient Greece and Rome, infanticide was condoned on eugenic grounds, and in these patriarchal societies it was usually the father who decided whether or not a sickly or female infant should be exposed, drowned, or otherwise disposed of. Rabbinical law forbade such killings, as did Christian teaching, and one consequence of the spread of Christianity in the Roman empire was the imperial edict by Constantine which led to the prohibition of infanticide by the end of the fourth century A.D. This law was, however, largely unenforceable as the Roman empire began to crumble in the face of the Barbarian invasion (Moseley 1986).

The Middle Ages in Europe were dominated by a mixture of Christian and pagan beliefs about the causes of deformity and disablement in children, thus leading their parents often to maltreat or even to kill them. For example, it was thought that such children were changelings, the real child having been stolen by fairies. Alternatively, it was believed that they were the victims of demoniac possession, and here the blame was shifted onto the mother because the only possible explanation was that she must have consorted with the devil. She was therefore suspected of being a witch deserving death, preferably by dreadful means. The *Malleus malleficarum* left an escape route open to parents of handicapped children who died of natural causes or in suspicious circumstances. Another person suspected of being a witch could be blamed for having caused the deformity and the death of the infant (Moseley 1986).

Disablement was, however, only one of several reasons behind the killing of infants: poverty, birth out of wedlock, the wish for male children were prominent risk factors (and still sometimes are; see e.g., Eisenberg 1981, Minturn 1984, U.S. National Academy of Science 1984). One common way of getting rid of an unwanted child was by suffocation; the parents often pleaded that one or both of them had accidentally "overlaid" the infant while they slept together in the same bed. The usual penance for such an offence, if the mother was a married woman, was a diet of bread and water for a year or so, but if the mother was unmarried she was liable to be condemned to death.

Not surprisingly, many desperate unwed mothers, facing the wrath of the church for bearing a bastard child, turned to desperate remedies. They attempted to conceal their pregnancies and then, having killed the newborn infant, they tried to secrete the corpse. A law was passed in 1623 ("Jacobean Bastard Act") which made concealment a capital offence, and in effect, it was an attempt to deter "lewd" women from bearing bastard children. One way round the law was for the mother to produce a witness who would confirm that the child had been stillborn, and then it was for the Crown to prove that there had been a live birth, a task that is sometimes even nowadays beyond the competence of skilled pathologists (Simpson 1979).

The Stuart Act of 1623 and the legislation that replaced it in 1803 did little to stem the appallingly high rate of infanticide. In Victorian England, public concern mounted not only over the regular and frequent discovery of infants' corpses, but also over the scandal of "baby farming" and "burial clubs." Nurses who acted as childminders for working mothers frequently took on more infants than they could manage. Not surprisingly, in overcrowded and unhygienic conditions, the death rate was high, and it was further boosted by the liberal use of opiates that were freely available in various sedative mixtures and cordials. Insurance premiums that were taken out on infants' lives with the laudable aim of avoiding a pauper's funeral brought in desperately needed financial returns, and the temptation to do away with the child was often too great for poverty-stricken parents (Behlmer 1979, Forbes 1986). Under growing public and medical pressure, Parliament eventually responded in 1872, by passing the first Infant Life Protection Act, the forerunner of present-day legislation, designed for the care and protection of children and for the prevention of cruelty.

It is against such a backdrop that one must place the development of legislation relating to infanticide by mothers while their balance of mind was disturbed. Although such cases were infinitesimally few in comparison with the mass of child murders that were related predominantly to social factors, they were in their own way just as important because they made a major contribution to the way in which the law evolved to deal with diminished responsibility. As trial by jury became established in England from the thirteenth century onward, so it became clear that some of the offenders were both guilty and of unsound mind. Should they be punished because they had, after all, committed a serious crime? Walker (1968) describes how a compromise solution was eventually found for dealing with such cases:

On the one hand the harm done must be acknowledged by the legal process; on the other hand the legal process could not be carried to its grim conclusion if the harm was unintentional. So there must be interference with the due process of the law by the one person who could properly interfere—the king. . . . the period during which it became the regular practice to acquit the insane accused instead of leaving him to be pardoned by the king cannot be identified with certainty. . . . the earliest clear case of acquittal which I have found belongs to 1505. "A man was accused of the murder of an infant. It was found that at the time of the murder the felon was of unsound mind (de non saine memoire). Wherefore it was decided that he should go free (qu'il ira quite). To be noted. Yearbooks of Henry VII, 21 Michaelmas Term, plea 16." (Walker 1968)

It is ironic that the defendant should be a man in what is thought to be the first known acquittal for child murder on the grounds of insanity.

Two cases, both heard in the year 1688 and both cited by Walker (1968) illustrate neatly the distinction in the minds of judges and juries between an unwed woman who attempted to conceal her pregnancy and a married woman of good reputation who unaccountably, and in "a temporary phrenzy," killed her newborn. Both were indicted of murder, the former was convicted, and the latter was found not guilty "to the satisfaction of all that heard it." Not all cases could be so easily placed into these two categories, a problem that persists to the present day (D'Orban 1979). For example, a case that was heard in Scotland in 1756 created some difficulties. A woman killed her bastard child at the age of a week, but she did not conceal either the pregnancy or the act, saying that the devil had tempted her to kill the baby. Because the jury could not be satisfied that she had in fact been of unsound mind, she was found guilty of murder but was saved by the royal mercy. Walker adds, "I have not been able to find a contemporary example of similar clemency in an English case. What probably saved the Englishwomen in such situations—in the cases in which they were saved—was the increasing reluctance of juries to convict for murder in such cases. They would grasp at any suggestion that the baby had been stillborn, or had died in the course of birth, or had been accidentally killed. . . . In the occasional case in which the facts pointed unmistakably to murder they could recommend the mother to mercy; and by the nineteenth century they usually did so, with the support of most judges." One of the last recorded executions of a mother for the poisoning of her own baby was in 1849 and what seemed to have weighed against her was the suspicion that she had already disposed of several other children in the same way.

Walker (1968) notes that "by the time of the Capital Punishment Commission 1864–66, it was 'established practice' in the Home Office to advise the commutation of the death penalty when a woman was convicted of murdering her own child when it was under or not much over the age of twelve months." A change in the law had meanwhile provided a loophole for the prosecution to bring a charge for a lesser offence that bypassed the possibility of a death sentence for murder. The Offences Against the Person Act (1861) had extended the offence of concealment to legitimate children, and because the penalty was imprisonment, this charge was often preferred even when the facts might point to murder (Osborn 1987). Twentieth-century legislation on infanticide has been used in the same way (D'Orban 1979). Women who kill their infants within a day of birth are not usually manifestly mentally ill, but they are often charged with infanticide. This charge contains a presumption of mental illness, and it avoids the possibility of conviction on a murder charge.

Acquittals on the grounds of insanity (e.g., Lancet 1848) set in train the process of law reform which was, eventually, to result in the Infanticide Act, 1922. In evidence to the Royal Commission on Capital Punishment 1864–66, Sir Fitzjames Stephens made one of the earliest references to *puerperal* insanity as a specific defence, "women in that condition do get the strangest symptoms of what amounts to temporary madness, and . . . often hardly know what they are about, and will do things which they have no settled or deliberate intention whatever of doing" (Osborn 1987).

Seaborne Davis (1938) commented that judges in the nineteenth century frequently found themselves in the anomalous position of sentencing to death women who had committed infanticide and who were manifestly not insane, in the sure knowledge that they would not be executed. Repeated attempts were therefore made to bring the law into line with actual practice and also to stop the use of the offence of concealment as a way of avoiding a charge of murder. Bills were placed before Parliament that attempted to rationalize the law on child murder, and in 1872 it was proposed that, if a woman murdered her child "at or soon after the birth and whilst deprived of her ordinary powers of self-control by the physical effects of the birth," the trial Judge should be given the option to impose a prison sentence of not less than five years. A year later the Infanticide Law Amendment Bill, 1873–74, tried to stop the use of concealment as an alternative charge to murder. Seaborne Davis (1938) notes that both bills eventually fell by the wayside, and in 1878 a new bill proposed that "a mother who killed her child at or immediately after its birth was to be punished as for manslaughter if she was at the time deprived by reason of bodily or mental suffering of the power of self-control." This provision also failed to reach the statute books because the prime need at the time was not to codify in this limited context the concept of diminished responsibility but rather to tighten up the law on concealment because of the difficulty the Crown frequently faced in proving a live birth. A new provision was introduced which stated that a life sentence should be imposed on women who "with the intent that the child should not live, neglected to provide reasonable assistance in the delivery, if the child died immediately before, during, or shortly after the birth, unless she proved that such death was not caused either by such neglect or by any wrongful act to which she was a party."

Infanticide Act

In 1922 Parliament finally passed the Infanticide Act, which stated "where a woman by any willful act or omission caused the death of her newly-born child, but at the time of the act or omission she had not fully recovered from the effect of giving birth to such child, and by reason thereof the balance of her mind was disturbed, she shall, notwithstanding that the circumstances were such that but for this Act the offence would have amounted to murder, be guilty of a felony, to wit of infanticide and may for such offence be dealt with and punished as if she had been guilty of the offence of manslaughter of such child."

It was not long before questions were raised by the defence about the definition of "newly born" in cases (Rex v. O'Donoghue 1927 and Rex v. Hale 1936) where the victims were aged thirty-five days and twenty-one days, respectively. Without any clear reasoning either way, the judge in Rex v. Hale settled on a period of one month. As Seaborne Davis (1938) observed, the time was of secondary importance, but rather, the crucial question was whether the mother had been mentally deranged after the birth and at the time of the offence. Nevertheless, there had to be some stipulated limit; otherwise, the infanticide defence could theoretically be open to any mother at any time in her life after bearing a child. Thus the option of simply removing the words "newly born" from the act was rejected, and in 1936 a bill was placed before Parliament proposing to extend the time limit to eight years, but it was lost in the Abdication crisis. Meanwhile, the pressure to modify the law did not abate, the main reason being less a reforming zeal on the part of the judiciary and more a need to save judges from the continuing mockery of solemnly passing death sentences, as they were obliged to do, when juries brought in verdicts of guilty on mothers who had killed their children aged a month or more. The judges sentenced these women to death knowing that they would be reprieved, just as they had been before the Act of 1922. O'Donovan (1984) reminds us that there had been no execution in such cases between 1849 and 1864 and only one in sixty cases of women sentenced between 1905 and 1921.

Eventually, an amendment to the 1922 Act was passed by Parliament which settled on a time limit of one year (Infanticide Act 1938). The new act contained an additional clause that appeared to provide a scientific rationale for the extension of the period of diminished responsibility—viz., "the balance of mind was disturbed by reason of her not having fully recovered from having given birth to the child *or by reason of the effect of lactation consequent upon the birth of the child.*" Medical authorities since the time of Hippocrates had ascribed puerperal insanity to both the consequences of the birth itself and to lactation, and experts such as Esquirol (1838) and Marcé (1858) had distingushed between puerperal, and the later onset of "lactational" insanity. However, the medical basis for the new legislation was, and still is, unproven, and as Walker (1968) later observed, the act was not *recognising* legally a link between childbirth and lactation and infanticide, but *creating* it.

Inevitably, there was going to be a reaction from the medical profession, and interestingly, this happened not in England, where doctors were reluctant to undo the work of many years that had gone into the introduction of humanitarian legislation, but in the United States, where such laws did not, and still do not, exist. A series of influential articles appeared in journals rejecting the proposition that there was an aetiological link between childbirth and psychosis or that there were any clinically distinguishing features that set puerperal psychoses apart from schizophrenia and manic-depressive disorders (Strecker and Ebaugh 1926, Kilpatrick and Tiebout 1926, Karnosh and Hope 1937, Foudeur et al. 1957). These conclusions are open to question in the light of more recent evidence, but they were to be echoed many years later in England by the Butler Committee (1975) as one of the reasons for doing away with the special provisions of the Infanticide Act. The problem was further compounded by the fact that the medical and legal professions were interpreting the act in a liberal manner, taking into account the effects of stress on the mother stemming from a variety of social and environmental pressures. The wheel had turned full circle since the original Jacobean Statute of 1623, which had sought to bring about social reform by *punishing* women who had tried to conceal neonaticide in circumstances of extreme social stress.

Homicide Act 1957 and Diminished Responsibility

The Homicide Act (1957) abolished the death penalty and Section 2(1) of the act also enshrined the doctrine of diminished responsibility. Until 1957, a mentally ill person charged with murder was judged against the M'Naghten rule, which was formulated in 1843: "every man is proved to be sane, until the contrary be proved, and that to establish a defence on the ground of insanity it must clearly be proved that at the time of committing the act, the accused was labouring under such a defect of reason, from disease of the mind, as not to know the nature and quality of the act he was doing; or if he did know it, that he did not know that what he was doing was wrong." Mothers who had killed their children had reason to be grateful for the Infanticide Act because if the prosecution brought a charge of infanticide, the burden of proof of insanity was automatically removed from the defence, and further, it was not necessary to prove that their mental condition had *caused* them to commit the offence, but simply that their balance of mind had been disturbed at the time. Of course, it was open to the prosecution to charge mothers with murder, and then, subject to a satisfactory defence, the jury could bring in a verdict of infanticide. Thus infanticide could be both a charge and a verdict; the result of such a verdict was avoidance of the death penalty and of the subsequent wait for a reprieve.

The Homicide Act (1957) was a major reform—a mandatory life sentence replaced capital punishment as the penalty for murder and in the case of a mentally ill offender, it was up to the defence to prove diminished responsibility, which if accepted, reduced the offence to manslaughter. The sentence for manslaughter could vary at the judge's discretion from discharge to life imprisonment. The Homicide Act defined diminished responsibility as follows: "where a person kills or is party to the killing of another, he shall not be convicted of murder if he was suffering from such abnormality of mind (whether arising from a condition of arrested or retarded development of mind or any inherent causes or induced by disease or injury) as substantially impaired his mental responsibility for his acts or omissions in doing or being a party to the killing." Although the terms of this act were wide enough to cover all capital offences, including infanticide, the 1938 legislation was not repealed. This had the result that mentally ill mothers could be charged and convicted of murder; they could alternatively be convicted of manslaughter with diminished responsibility or of infanticide. They could also, if the prosecution so wished, be charged with infanticide, in which case, apart from acquittal, the only possible verdict was infanticide.

Both options (i.e., to bring a charge of murder or of infanticide) are still open to the prosecution, and a survey by D'Orban (1979) showed that, like the concealment law, the Infanticide Act was being used to protect many unfortunate women, particularly those who had committed neonaticide. Virtually none of them were diagnosed as suffering from a mental illness at the time of the offence, but the verdict was infanticide. Although D'Orban does not specify the numbers, it is possible that infanticide had also been the charge in most of these cases, i.e., the prosecution may have felt it unnecessary and inappropriate to press for, and obtain, a conviction for murder.

Paradoxically, among women who had clearly been mentally ill (mainly with psychotic illness), the most common verdict was of manslaughter with diminished responsibility; therefore, the charge must have been murder. Many of the women for whom the Infanticide Act had originally been intended were being charged with murder, and women who were not obviously mentally ill were being charged with infanticide. Yet others who fell into that most difficult of all categories, disorder of personality, were open to either charge. The logic behind the choice of charge by the prosecution seems, at best, unclear.

Infanticide or Manslaughter—Butler Report

It is confusing to have two laws covering the same offence, but even more puzzling is the way in which these laws are being used. A committee appointed by Parliament and chaired by Lord Butler reviewed the problem of dealing with mentally ill offenders, and in its report (1975) the committee devoted a section to infanticide. The Butler Committee was in favour of removing the mandatory life sentence for murder, in which case the provision for a plea of diminished responsibility would be unnecessary. If this proposal was rejected (which it was) the committee was still in favour of rationalising the law by abolishing the Infanticide Act, and it proposed that where medical opinion was unanimous in showing plainly that the case was one of diminished responsibility, it should be open to the prosecution, if the defence agreed, to charge manslaughter in the first instance. Although this recommendation was a general one (and it was not accepted), specifically in relation to the Infanticide Act it was no more than a proposal for a cosmetic change. Only the name of this offence would be altered, from infanticide to manslaughter (with assumed diminished responsibility).

The Butler Committee was critical of the Infanticide Act on other grounds: the law was arbitrary in its setting of a limit of one year and did not allow for a woman who killed two children, one older than a year, in which case she would have to be charged with murder for one offence and could be charged with infanticide for the other. The act also did not cover women who attempted to kill but only injured their infants; there was no offence of attempted infanticide, and such women were charged with attempted murder.* The medical principles upon

*Wilkins (1985) does however describe a case that sets a precedent in which a plea of guilty to attempted infanticide was accepted by an English court.

which the act was based might no longer be relevant: puerperal psychosis was not any more regarded by psychiatrists as different from other psychoses, its hormonal basis was unproven and childbirth was only a precipitant. The relationship to incomplete recovery from the effects of childbirth or lactation specified in the act was somewhat remote. Mental illness was probably no longer a significant cause of infanticide; most cases coming before the courts were about "battered babies" where a combination of environmental stress, personality disorder, and low-frustration tolerance were the usual aetiological factors. Nevertheless, the act was almost always invoked in cases of maternal filicide when the child was under a year old. Taken together, all these reasons added up to a powerful argument for abolishing infanticide as a special case in the law. But how valid were the medical opinions that impressed the Butler Committee? In the final section of this review it will be argued that the committee was erroneously persuaded that there was no such illness as puerperal psychosis, and D'Orban's (1979) study shows, as does Figure 20.1, that the Infanticide Act was not "almost always" invoked in such cases. It seems that the committee was looking for reasons to justify tidying up the law.

Although the law was not changed, it seems reasonable to assume that the gradual fall in verdicts of infanticide following publication of the report was not just a coincidence (see Figure 20.1). It is less easy to explain the increase in the recorded rate of all homicides involving infants up to one year of age, which was evident within a year of the publication of the Butler report. Perhaps greater awareness of the problem resulted in more prosecutions, but it is difficult to be sure.

A working party was set up by the Royal College of Psychiatrists to report to the Criminal Law Revision Committee, specifically to give its opinion on the medical principles underlying the offence of infanticide and to offer any general thoughts on the advantage or otherwise of there being a separate offence of infanticide. In its report (Bluglass 1978) the working party lamented the lack of epidemiological studies relating the incidence of mental disorder to childbirth but failed to refer to the most important available research which was by Paffenbarger (1964). The working party concluded that there was little hard evidence to support theories of a hormonal basis for puerperal psychosis. It also noted, without citing evidence, that "some have regarded psychological and social factors as equally or even more important." The working party was not impressed by the contribution of lactation to mental illness, and it advised removal of the clause that had been put into the 1938 amendment of the earlier act. The killing of a second child up to five years could be incorporated into an amended act, and the working party concluded that the act should be retained but with a

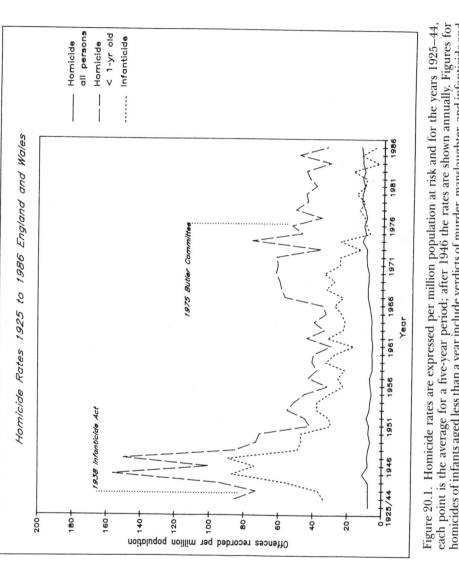

Figure 20.1. Homicide rates are expressed per million population at risk and for the years 1925–44, each point is the average for a five-year period; after 1946 the rates are shown annually. Figures for homicides of infants aged less than a year include verdicts of murder, manslaughter, and infanticide and may also include some cases where the offender may not have been the mother. A persistent fall can be seen in the infanticide verdicts after the report of the Butler Committee in 1975.

wider ambit as long as the offence of murder carried a life sentence. It suggested changing the wording linking disturbance of balance of mind with incomplete recovery from childbirth or the effect of lactation to a more general form of words. Such disturbance might occur "by reasons related to childbearing," thus giving an official blessing to the inclusion of "cases resulting from the effects psychological and environmental stress and incidental mental illness as well as cases resulting from *true* puerperal illness." This last phrase is a telling one because it amounts to a recognition that there was, in the working party's opinion, such an illness (puerperal psychosis) and that, contrary to the evidence cited by Butler (1975), childbirth was not just a precipitant. This is a key issue because the infanticide law, however it is interpreted or works in practice, rests on the assumption that there is an underlying and specific relationship between childbirth and mental illness. If this assumption is false, then the law is manifestly unsound.

The working party also recommended that provision should be made for charging women with attempted infanticide. Finally, it suggested that there should be further research into the incidence of neonaticide, into the effects of hormonal changes on mental state, into the balance between hormonal changes and psychological and environmental changes, and also into the relationship between a failure of attachment and bonding and the development of mental illness.

The Criminal Law Revision Committee (CLRC) examined the proposal (Butler 1975) to abolish the offence of infanticide and, in its fourteenth report (1980), decided against making any changes. As Walker (1981) observed, this committee was probably impressed by the large number of organisations that supported the status quo. More importantly, however, it recognised that the wording of the Infanticide Act (1938) was allowing flexible and lenient interpretation of the mother's mental disturbance. The CLRC presumably felt that it was better not to tamper with a law, which although imperfect, was nevertheless being operated humanely and in favour of the great majority of mothers who killed their infants. Major changes along the lines proposed by Butler (1975), i.e., removal of the mandatory life sentence for murder and permission to charge manslaughter (in cases of "recognised" diminished responsibility) had not been found acceptable, and the CLRC commented that the further suggestion that the term "mental disorder" as then defined in the Mental Health Act (1959) be substituted for "abnormality of mind" might put "too great a strain upon the professional consciences of expert witnesses." They were, nevertheless, as Walker (1981) comments, prepared to continue to turn a blind eye to expert (mis)interpretations of "disturbed balance of mind" because, in practice, psychiatrists were going beyond the letter of the infanticide law and using it to cover "stresses" related to social difficulties.

The two relevant pieces of legislation in current operation in England and Wales therefore still are the Homicide Act (1957) with its provision for diminished responsibility and the Infanticide Act (1938), which states:

Where a woman by any wilful act or omission causes the death of her child under the age of 12 months, but at the time of the act or omission the balance of her mind was disturbed by not having fully recovered from the effect of having given birth to the child or by reason of the effect of lactation consequent upon the birth of the child, then notwithstanding that the circumstances were such that but for this Act the offence would have amounted to murder she shall be guilty of an offence, to wit of infanticide, and may for such offence be dealt with and punished as if she had been guilty of the offence of manslaughter of the child.

Comments

Two Laws

The law is confusing in its current application to the question of diminished responsibility in the case of mothers who kill their infants. There are two sets of relevant legislation, and the one that was specifically intended for psychotic mothers (Infanticide Act 1938) is being used by lawyers and doctors to obtain lenient treatment for mothers who are either not mentally ill or who have personality disorders and where there is usually evidence of environmental and social stress. Psychotic mothers are, paradoxically, commonly being charged with murder (D'Orban 1979). There is considerable overlap between the provisions of the Homicide Act (1957) and the Infanticide Act, but the latter affords women special protection—because infanticide can also be a charge and, uniquely, because demonstration of cause and effect between mental illness and the offence is not required. This added protection is not written into the act, but seems to have arisen out of the way in which the act was drafted.

Puerperal Psychosis

The infanticide law assumes a link between childbirth and lactation (possibly as a result of some hormonal dysfunction) and disturbance of balance of mind, but it does not require proof of any physiological basis either for the offence or for the occurrence of illness. This law has been criticised because puerperal psychosis cannot easily be distinguished from other severe mental illnesses and because the very existence of such a condition is in doubt. Neither "official" system for classifying mental disorders (*ICD-9* or *DSM-III-R*) currently has any place for puerperal psychosis (see Kumar 1989 for review of changing medical attitudes toward the existence of "puerperal psychoses"). In some states in the United States, the rejection of the concept of an independent syndrome related to childbirth has had the consequence that women are serving prolonged prison sentences for infanticide because an inexpert defence was discredited on the grounds that their supposed illness did not exist. However, there is inescapable epidemiological evidence for a strong link between childbirth and the incidence of psychosis (Paffenbarger 1964, Kendell et al. 1987), and the studies that failed to distinguish between puerperal and other psychoses can be criticised on methodological grounds and because the conditions from which the differentiation is being made are by no means sharply defined syndromes in themselves (Kendell 1975, Kumar 1989).

There is circumstantial evidence that the likely causes for puerperal psychosis are in the physiological, rather than in the social and environmental domain (Kumar 1989). There is therefore a better rationale for preserving the infanticide law as a special case—at least for psychotic mothers—than there is for repealing it. Walker (1968) gives another important reason for retaining this legislation: removing the label of murder from this form of homicide and substituting a different and more technical term has the effect of reducing the stigma that attaches to the offence, and it changes not only the attitudes of judges but also those of society.

Self-Control and Mitigation Based on Internal versus External Factors

A fundamental question must, however, be addressed. Why should there be any greater mitigation if there is a presumed physiological dysfunction than if there is a similar presumption of social and environmental stress? As the wording of the law is currently (correctly) interpreted, postnatal depression is as valid a defence as is puerperal psychosis, yet the aetiology of the former is predominantly psychological and social (Kumar 1982, O'Hara and Zekoski 1988). A serious consideration of this question poses other questions about special treatment of women. If mothers can be defended in this way why not fathers?

Infanticide will not go away, and the majority of offenders will continue to be mothers, a few of whom are psychotic, some depressed, some with personality disorders, and others who have no mental disturbance or disorder but who may have an unwanted child or other motive such as displaced revenge (Resnick 1969). It is interesting to note in passing that the Abortion Act (1967) has made no difference to the overall recorded rate of infant homicides. Also, while the general homicide rate is rising slightly and steadily, homicides of children under 1 year of age are at a more or less constant rate per million "at risk" (see Figure 20.1). However, there are obvious imperfections in statistics of recorded offences.

The motives for infanticide are poorly understood, and there does not seem to have been any study of why a woman kills one of her children and not another, nor any follow-up investigation of the likelihood of reoffending, possibly related to the type of disorder or disturbance manifested at the time of the original offence. Virtually nothing has been written about the psychopathology of neonaticide. Such cases continue to occur despite the greater emancipation of women, the availability of contraception, and since 1967, of abortion on psychosocial grounds. Criminal statistics that are published by the Home Office usually give the age of the victims as under 1 year, 1 to 4 years, 5 to 15 years, and so on, and more detailed information on the epidemiology and psychopathology of neonaticide may be revealing. Is it less the product nowadays of an unwanted pregnancy and more likely the extreme end of a condition that is sometimes described as a failure of "bonding"? In a series of self-selected cases collected by the author in which the mothers reported severe problems of attachment to their newborn, many were tormented by infanticidal ideas. Are the cases of neonaticide and abandonment of infants the visible tip of a much larger and poorly understood problem?

There is little doubt that the existing Infanticide Act is imperfect and, in some ways, arbitrary. It is not clear what leads the prosecution to charge murder in some cases when the appropriate charge might have been infanticide. It could be argued that the opposite is also sometimes the case, but a detailed investigation of a consecutive series of cases is the only way of answering such questions. If the Infanticide Act continues to be preserved, as it probably should be, as a piece of reforming and humanitarian legislation, such research may help in laying down guidelines about when it may be appropriate to charge murder and when infanticide.

Suggested Changes

The recommendations of the Working Party of the Royal College of Psychiatrists for additions and changes in the wording of the Infanticide Act, were intended to remove anomalies. Changing the reference from "incomplete recovery from childbirth and lactation" to "by reason of childbearing" would simply reflect the current practice of recognising that childbearing women may also be peculiarly vulnerable to social and environmental adversity. There is no evidence of increased rates of psychosis or nonpsychotic depression soon after men become parents, and therefore, the grounds for including fathers as a special case are not strong. It is open for a man to plead diminished responsibility to a charge of murder. The time limit of one year is arbitrary, but as Figure 20.1 shows, the first year is the time of maximum vulnerability. A child under 1 year of age is four times more likely to be a victim of homicide than afterward. In the years 1978–87, the average rate for homicide of children age 12 months or less was forty-two per million "at risk," and for the total population, the rate was eleven per million. Therefore, on empirical grounds, the existing limit makes sense. Similarly, extending the age limit for other child victims to five years is also based on evidence from criminal statistics (Bluglass 1978), and this type of change would remove the majority of anomalies when two or more children are victims.

The current rate of recorded homicide of infants is about one per 30,000 births, i.e., about twenty-five cases per year in England and Wales. This offence, although rare in absolute terms, is nevertheless of considerable medicolegal importance, and yet, despite the protracted and learned legal arguments and the many expert witnesses who have given evidence to innumerable committees over the past 100 years or so, it is striking how little serious research has been done into the psychopathology of infanticidal mothers. How should they be categorized: by motive (e.g., Resnick 1969), by diagnosis (D'Orban 1979), or by source of impulse (Scott 1973)? How do they fare after the offence, and are there data to show that probation and, where necessary, medical treatment have a good outcome both for the mother herself and for the prevention of reoccurrences? What purpose is served, except in rare instances, by meting out long prison sentences? Is there a continuum of severity, that is, are some women (and their partners) prone to repeatedly harm their children, only a few of whom die? Are there others who only act impulsively and decisively in the throes of a mental illness, and are their actions in any way related to a disorder of attachment?

References

Behlmer, G. K. (1979). Deadly motherhood: Infanticide and medical opinion in mid-Victorian England. *J. Hist. Med. Allied Sci.*, 34(4):403–27.
Bluglass, R. (1978). Infanticide. *Bull. R. Col. Psychiatr.*, (August):130–41.

Butler Committee (1975) Report of the Committee on Mentally Abnormal Offenders. Chairman: Lord Butler of Saffron Walden. Cmnd 6244:HMSO.

Criminal Law Revision Committee, 14th Report (1980). Offences against the person. Cmnd 7844:HMSO.

Darbyshire, P. (1985). Lambs to the slaughter. *Nursing Times* (August 14), (33):32–35.

D'Orban, P. T. (1979). Women who kill their children. *Br. J. Psychiatry*, 134, 560–71.

Eisenberg, L. (1981). Cross-cultural and historical perspectives on child abuse and neglect. *Child Abuse and Neglect*, 5:299–308.

Esquirol, E. (1838). *Des maladies mentales*. Paris: Ballière.

Forbes, T. R. (1986). Deadly parents: Child homicide in eighteenth- and nineteenth-century England. *J. Hist. Med. Allied Sci.*, 41:175–99.

Foudeur, M., Fixsen, C., Friebel, W. A., and White, M. A. (1957). Postpartum mental illness. *Arch. Neurol. Psychiatry*, 77:507–12.

Karnosh, L. J., and Hope, J. M. (1937). Puerperal psychoses and their sequelae. *Am. J. Psychiatry*, 94:537–50.

Kendell, R. E. (1975). *The Role of Diagnosis in Psychiatry*. Oxford: Blackwell.

Kendell, R. E., Chalmers, J. C., and Platz, C. (1987). Epidemiology of puerperal psychoses. *Br. J. Psychiatry*, 150:662–73.

Kilpatrick, E., and Tiebout, H. M. (1926). A study of psychoses occurring during the puerperium. *Am. J. Psychiatry*, 6:145–59.

Kumar, R. (1982). Neurotic disorders. In I. F. Brockington and R. Kumar (Eds.), *Motherhood and Mental Illness*, pp. 71–118. London: Academic Press.

———. (1989). The concept of puerperal psychoses. In preparation.

Lancet (1848) (ⁱ). Lord Demman on a case of infanticide, pp. 318–19.

Langer, W. L. (1974). Infanticide: A historical survey. *History of Childhood Quarterly*, 1:353–65.

Macfarlane, A., and Mugford, M. (1984). *Birth Counts*. London: Her Majesty's Stationary Office.

Marcé, L. V. (1858). *Traité de la folie des femmes enceintes, des nouvelles accouchées et des nourices*. Paris: J. B. Ballière et Fils.

McKenna, J. J. (1983). Primate aggression and evolution: An overview of sociobiological and anthropological perspectives. *Bulletin of the American Academy of Psychiatry and the Law*, 11(2):105–30.

Minturn, L. (1984). Changes in the differential treatment of Rajput girls in Khalapur: 1955–1975. *Medical Anthropology*, 82:127–32.

Moseley, K. L. (1986). The history of infanticide in Western society. *Issues in Law and Medicine*, 1(5):345–61.

O'Donovan, K. (1984). The medicalisation of infanticide. *Criminal Law Review*, 259–64.

O'Hara, M. W., and Zekoski, E. M. (1988). Postpartum depression: A comprehensive review. In R. Kumar and I. F. Brockington (Eds.), *Motherhood and Mental Illness*, Vol. 2, pp. 17–63. London: Wright.

Osborne, J. A. (1987). The crime of infanticide: Throwing the baby out with the bath water. *Revue Canadienne de droit familiale*, 6:47–59.

Paffenbarger, R. S., Jr. (1964). Epidemiological aspects of postpartum mental illness. *Br. J. Preventive and Social Medicine*, 18:189–95.

Resnick, P. J. (1969). Child murder by parents: A psychiatric review of filicide. *Am. J. Psychiatry*, 126:325–33.

Scott, P. D. (1973). Parents who kill their children. *Medicine, Science and the Law,* 13:120–26.

Seaborne Davies, D. (1938). Child killing in English law. *Modern Law Review,* (March) 269–87.

Simpson, K. (1979). *Forensic Medicine,* 8th ed. London: Edward Arnold.

Strecker, E., and Ebaugh, F. C. (1926). Psychoses occurring during the puer-perium. *Arch. Neurol. and Psychiatry,* 15:239–52.

Taylor, E. M., and Emergy, J. L. (1982). Two-year study of the causes of post-perinatal deaths classified in terms of preventability. *Arch. Dis. Child.,* 57:668–73.

Walker, N. (1968). *Crime and Insanity in England,* Vol. 1. Edinburgh: Edinburgh University Press.

———. (1981). Butler v. the CLRC and others. *Criminal Law Review,* September, 596–601.

Wilkins, A. J. (1985). Attempted infanticide. *Br. J. Psychiatry,* 146:206–8.

World Health Organisation (1978). Mental disorders: Glossary and guide to the classification in accordance with the ninth revision of the International Classification of Disease. Geneva: World Health Organization.

U.S. National Academy of Science (1984). Chinese census: Demographic transition under way. *Nature,* 310:177.

Chapter 21
Postpartum Psychosis, Infanticide, and Criminal Justice

Daniel Maier Katkin

In the past few years, postpartum psychosis has been offered as a legal defense in a few deeply disturbing infanticide cases in several American jurisdictions. These cases have attracted a great deal of media attention and fueled public discussion about the mental health of mothers who kill their own babies. From the perspective of the criminologist, these cases present an extraordinary pattern of criminal behavior. Not merely a few isolated incidents, but a recurring pattern of the destruction of planned-for, wanted children by their own mothers with no apparent motive and under circumstances that suggest transitory mental illness. Are these women insane at the time of the act? Is their behavior the product of a diseased state of mind, or is it premeditated and willful? Court decisions and sentencing practices indicate great diversity of opinion about these issues that lie at the core of the concept of criminal responsibility.

It is an established principle of justice in the Western world that criminal punishment—the deprivation of life, liberty, or property—is an appropriate response to harmful acts only if they are accompanied by a bad state of mind. This is the boundary between tort law (the law of accidents) and criminal law. As Justice Oliver Wendell Holmes observed: "even a dog knows the difference between being kicked and being stumbled over." Tortfeasors are required to set right the wrong they have caused, but they are not deprived of life or liberty as felons.

The absence of a bad state of mind may constitute a defense against criminal conviction in cases where there is no claim of accidental misbehavior. A defendant who claims self-defense, for example, concedes the commission of the act but denies moral culpability: arguing, in essence, "I did not wish to kill nor to do any harm; my state of mind was that I did not want to be killed myself." Duress is another example of a defense in which the commission of a criminal act is conceded, but the innocence of the defendant's state of mind is asserted: the banker, who unlocks the vault in which depositors' funds are kept when threatened by a gunman will argue that the act was not a product of free will, but of an overwhelming external force.

The insanity defense raises the possibility that free will may be overwhelmed by internal forces, but it creates difficult problems because insanity is so hard to define. In antiquity the law treated as insane only those who had "no more reason than a wild beast" (Goldstein 1967, Walker 1968). Such people may have existed in the dark ages, e.g., a mentally retarded child abandoned early, barely learning to talk or think, but this is hardly the modern conception of insanity. In 1843, after an attempt by Daniel M'Naghten on the life of Prime Minister Robert Peele, a panel of Britain's top judges formulated a definition of insanity that has dominated legal thought ever since. Under the M'Naghten rule a defendant is not guilty by virtue of insanity if, at the time of the commission of the act, he "was labouring under such a defect of reason, from disease of mind, as not to know the nature and quality of the act he was doing; or, if he did know it, that he did not know he was doing what was wrong" (M'Naghten 1843). Many jurisdictions have added an "irresistible impulse" clause to the definition of insanity. A defendant, it is argued, may have known that what he was doing was wrong but may have been unable to control his behavior. But this is problematic because it may be a very fine distinction between one who is unable and one who is unwilling to control his behavior.

By the mid-1950s there was deep dissatisfaction with the received definitions of legal insanity. Psychiatry and psychology had made great strides in advancing scientific knowledge about mental illness, but the law was still relying on antiquated principles of moral philosophy. What seemed to be needed was a definition of insanity that allowed the incorporation of modern scientific knowledge about schizophrenia, obsessive compulsions, multiple personalities, and other mental disease. In Durham v. United States (D.C. Cir. 1954), Judge Bazelon of the Federal Circuit Court of the District of Columbia held that a defendant "is not criminally responsible if his unlawful act was the product of mental disease or mental defect." But this is tautology rather than a definition. The Durham rule places no restrictions on the testimony of experts, and thus it may bring more complete scientific evidence into the courtroom, but it fails to provide jurors with comprehensible standards to guide their judgment. In 1962 the American Law Institute offered a definition of legal insanity that combines elements of the M'Naghten, irresistible impulse, and Durham rules: "A person is not responsible for criminal conduct if at the time of such conduct as a result of mental disease or defect he lacks substantial capacity either to appreciate the criminality (wrongfulness) of his conduct or to conform his conduct to the requirements of the law" (American Law Institute 1962).

Applying these rather abstract principles of justice to real cases is no easy matter. How are courts to determine whether a particular mother was legally insane at the moment in which she extinguished life in her own newborn child? To some extent, the issue of sanity may be illuminated by the circumstances of the killing. Unfortunately, in the United States, unlike Britain, there is no systematic registry of data about infanticide cases; as a consequence, scientific analysis of the phenomenon is virtually impossible for American scholars. Since 1986, I have collected the accounts of thirty-five infanticides that appear to be related to postpartum psychoses. While this does not constitute a probability sample from which generalizations may be drawn with confidence, it is almost certainly among the most complete data bank about infanticide litigation in American jurisdictions.

In a substantial majority of these cases, the women were in comfortable circumstances, with no history of abuse or criminality; they gave every indication of wanting to have children. Indeed, the homicidal acts frequently followed the birth of a planned second child. In one such case, a New York City family had actually spent more than $20,000 over a four-year period on fertility assistance. When the son thus conceived was two months old he was drowned in the bathtub by his mother; shortly thereafter, she transported the body in a plastic bag to a garbage can a few blocks from home, and then called the police to report a kidnapping. Death by drowning is a recurrent theme in these cases, and so too are fabricated stories of kidnapping. Other means of producing death have included suffocation, defenestration, shooting, and in one case, placing the infant behind a rear wheel of an automobile and driving over it. In some of the cases, the mother appears to have heard voices or suffered delusions. In a few cases, the homicidal acts were followed by suicide attempts.

These cases are shocking, in part, because the compelling nature of motherly love is associated in our minds with joy. The tribulations of motherhood may be great—particularly as children grow older—but the period of bonding between mother and baby is generally regarded as a happy time of affectionate and protective feelings. The medical reality, documented extensively in other chapters of this book, is that depression is also an aspect of the early stages of motherhood. Pregnancy is hard work, and women may grow tired near the end. Perhaps the delivery is protracted and exhausting, or the baby is not quite what was expected. The responsibilities that lie ahead may seem insurmountable, or some image of contentment may seem unattainable.

Perhaps there is a touch of melancholy about one's own inexorable passage through the stages of life. Alterations in body chemistry associated with pregnancy and childbirth may also influence moods. Whatever the causes, transitory postpartum "blues" affect as many as 80 percent of all new mothers in the Western world during the first few days after delivery. Symptoms include sadness, heightened emotional lability, weeping, irritability, and fatigue. Deeper and longer lasting depressions are experienced by a smaller, but still considerable percentage of all new mothers. The weight of expert opinion suggests that more than 10 percent of all mothers experience depression lasting from a few weeks to a few months during the year after giving birth.

Postpartum psychosis is a rare disorder occurring in fewer than 2 cases per 1,000 births. These women experience terrifying delusions and hallucinations. There is personality change; mood swings occur very quickly. Sometimes voices are heard; sometimes there are overwhelming impulses. This is not a new phenomenon; the syndrome was described by Hippocrates and again by Galen in the earliest medical treatises. A comprehensive study of postpartum psychoses was published by the French physician Louis Victor Marcé in 1858. Epidemiological studies conducted in several nations have confirmed the characteristics and the steady incidence of postpartum psychoses in the intervening years (Kruckman and Asmann-Finch 1986).

A considerable body of research literature focuses on biological factors in the etiology of postpartum psychosis. The revolution of psychopharmacology that began in the 1950s increased interest in the relationship between postpartum depression and hormonal changes. It has been consistently noted that the onset of symptoms follows a precipitous fall in levels of estrogen, progesterone, and other female reproductive hormones that can increase tenfold during pregnancy and then plunge to prepregnancy levels in a matter of days. Studies indicate that women with the greatest fluctuation in the levels of these hormones are most likely to experience depression; this is consistent with other research on chemical dependency and withdrawal (Aytten and Leitch 1964, Brockington and Kumar 1982, Dalton 1988).

Other studies indicate that the onset of postpartum disorders may also be associated with psychosocial factors. Feelings of inadequacy are cited. Role confusion and role conflict in a society with changing expectations for women have been identified as predictive of emotional distress among new mothers. There appears to be a relationship between depression and low socioeconomic status, but this has much stronger predictive value for postpartum depression than for full-blown cases of postpartum psychosis. On the other hand, family dynamics, including the repression of feelings and patterns of passive aggressive personality disorder may be factors in the etiology of both depression and psychosis (Kruckman and Asmann-Finch 1986).

There is disagreement among the experts about whether these psychoses constitute an independent diagnostic category or whether they are manifestations of other disorders, such as manic-depressive psychosis with onset occurring at childbirth. Some psychiatrists argue that childbirth is a period of emotional lability, during which all forms of psychiatric disturbance may occur, and that this diversity of syndromes should not be lumped together into an artificial category called postpartum psychiatric illness. In 1952, the *Diagnostic and Statistical Manual* excluded "psychosis after childbirth," as a distinct diagnostic category; this does not mean that the psychiatric profession doubts the existence of insanity during the postpartum period, but only that there is disagreement about the importance of childbirth as the precipitating factor (Hamilton 1989).

It is clear that the scientific evidence is in conflict. Thus, judges and legislators are left to formulate policy in the absence of definitive knowledge. The legal situation in America is confused. There are no appellate court decisions addressing the status of postpartum psychosis as a defense in infanticide cases, and the record of trial court decisions is spotty, incomplete, and equivocal: the courts are divided on the disposition of cases and inconsistent in the imposition of sentences.

Of the thirty-five cases I have been able to follow, eleven are still in process at the time of this writing. Consequently, there are only twenty-four cases that offer observations about the behavior of courts. The most striking characteristic of these cases is the disparity of result. One-third of these cases (eight) concluded in verdicts of not guilty by reason of insanity. Among the sixteen homicide convictions one finds sentences of probation (four), terms of incarceration of less than five years (three), a term of incarceration of not less than five nor more than twenty years (seven), and life imprisonment (two).

One is hard-pressed to find a rational basis for this disparity in the facts of the cases. Although it appears that women who kill more than one child, women who attempt suicide after committing murder, and women who claim to have heard voices are most likely to be found to have been insane. On the other hand, women who fabricate misleading stories (such as claims that their babies have been kidnapped) are more likely to receive long terms of incarceration. The success of prosecutors in asserting that women who tell self-serving lies cannot be insane is particularly distressing because it flies in the face of psychiatric experience—insanity is by no means a guarantee of honesty, nor of simple-mindedness.

While American justice tolerates extensive disparity in the disposition of infanticide cases—leaving the problem open to the discretion of judges and juries, many other jurisdictions appear to have established uniform and nonpunitive practices. The general trend in Britain, Canada, and several European nations is to treat these cases as instances of mental illness (Kumar 1989). The British Infanticide Act of 1938 (1 & 2 Geo 6 c36), for example, authorizes leniency for a woman convicted of killing her own child under the age of twelve months "if at the time of the act or omission the balance of her mind was disturbed by reason of her not having fully recovered from having given birth to the child or by reason of the effect of lactation consequent upon the birth of the child." Studies of the implementation of this act indicate that the overwhelming majority of infanticide cases in Britain result in suspended sentences, probation, and/or mental health commitments, with a small percentage resulting in short terms of imprisonment (D'Orban 1979, see also Chapter 20).

The challenge facing American jurisdictions is to establish a rationale for more humane treatment of a group of offenders whose emotional condition can be characterized as troubled, whose misbehavior borders on self-destructiveness, and for whom the traditional legal values of deterrence, retribution, and incapacitation are of questionable appropriateness. The confusion in American law appears to be related to the confusion within psychiatry. Reformulation by the mental health professions of the standards for diagnosis contained in the *Diagnostic and Statistical Manual of Mental Disorders* to reincorporate the ancient knowledge that insanity is sometimes produced by parturition would strengthen the legal defense of women who kill their children while suffering from postpartum psychosis. Disparity in the law is partly the result of ambiguity in psychiatry.

On the other hand, however, it may be that outright findings of legal insanity are not always appropriate in these cases, or at least the courts cannot be expected to understand the dimensions of mental illness well enough to reach proper results consistently. Consequently, it may be best to encourage lawmakers in America to consider a middle ground solution that allows for findings of guilt, while authorizing lenient and humanitarian treatment. On the surface, it appears that the verdict of guilty but mentally ill, which has been adopted by thirteen states during the past decade offers such a solution. This approach permits conviction when a court finds that a defendant has committed an offense under circumstances that indicate mental illness of lesser severity than the legal standard of insanity (Callahan et al. 1987). In practice, however, there is reason to fear that verdicts of guilty but mentally ill result in the same level of punitive sanctions as regular guilty pleas (Perlin 1989).

Among the cases I have followed the one that was resolved with a plea of guilty but mentally ill resulted in a prison sentence of ten to twenty years. This suggests that advocates of reform will have to pursue another strategy. Perhaps the best that can be hoped for is that American jurisdictions will follow the British example of special legislation dealing with infanticides perpetrated by mentally ill mothers. But it must be remembered that America is a federal republic, and that criminal law and criminal justice administration are among the powers reserved to the states. With such great diversity among jurisdictions, it does not seem likely that a uniform policy of humanitarian response to infanticides resulting from postpartum psychosis will soon emerge. This is not to suggest that reformers should despair, but only that they should have a realistic perception of the magnitude of the task at hand.

References

American Law Institute (1962). *Model Penal Code.* Section 4.01.

American Psychiatric Association. APA. (1952). *Diagnostic and Statistical Manual of Mental Disorders.* Washington, D.C.: American Psychiatric Press.

Aytten, F. E., and Leitch, I. (1964). *The Physiology of Human Pregnancy.* London: Blackwell.

Brockington, I. F., and Kumar, R. (Eds.) (1982). *Motherhood and Mental Illness.* London: Academic Press.

Callahan, L., Mayer, C., and Steadman, H. J. (1987). Insanity defense reform in the United States—post Hinckley. *Mental and Physical Disability Law Reporter,* 11:54.

Dalton, K. (1988). *Depression after Childbirth: How to Recognize and Treat It.* Oxford: Oxford University Press.

D'Orban, P. T. (1979). Women who kill their children. *Br. J. Psychiatry,* 134: 560–71.

Durham v. United States. 1954. 214 F. 2d 862 (D.C. Cir. 1954).

Goldstein, A. (1967). *The Insanity Defense.* New Haven: Yale University Press.

Hamilton, J. A. (1989). Postpartum psychiatric syndromes. *Psychiatr. Clin. North Am.* 12(1):89–103.

Kruckman, L., and Asmann-Finch, C. (1986). *Postpartum Depression: A Research Guide and International Bibliography.* New York: Garland.

Kumar, R. (1989). Presentation at the Second Conference on Postpartum Psychosis, Infanticide and Criminal Responsibility at the Pennsylvania State University.

Marcé, L. V. (1858). *Traité de la folie des femmes enceintes, des nouvelles accouchées et des nourrices.* Paris: J. B. Ballière et Fils.

M'Naghten, D. (1843). Daniel M'Naghten Case 10 Cl. & F 200, 8 Eng. Rep. 718 (H.L. 1843).

Perlin, M. (1989). *Mental Disability Law, Civil and Criminal* 3(15.27):360.

Walker, N. (1968). *Crime and Insanity in England.* Edinburgh: Edinburgh University Press.

Chapter 22
Postpartum Disorders and the Law
Susan A. Hickman and Donald L. LeVine

Newspapers carry a sensational story about an infant kidnapping and later feature police discovery of what is suspected of being a "baby blues" infanticide.

A new mother with "everything to live for" is reported to have jumped from a bridge, a victim of unexplained suicide.

Infanticide and suicide are two catastrophic outcomes of postpartum psychiatric illness. Although reliable statistics are not available on the incidence of these tragedies, statistical inferences have been made. An Advisory Task Force on Postpartum Psychiatric Illness, called by California State Senator Robert Presley (1989), made an estimate that between 80 and 120 infanticides are committed by psychotic new mothers each year in the United States. This estimate excludes cases of child abuse and murder with criminal intent. The number of suicides by new mothers with postpartum illness is estimated with even less certainty, but it is substantial. Suicide is mentioned occasionally in this chapter because the causes are often similar to the causes of suicide, and suicide attempts are often associated with infanticide.

The legal defense of infanticide cases has some unusual difficulties. One is that jurors and other decision-makers may have deep feelings about the nature of the crime and its perpetrator. Another difficulty when the defense is insanity is that most patients recover from psychiatric illness, and most are likely to appear sane by the time of the trial. A third reason is that the terminology commonly used to designate these cases does not convey the degree and quality necessary to establish a credible position for the legal concept of insanity. Also, the unique qualities of psychosis after childbirth, the confusion, and the striking changeability of the disorder are difficult to convey.

Among psychiatrists knowledgeable about psychiatric illness after childbirth, there is fairly good agreement that the severe cases of postpartum illness divide themselves into two categories. These are described briefly, particularly with regard to the unique features that can lead to violent behavior.

The first is an agitated psychosis that presents itself usually between the third and the fifteenth day after delivery. This is called postpartum psychosis or puerperal psychosis in the unofficial jargon of psychiatry. This psychosis of early onset has a variety of different presentations or syndromes, such as extreme anxiety and agitation, delirium, mania, hallucinations, delusions, and depression. Confusion is pervasive. Sometimes the patient appears to be calm and rational. Sometimes the different presentations change rapidly from one to another, or back to normal for a time.

The postpartum psychosis of early onset may rise to a peak in a few days, last for days or a few weeks, and then recede to a state of *apparent* recovery. Sometimes the florid, agitated forms of the presentation diminish or appear to go away, leaving the patient with a dull, confused depression of mild to moderate severity which may go on for many months. An important feature of this dull depression is that it may sometimes explode into an episode of violent, psychotic behavior which may last for a few hours or days. This exacerbation of psychosis is usually unpredictable, but sometimes it occurs premenstrually. Patients are usually unclear about or have amnesia for their thinking and actions during these episodes of acute psychosis. A small sample of infanticides suggests that at least half of them occurred during these late exacerbations.

Among psychiatric and psychological examiners, there is a predisposition to designate disorders or conditions by the symptoms and signs apparent at the time of the examination. This may result in case histories where the diagnosis changes from psychosis to depression over the course of an illness, as the predominant presentation appears to change. Bernhard Pauliekhoff in Chapter 18 suggests that a change of diagnosis is a serious mistake, since it may lead to neglect of the continuing hazards of the psychosis. He suggests the term "postpartum psychotic depression," since this acknowledges the persistence and the hazard of episodes of frank psychotic behavior throughout the course of the illness.

The second major disorder occurring after childbirth is a slowly developing depression that begins after the second or third week postpartum. It is often accompanied by concurrent physical complaints. The rapidly changing distortions of consciousness of postpartum psychotic depression are absent, although a patient's preoccupation with futility and failure may be so great that this is considered a distortion of reality. The mental state of the patient with this postpartum depression may resemble that of the major depression unrelated to childbearing, although confusion is more apparent and the physical complaints are likely to be more apparent in the postpartum case. The term "major postpartum depression" has been suggested in Chapter 19 for this disorder.

Infanticide is infrequent with major postpartum depression, although planned suicide is a real risk. Cases of infanticide diagnosed as depression, when their histories are subjected to detailed retrospective examination, usually turn out to have had definite psychotic symptoms early in their illness.

Among hospitalized cases of postpartum illness, about five out of six are postpartum psychosis, i.e., the patients have had psychotic symptoms sometime during their illness. The hospitalized cases of major postpartum depression tend to be the severe, sometimes the moderately severe, cases. Instances of moderate to mild major postpartum depression, i.e., women who are office patients with depressive postpartum complaints, may exceed the hospitalized depressive patients by a factor of five to ten. This would not bring them to an incidence of more than ten per 1,000 of the obstetrical population.

The matter of incidence becomes important in court, where a cited incidence of "one postpartum depression in every ten deliveries" may confuse decision-makers. The figure of one in ten comes from a count of yes answers to symptom questions on a written questionnaire, not clinical cases of depression.

The nomenclature manual of the American Psychiatric Association, the *DSM-III-R* (1987) is of little help in elucidating the special qualities of postpartum illness for court decision-makers. Decisions made forty years ago resulted in the elimination of the term and special classification "postpartum," together with any acknowledgment of special qualities or relation to childbearing. Wide latitude is allowed in selecting diagnostic terms. Most common designations are psychosis not otherwise specified (atypical psychosis) (298.90), schizophreniform disorder (295.40), and bipolar disorder, mixed (296.60). None of these named categories nor their official descriptions convey any indication of the unique qualities and hazards of postpartum illness.

An important distinction can be made between the two principal postpartum disorders and the antisocial personality, otherwise known as the sociopath and historically as the psychopath. These are individuals with lifelong histories of violence, impulsive and irresponsible behavior, and conflict with others and with the law. They are the principal offenders in crimes of child abuse. The term antisocial personality designates a defect in character and personality, not an illness.

This discussion of postpartum disorders and the law turns now to matters related to criminal responsibility and defense. A hypothetical case is presented. This case, while it has elements fairly common to many infanticide cases, is not based on a single individual.

Case Study

Marie and Thomas Rogers had been married for three years when Marie became pregnant for the first time with a planned pregnancy. The couple was delighted, and elaborate plans were made for the child's arrival. Marie's pregnancy was somewhat difficult during the third trimester, but delivery was normal. By the second day after delivery, Marie felt fine. She returned home on Day 3. Nursing was somewhat of a problem, with some concern that she did not have enough milk for the baby. On Day 5 she felt intense anxiety for several hours. She was troubled by the anxiety, especially because there seemed to be no reason for it. She called her obstetrician and described a feeling of fear, dread, and an ominous feeling of evil. The obstetrician told Marie not to cry, that occasionally new mothers have strange feelings, and to get some rest. Marie slept poorly that night and was exhausted the following day. Sleep and energy problems continued. She worried about the baby and his health, and it seemed to her that the baby cried a lot. She reported her concern to the pediatrician, but he could find no basis for the mother's worries.

For the next five weeks, Marie spent a great deal of time in bed. She was examined twice by her physician, but no physical ailment could be found. She was prescribed psychotropic medication, but later said that she had not taken it because her husband had said, "How can you ever consider giving up nursing this little boy to take medication?" Marie cried a lot but could never give a reason for her tears. She said that she often had bad dreams, but said that she could not remember the content of the dreams. On several occasions, when friends called, she did not recognize them at first. She often seemed confused. Occasionally, she had spurts of energy, got up and worked for several hours and then returned to her bed.

Gradually she seemed to get better. She spent more time with housework and with the baby. Three months after delivery, Marie weaned the baby and again took him to the pediatrician, again concerned about his health. The pediatrician could find little basis for her concern. Marie began to be unable to sleep even when someone else was caring for the baby. She began to read her Bible several times daily and was singing hymns around the house.

One morning Marie went shopping for groceries, returned home, and telephoned her husband that the baby had been kidnapped from the car while she was in the store. A police hunt was organized, and the baby's body was found in a dumpster. When Marie was interrogated, she said that she may have killed the baby but wasn't sure.

Newspapers that had carried the earlier story of the kidnapping now featured police discovery of the baby's body and the possibility of a "baby blues" infanticide. Examination by a psychiatrist the day after Marie's arrest indicated that Marie was depressed but not psychotic at the time of the examination.

After spending six weeks in jail, Marie was moved to the psychiatric service of a general hospital on bail. Notes of physicians, nurses, and other therapists mentioned a general trend toward reclusiveness and depression, with occasional episodes of gross confusion and bizarre behavior. The discharge diagnosis was major depression.

Five months after the baby's death, Marie has improved somewhat, and the defense counsel prepared the case.

Initial Considerations

The defense attorney needs many critical pieces of information in order to plan an optimal strategy. This information is rarely available without search by an individual familiar with the unique qualities of postpartum illness, ordinarily a health professional. The important areas of information, and the reasons for their importance are discussed below.

Prepregnancy, Prechildbirth Personality

Most cases of infanticide are committed by one of three types of individual: a woman with a postpartum psychosis, one who has an antisocial personality who is inclined toward impulsiveness and violence, and new mothers whose capacity to function is limited by such factors as stress, anxiety, exhaustion, depression, mental retardation, or drugs.

If a defense of not guilty by reason of insanity (NGI) is considered, the investigator is unlikely to find indications of psychotic or prepsychotic behavior prior to pregnancy. (An exception is the rare case of the infanticide by a chronic schizophrenic.) What is important is for the defense to be quite certain that the prosecution has no basis for making a case that the defendant is an impulsive, antisocial personality.

A typical prosecution argument against an insanity defense is that the defendant became angry at the infant because of the continuing and urgent requirements of infant care, and perhaps because of persistent crying or other disturbing features of infant care and responsibility. Finally, goes the argument, the new mother lost her temper and attacked the infant. In effect, the argument represents an effort of the prosecution to portray an infanticide as an example of extreme child abuse. The defense needs ample positive evidence that the character and personality of the accused would make this theory an impossibility. Such evidence is best obtained from old acquaintances, school friends, and work associates. Open-ended questions may yield convincing quotations. School records and teacher evaluations may contribute substantially to the background evaluation.

Behavior Standards and Social Environment

Interviews with former associates lead readily to the determination of whether the defendant was part of an environment that accepted violent behavior for the solution of problems. Examination of the defendant's early history, personality, and environment may lead to information that indicates personality traits, habits, and standards quite contrary to the hypothesis of an explosion of anger: sensitivity, patience, religious faith and beliefs, and actions of social responsibility.

Detailed History after Childbearing

A detailed history of the defendant from delivery to the time of the trial is highly pertinent to the defense. This information includes the events of childbirth, and a day-to-day, detailed account of the first days and weeks after childbirth. Hospital and all medical records, including those of the pediatrician, are very valuable.

Detailed interrogation of those who came in contact with the defendant is important. Different individuals may have seen different clues to abnormal behavior and psychosis, but these clues may not be put together; often they are put aside and forgotten. Confusion, failure to identify friends, periods of uncommunicativeness, and bizarre or irrational statements are all observations that can be overlooked or misinterpreted. Increased or changed activity of a religious nature is often recalled, as in the foregoing case study. Deviations of religious expression that are accepted as normal and appropriate in this society become a matter for analysis when an individual's mode of religious expression changes abruptly after childbirth.

Interrogation of the defendant herself may lead to general statements regarding "feeling badly," "frantic with the baby's illness," "depressed," and "bad dreams." Details may be conspicuous by their absence. Even persistent inquiry may fail to elicit details. It is a general characteristic of postpartum illness that the details, and even major events that occur during psychosis, are forgotten quickly. Memories are like the events of a dream. Whatever is remembered is easily distorted or added to by subsequent discussion or interrogation. Many nineteenth-century physicians tried to describe these states or find similarities to more familiar kinds of behavior. One of the best of the classic treatments was that of H. Hoppe, who compared the mental state to that of a sleepwalker.

Sometimes interrogation of a friend or family member reveals a fragment of conversation or abnormal behavior that may be useful to stimulate the defendant's recall. For example, an informant may remember a reference to the devil. A recurrent hallucination is the change of the infant into a devil. Repetition of the hallucination may give it qualities of a delusion. Such a thought is likely to be unacceptable to the thinking of the new mother, so it is repressed during more lucid intervals.

The investigator is likely to find repeated indications of the unique and remarkable changeability of postpartum psychosis. The defendant in the case study appeared at times to be quite out of contact, hallucinating or grossly delusional, and then exhibited a remission during which she talked at length about practical matters and the infant's health. This is a phenomenon that gives false hope to family members, who interpret it as part of the process of improvement. It is also a phenomenon confusing to those who are concerned with the enforcement of justice. The ordinary concept of severe mental illness is that if one is psychotic, one is always psychotic. The stereotype image of the insane person is an individual who is "crazy all of the time," and obviously so.

The changeable, mercurial quality of postpartum psychosis is often apparent during the hours and days after an infanticide is committed. The death of the infant has the potential of tremendous shock, and an individual who is psychotic is not immune to this shock. The effect of the shock may be a change of the pattern of theme of psychotic thinking, coupled with terror, disorganization, and depression. Thinking may continue to be psychotic, but the theme may be denial and escape. If a suicidal instrument is at hand, it may be used. The psychotic theme may turn to the creation of a reason for the absence of the child. This is usually a bizarre or unbelievable reason, far from a sophisticated alibi. It is a psychotic escape from the result of another psychotic theme. Eventually, the psychosis is likely to evolve into a state of confused depression.

Special Defense Problems

When the personal history, the interviews that illuminate personality, the pregnancy history, the obstetrical and other medical records, and the detailed history of psychiatric events and observations from the date of delivery are assembled, the defense has still other matters to consider.

Psychiatric and Psychological Examinations

The timing of examinations is critical. Most cases of psychiatric illness after childbearing evolve in their symptoms and severity. In general, the symptoms move from psychosis to depression, and then toward recovery. The usual psychiatric examination, and almost all psychological examinations, are designed to determine the mental status at the time of the *examination*. The concern of the criminal justice system is the mental status at the time of the *commission of the crime*. Trials for infanticide often have no psychiatric assessment made in temporal proximity to the crime. The achievement of such an assessment is the first goal of the program of the California legislation initiated by Senator Presley (1989). The defense requirement without this is to look back to the time of the commission of the crime, make inferences from available information regarding the mental state that obtained then, and encourage the court to look at the case from this time frame.

Terminology Confusion

The official terminology is based on patterns of symptoms, and it avoids the important unique features of postpartum illness, the special biological and psychological factors, and the changing illness patterns with time, all of which define postpartum illness. This creates enormous problems in legal proceedings and decisions and may be responsible for the erratic nature of criminal justice decisions in this field. It is not unusual for a defendant who was unquestionably psychotic at the time of infanticide to be sentenced to many years in prison, while a case with less defined criteria of psychosis may receive no penalty at all. Rather than use terms likely to confuse the court, the defense attorney may find it preferable to define and use terms appropriate to psychiatric illness after childbearing. (See Chapter 3.)

The Memory Problem

Memory for events that take place during acute episodes of postpartum psychosis, like the memory of a dream, may be very incomplete, hazy, and sometimes totally absent. Usually, when a new mother is suspected of infanticide, she is subjected to intensive interrogation. The interrogator is likely to have some details regarding the crime and may infer others. Prying for information and admission of guilt, the interrogator may easily firm up, and even reconstruct, the defendant's memory. Events that never happened may be inserted into the clouded memory of the defendant.

More serious, the interrogator can introduce seemingly rational motives for the infanticide into the mind and memory of the defendant, when in truth the infanticide may have had no motive other than the voices, commands, or demands of hallucination and delusion. Later on, even at the time of the trial, the defendant may not be able to distinguish between what took place and what was introduced in the course of interrogation. There is no magic preventive for this kind of memory distortion. Hypnosis and "truth-drug" interrogation have been tried, but their efficacy is far from proved.

The Changing Symptom Pattern

Psychiatric illness after childbearing tends to evolve and change in tandem with the return of female physiology to the nonpregnant state. An agitated psychosis may evolve into a state that may appear to be a mild to moderate depression most of the time. Then *this* may clear. At the time of the trial, the defendant may appear quite normal. This aspect of postpartum illness needs to be explained to every jury.

Prudence in the Choice of a Charge

Other than cases obviously attributable to criminal motives, such as revenge, most cases of infanticide are probably the result of psychosis. Were it realistic to expect decisions based only on principles of criminal law, the kind of psychosis that leads to infanticide probably qualifies, in the great majority of cases, as legal insanity.

Factors such as the confusion in terminology and in records and the difficulty in proving a diagnosis of psychosis when it was not appreciated or was concealed at the time it was acute may make it prudent for the defense attorney to bargain for a charge that does not depend completely on proof of psychosis. The following discussion indicates why this may be the case.

Basic Concepts of Criminal Law

The law of homicide follows this principle: a homicide, in and of itself, simply means the killing of one human being by another. Whether the homicide is first-degree murder, second-degree murder, or some lesser charge such as manslaughter depends on what was going on inside the mind of the accused.

Murder is generally divided into first- and second-degree murder. First-degree murder is "an unlawful killing, the commission of which is willful, deliberate, premeditated and with express malice aforethought" (People v. Anderson 1968). The essence of first-degree murder is the definite cold-blooded intent to kill. Certain types of crime, such as murder by an explosive device, may be determined by statute to be first-degree murder.

The term "malice" as used in the law of homicide does not require hatred, ill will, or spite as it may be interpreted by common usage; rather, the phrase "malice aforethought" encompasses the element of the intent to kill on behalf of the perpetrator. This intent may be expressed or implied. Malice is expressed when there is a conscious, premeditated intent to kill. This is the criterion for first-degree murder. Malice is implied when the killing results from an intentional act involving a high degree of probability that it will result in death. This distinguishes second-degree murder.

The term "aforethought" does not imply deliberation or the lapse of a considerable period of time; it only requires that the required mental state must precede rather than follow the act.

The law searches constantly for precise indicators to facilitate decisions. "Malice aforethought" is such an indicator, but in this case, the indicator overreaches the knowledge upon which it depends for support. This becomes particularly apparent in legal proceedings that seek to pin down and describe the mental state of a woman immediately preceding the act of infanticide. Was this a moment of sane intent?

This is a question to which no valid affirmative answer is possible. As pointed out by Bernhard Pauliekhoff in Chapter 18, if postpartum psychotic depression is present, the psychosis continues from its inception to its cure. It is the symptoms that change. Also, with the characteristic confused, nightmarelike mental state of the psychosis, the determination of mental content at a definite past moment in time would be impossible.

If the element of malice aforethought is missing, then the charge may be that of manslaughter. Various types of manslaughter are designated, but voluntary and involuntary manslaughter are particularly important charges. Voluntary manslaughter is intentional. It is an act committed in anger or upon provocation. Involuntary manslaughter is homicide resulting from gross negligence. The severity of a charge may be reduced because of voluntary intoxication, drugs or mental state, stress, or mental disorder. A murder charge can be reduced to either voluntary or involuntary manslaughter. If the mental disorder is such that it meets the criteria for not guilty by reason of insanity, this will undermine a conviction for murder or manslaughter.

In the foregoing case study, the defendant Marie Rogers might be charged with either second-degree murder or manslaughter. If the investigation of her personal history, background, and personality revealed no indications of antisocial personality or a predilection for violence, and if the investigation accumulated a substantial amount of information pointing toward the defendant having had a postpartum psychosis, a defense of not guilty by reason of insanity may be appropriate. If the information does not provide substantial support for establishing a case for the retrospective diagnosis of a psychosis, the defense may find it prudent to seek a charge of manslaughter and then present mitigating evidence such as depression, confusion, exhaustion, or anxiety. Evidence favoring the hypothesis of a psychosis may be presented, but the proof of insanity is not an absolute requirement.

Competency to Stand Trial

If a defendant continues to exhibit psychosis symptoms, it may be necessary to determine whether or not she is competent to stand trial. The rule in most jurisdictions holds that a person cannot be tried or adjudged to punishment while that person is mentally incompetent.

A person is mentally incompetent if, as a result of mental disorder, that person is unable to understand the nature of the criminal proceeding or to assist in the conduct of his or her own defense. The standard of competency is a very minimal standard. If a defendant in an infanticide case is found to be incompetent, she will be sent to a mental institution, but she will not receive treatment in the usual sense of the word. Rather, she may be given medicine to stabilize her condition and be taught who the parties are in a court proceeding and what each does. Once she knows the role of the judge, the prosecutor, and her own attorney and is taught to cooperate with counsel, she can be certified as competent. When this occurs, criminal proceedings can be reinstated, and the defendant will proceed to trial.

If a person has been adjudged to be incompetent, this has no direct bearing on the issue of NGI. However, the finding of incompetence could assist the defense attorney in arguing for that decision. Since the trend of most cases of postpartum psychosis is toward recovery, the need for competency training is rare. That it is considered at all is close to prima facie evidence that the diagnosis of a chronic disorder with psychosis, such as Sheehan's syndrome, has been missed.

Insanity at the Time of the Offense

The word "psychotic" is a medical term that indicates gross impairment in the testing of reality. The expression "gross impairment in the testing of reality" implies incorrect evaluation of perceptions and thoughts, and incorrect inferences about external reality, even in the face of contrary evidence. Direct evidence of psychotic behavior is the presence of either delusions or hallucinations without insight into their pathological nature. A hallucination is an apparent sensory perception without external stimulation of the relevant sensory organ (hearing voices, seeing visions, or perceiving things as grossly distorted). A delusion is a false belief based on incorrect inference about external reality and maintained firmly despite incontrovertible evidence and general acceptance of a contrary inference (belief that God personally directs one's own actions; belief that one must take certain actions to save the world).

Although the medical definition of psychosis differs from the legal definition of insanity, the establishment of firm evidence for a psychosis can be a long step toward the legal establishment of insanity. A Work Group of the American Psychiatric Association developed useful concepts on bridging the gap between psychosis and insanity (Insanity Defense Work Group 1983).

Two legal definitions of insanity are current, and the defense attorney will know which is operative in a given jurisdiction. The first is the M'Naghten rule, which holds that a person was insane at the time of an offense if she had a disorder that makes a person incapable of knowing or understanding that her act was wrong. The thrust of the M'Naghten rule is in the word "knowing," and the application of the rule is said to be a cognitive test.

The second definition is in the Federal rule, a policy adopted by most jurisdictions in the United States. This rule holds that a person is not responsible for criminal conduct, as a result of severe mental disease or defect, if he or she was unable to *appreciate* the wrongfulness of the act. The term "appreciate" goes beyond the simple knowledge of whether an act is "right or wrong," and requires a deeper understanding at a level of feelings and emotions regarding the act. The implications of this are ably discussed by R. L. Goldstein (1989), who subsumes postpartum psychotic behavior under the general rubric of postpartum depression.

Despite various differences in the application of these tests, the situation of psychotic postpartum patients is likely to qualify as insanity under either rule. The common element is *control*. If, at the time of the infanticide, the accused was suffering from a disorder characterized by grossly distorted reality, by perceptions dominated by hallucinations, or thinking dominated by delusions, it follows that she would have no capability to control her knowledge of the act, to control her judgment whether it was right or wrong, or to control her feelings about the crime. On the contrary, the psychotic state that predisposes to infanticide almost always includes the mandate that the act *must* be done for some high purpose, the welfare or salvation of the infant or the salvation of the world. The control feature is very characteristic of the psychosis that predisposes to infanticide. An eerie quality of the psychosis, in women with strong religious backgrounds or beliefs, is that the hallucinations and delusions often take the form of commands by the deity that the act of infanticide be done.

The expert witness in a postpartum case must bear in mind that he or she is dealing with a psychosis, the symptoms and patterns of which may change from time to time, and they may change rapidly. Also, the symptoms may diminish spontaneously, or they may appear to be interrupted by human intervention, a telephone call, a visitor, or such routine events as stopping at a traffic signal or making a purchase in a store. These are not recoveries from the psychosis; they are interruptions of symptoms. (See Chapter 18.)

A jury may be influenced by its estimate of the social hazard of releasing the accused. A recovered psychosis after childbearing has little chance of recurrence except after another pregnancy. The mental health expert can state correctly that prophylactic measures for such patients are available. (See Chapter 17.)

Many reasons may influence the defense attorney to seek a charge of lesser degree than murder and to construct a case based on mitigating circumstances: depression, exhaustion, marital stress, physical disability, or limited capability. This decision depends on the individual case and need not be discussed here. This chapter purports to be neither a guide for the defense witness nor a manual for the defense attorney. It outlines some of the problems of each, for the other. The details of evolving legal thinking and strategies are followed and reported by Vivian M. Keller, J.D.*

The possibility that new mothers can be involved in violent activity and infanticide received little attention, perhaps consistent avoidance, for many years. The taboo is lifting. The new openness is attributable to several factors:

Criminal Practice Manuals. Bureau of National Affairs, Inc., 1231 Thirty-Fifth St., N.W., Washington, D.C. 20037.

1. Many women in support groups have begun to talk about these matters and to guide sick new mothers toward help.
2. Conferences on criminal responsibility of new mothers have been held in 1987 and 1989, sponsored by the Administration of Justice Department, Pennsylvania State University. Professor Daniel Maier Katkin of this university is the author of Chapter 21.
3. Media coverage has resulted in widespread awareness.

Now, physicians, patients, and families can talk about postpartum illness and take precautions. Patients, by talking about bizarre, dreamlike ideas, may defuse the translations of thoughts into actions. With the new and open attention directed toward postpartum psychiatric illness, it is likely that the incidence of the disasters of infanticide and suicide, and the incidence of erratic case dispositions, will decrease markedly.

References

American Psychiatric Association (1987). *Diagnostic and Statistical Manual of Mental Disorders,* 3rd ed., revised. Washington, DC: American Psychiatric Press.

Goldstein, R. L. (1989). The psychiatrist's guide to right and wrong: Part III: Postpartum depression and the "appreciation" of wrongfulness. *Bull. Am. Acad. Psychiatry Law,* 17:121–28.

Insanity Defense Work Group (1983). American Psychiatric Association statement on the insanity defense. *Am. J. Psychiatry,* 140:681–88.

People v. Anderson 1965. 70 Cal. 2d 15, 73 Cal. Rptr. 550, 447 P. 2d 942.

Presley, R. (1989). Senate Concurrent Resolutions (Cal.) No. 23 and 39, February 9 and May 30, 1989.

Chapter 23
Medical Insurance Litigation Problems of Postpartum Patients

Mark D. DeBofsky

Introduction

One of the most tragic consequences of postpartum psychiatric illness is the wrongful deprivation of insurance reimbursement for the medical and hospital expenses incurred in the treatment of the disorder. This occurs despite substantial legal precedent that supports payment of such claims.

The grounds for denial of benefits are twofold. The first reason is due to the nature of insurance coverage that is available in the United States. While some policies of insurance will pay substantial indemnity for treatment of mental or nervous disorders, the majority of insurance policies either provide no coverage or drastically limit payment for mental illness. Even with such policies, though, based upon strong legal precedent, postpartum psychiatric illness should be covered in the same manner as any other disease or illness. That is because of the organic etiology of the disorder and its relationship to the physiology of pregnancy. Unfortunately, physicians treating patients with such conditions fail to stress this fact in their diagnoses; and instead, follow the terminology of the *Diagnostic and Statistical Manual of Mental Disorders*, which lacks an accurate, descriptive portrayal of what medical science now knows about postpartum psychiatric illness. This ignorance encourages insurers, who are themselves uninformed of the disorder, to refuse payment of benefits.

The consequences of the insurers' denial of coverage for postpartum psychiatric illness are tragic to sufferers of the condition who are suddenly faced with enormous expenses that their insurers will not reimburse. As will be explained below, such misfortune can be avoided, and postpartum psychiatric illness should be indemnified regardless of limitations or exclusions in insurance policies. But if a claim is denied, there should be no reluctance to challenge the insurer's determination, even in the courts, if necessary.

Principles of Insurance Law and Coverage

Insurance coverage for psychiatric treatment is not always available. Some states, such as Massachusetts, have required insurers writing health insurance policies in that state, to provide at least minimal coverage for psychiatric treatment. Such an approach has been approved by the United States Supreme Court. In Metropolitan Life Insurance Company v. Massachusetts, 471 U.S. 724 (1985), the court ruled that it was within the power of a state's regulation of insurance companies to impose a requirement that psychiatric benefits be provided. Not every state requires insurers to issue such coverage, though, and to limit claims for psychotherapy and psychiatric hospitalizations, many insurance carriers have limited, if not excluded, coverage for mental or nervous disorders which would be defined in the typical insurance policy as "neurosis, psychoneurosis, psychopathy, psychosis, or mental or emotional disease or disorder of any kind."

Even if insurance coverage is available, however, it may not be sufficient to pay for the entire expense of treatment of postpartum psychiatric illness. Accordingly, it is necessary to construct a strategy to qualify postpartum psychiatric illness as a complication of pregnancy, which is commonly described in insurance contracts as

(1) Conditions requiring medical treatment prior or subsequent to termination of pregnancy whose diagnoses are distinct from pregnancy but are adversely affected by pregnancy or are caused by pregnancy, such as acute nephritis, nephrosis, cardiac decompensation, missed abortion, disease of the vascular, hemopoietic, nervous or endocrine systems, and similar medical and surgical conditions of comparable severity, and shall not include false labor, occasional spotting, physician-prescribed rest during the period of pregnancy, morning sickness and similar condition associated with the management of a difficult pregnancy not constituting a classifiably distinct complication of pregnancy;
(2) Caesarean section, ectopic pregnancy which is terminated, and spontaneous termination of pregnancy which occurs during a period of gestation in which a viable birth is not possible; and
(3) hyperemesis gravidarum and pre-eclampsia

When it can be shown to the satisfaction of the insurer that the claim indeed involves a complication of pregnancy and not a mental disorder, the claim should be paid in full because it is the rare insurance policy that would limit coverage for physical illness in the same manner as psychiatric coverage is restricted.

The problem, of course, is with the terminology. The *Diagnostic and Statistical Manual of Mental Disorders,* third edition (*DSM-III*), does not clearly describe the nature of postpartum psychiatric illness. While the index to the *DSM-III* lists several possible categories under which such conditions may be classified, there is no discrete listing for postpartum psychiatric illness, which is now recognized by those knowledgeable in the field to represent several illnesses, of which postpartum psychosis is the most serious. Worse, though, is the recent revision to the *DSM-III,* the so-called *DSM-III-R,* which does not even contain a reference to postpartum psychiatric disorders in its index, but groups the condition under atypical psychosis. Because of the lack of a definite classification, physicians admitting patients suffering from postpartum psychiatric disorders will often record a diagnosis of atypical psychosis without any further explanation. When the claim is later sent to the insurer for reimbursement, the insurer reads such a diagnosis as falling within its definition for mental or nervous disorders, and the claim is often subsequently denied.

To avoid refusal of benefits for treatment of postpartum psychiatric illness, it is necessary for the physician to be cognizant of nomenclature and insurance claims practices. One possible approach that can be used at present given the current state of the *Diagnostic and Statistical Manual,* is to diagnose the illness under Axis I as an organic mental disorder not otherwise specified (294.80). Under the Axis III diagnosis, childbirth should be listed in order to stress the relationship of postpartum psychiatric illness to childbirth and to emphasize the hormonal involvement.

This strategy will bring the claim closer to other cases in which courts have ordered organic mental disorders to be indemnified by insurers even when the insurance policy excludes mental or nervous illnesses. Thus, in Sachs v. Commercial Insurance Company of Newark, N.J., 119 N.J. Super. 226, 290 A.2d 760 (1972), the court determined:

The limitation [on payment for mental or nervous disorders] was intended to apply to purely mental disorders involving functional etiology, and not to mental symptomology produced by organic disease.

The court explained its ruling by stating:

It is reasonable to assume that the limitation [on payment for mental or nervous disorders] was intended to delimit claims in cases of insanity or other degrees of mental aberration which are functional in origin. The public would not expect that such a limitation would control merely because the end result of an organic disease may affect the mental function of an individual.

The *Sachs* decision was based on an earlier decision of the New York Court of Appeals, the highest court of that state. In Prince v. United States Life Insurance Company in the City of New York, 42 Misc.2d 410, 248 N.Y.S.2d 336 (1964); *affirmed* 23 A.D.2d 723, 257 N.Y.S.2d 891 (1965); *affirmed* 17 N.Y.2d 742, 270 N.Y.S.2d 891 (1966), suit was brought against an insurer by an individual who had suffered an emotional disturbance as a result of a traumatic injury. Citing a policy exclusion for mental disorders, the insurer had refused to reimburse the policyholder for his medical expenses, and litigation was brought to force the insurer to indemnify the claim. The claimant was able to successfully argue that since there was coverage for accidental bodily injury and sickness or disease, an organically induced mental disorder should also be a covered expense. The court agreed with the argument and found:

The average person is not familiar with mental disease from the strictly medical point of view—and a layman is not required to read his policy as if he were a psychiatrist [citation omitted]. A layman would read the exception as applying to mental disorders unconnected with bodily injury.

This decision was also in accord with a ruling of the Supreme Court of Minnesota. In Gareis v. Benefit Association of Railway Employees Insurance Company, 169 N.W.2d 730 (1969), a trial court had found against an insurer and in favor of an individual who suffered a disease that damaged his nervous system causing memory loss and incoherence. The insurance company appealed, contending that the loss was a mental disorder and not a covered expense. Affirming the trial court, the Minnesota Supreme Court determined that

"mental disorder" in medical terminology, may be either organic or functional. But the meaning of the term medically is not necessarily the meaning assigned to this language by common usage. It is the meaning ordinarily conveyed to the popular mind that controls in construing the language of policies of insurance made available to the general public. We believe it is as likely as not that people would consider "mental disorder" refers only to a situation where an individual's mental functions are abnormal due to causes which cannot be explained in terms of the physiological changes attributable to the disease. (169 N.W.2d at 731.)

Then, following generally established principles of insurance law, the court ruled:

In the absence of evidence clarifying this ambiguity [between the term "mental disorder" as it would commonly be understood and a functional "mental disorder"], it should be resolved in favor of the insured, the insurer having chosen the language of the policy and being the one best able to make clear the meaning of the words used. Upon this principle, we believe that the trial court's determination that the disease suffered by the insured was not a "mental disorder" within the meaning of the policy even though this disease produced neurological changes resulting in loss of memory, was right as a matter of law. (169 N.W.2d at 732)

In each of these cases, the courts found that there was a conflict between insurance contract provisions insuring for bodily injury, sickness and disease, and the exclusion for mental disorders, and the courts resolved the conflict in a manner that the ordinary person would understand, which distinguished between functional and organic disorders to find coverage for organic disorders.

For many years, these cases provided the only guidance to resolving disputes over coverage for physiologically caused mental disorders. Recently, though, there has been a spate of decisions that have considered this issue. Indeed, in one case, the court went as far as ruling that treatment for chemical dependency would not be subjected to limitations for mental or emotional illness. In Hayden v. Guardian Life Insurance Company of America, 500 So.2d 811 (La.App. 1986), the court ruled that since there is substantial legal, medical, and scientific support for the propositions that alcoholism and drug dependency are sicknesses, it would be improper not to pay for treatment of such disorders in the same manner as other sicknesses are compensated. Another recent decision reasoned that in reviewing a claim for bipolar affective disorder it is improper for the insurance company to classify the illness by symptom rather than cause. Accordingly, in Arkansas Blue Cross and Blue Shield v. Doe, 733 S.W.2d 429 (Ark.App. 1977), the court disregarded the insurer's argument that psychotherapy was used to treat the illness, and found that treatment for a bipolar affective disorder is compensable in the same manner as other illnesses. The psychotherapy, according to the court, was merely part of getting the patient to accept the illness and to cope with her disorder, and that the psychotherapist needed to monitor the patient's medications.

Finally, the decisions cited above, Sachs and Prince, were followed in Malerbi v. Central Reserve Life of North America Insurance Company, 225 Neb. 543, 407 N.W.2d 157 (1987). The Nebraska Supreme Court reviewed a lower court decision awarding insurance benefits to the parents of a youth who was diagnosed as suffering from atypical organic brain syndrome with obsessive-compulsive features. The illness had been diagnosed by computerized tomography and by neuropsychological testing, and there was substantial evidence before the court that the patient was suffering from a dysfunction of the temporal lobe of his brain which was causing seizures and behavior problems. Following the earlier decisions, the court ruled that the plaintiffs would have generally understood an organically caused psychological disorder to be compensable in the same manner as any other physiological illness. Because the language of the insurance policy did not clearly delineate any difference between organic and functional disorders, the court ordered the insurer to pay the expenses of treatment.

The cases cited above represent virtually the entire sum and substance of reported decisions on the issue of insurance coverage for psychiatric illness of organic cause, which would be applicable to postpartum psychiatric illness. No specific ruling, however, has ever been issued concerning coverage for postpartum mental disorders. These decisions, which are based on established propositions of insurance law, point the way to finding coverage whenever there can be two interpretations of an insurance policy—one favoring coverage and the other denial of benefits. Generally, the more restrictive interpretation that would bar recovery will be overlooked by the courts.

Expectations of the average consumer support a finding that postpartum psychiatric illness would be a covered disease not excludable as a mental or nervous disorder since the condition is so closely related to the pregnancy. As a disease of the body, there can be no distinction between postpartum psychiatric illness and cardiovascular disease that causes, for example, a cerebrovascular accident or stroke. Both conditions, caused by physiological factors, have emotional consequences. Moreover, denial of insurance coverage for postpartum psychiatric illness, while allowing benefits for other bodily disorders, creates a conflict between the provisions of the insurance contract. Under general principles of insurance law that favor indemnification of losses where conflicts exist, claims for postpartum psychiatric illness must be paid in the same manner as payment for other complications of pregnancy.

Federal Legislation Affecting Coverage

The foregoing principles, however, are limited in a new area of insurance litigation that is becoming more prevalent. As part of the federal pension reform legislation passed in 1974, known as the Employee Retirement Income Security Act (ERISA), the statute regulates any employee welfare plan that, through the purchase of insurance or otherwise, provides medical, surgical, or hospital care or benefits in the event of sickness, accident, disability, or death. 29 U.S.C. §1002(1). Interpretive decisions issued by the United States Supreme Court have indicated that any form of health insurance provided by an employer will be governed by ERISA. Pilot Life Insurance Co. v. Dedeaux, 481

U.S. 41, 95 L.Ed.2d 39 (1987); Metropolitan Life Insurance Company v. Taylor, 481 U.S. 58, 95 L.Ed.2d 55 (1987). These rulings make it clear that suits for denial of insurance benefits, claims ordinarily brought as actions for breach of contract, will be replaced by ERISA. Until recently, this meant that the policyholder who is denied benefits faced a much more difficult standard of proof before denial of a claim will be overturned. A suit for denial of benefits brought under ERISA previously was reviewed only to determine whether the refusal to pay the claim was arbitrary and capricious, and the courts upheld the insurer unless its decision was arbitrary, capricious, or motivated by bad faith. What this meant was that so long as the insurer was able to provide a satisfactory explanation for its decision that includes a rational connection between the facts found and the choice made, the decision would be upheld. On February 21, 1989, this standard of review was overturned by the United States Supreme Court. In a surprising decision, the court held in Firestone Tire and Rubber Company v. Bruch, 109 S.Ct. 948 (1989) 57 U.S.L.W. 4194 (2/21/89), that courts should no longer apply the arbitrary and capricious standard, but instead must conduct a searching examination of the decision denying benefits, known as a de novo review. The court left open the possibility that employer-provided insurance plans could be redrafted to impose a higher standard of review, but unless that is done, a claimant need merely show that the denial of benefits was in error.

Although the impact of the ERISA statute has been minimized by the recent ruling of the Supreme Court, it can be anticipated that employers will seek to exploit the loophole left open by the court and amend their plans to impose a requirement that denials of benefits are to be reviewed only to determine if the decision was arbitrary and capricious. Accordingly, medical practitioners in this area should be especially careful to demonstrate the organicity of the condition. It is up to the medical profession to educate the insurers of the cause of postpartum psychiatric disorders and that, in fact, such illnesses are a complication of pregnancy in the same way as the other complications of pregnancy enumerated at the outset of this chapter in the sample definition provided.

Putting aside the issue of the standard of review, the ERISA statute probably has its greatest impact on insurance claims for coverage of postpartum psychiatric illness on the issue of damages, which are limited in ERISA claims. Many states allow damages against insurers for their "bad faith" in denial of claims or for the infliction of mental distress caused by the wrongful denial of claims. If a postpartum psychiatric illness claim is raised and the insurance policy involved is not provided by an employer, an argument can be made that the insurer's failure to pay the claim was a bad faith action, and damages can be awarded in excess of the medical expenses at issue to compensate for such consequences and to punish the insurer for having engaged in wrongful conduct. Under ERISA, though, the United States Supreme Court has interpreted the statute to totally reject payment of any damages other than compensation for the charges that have been incurred for treatment of the postpartum psychiatric disorders, along with payment of attorneys' fees, which are generally allowed.

Conclusion

The import of the foregoing discussion is that a claim for postpartum psychiatric illness can and should be covered by insurance even if the insurance policy at issue contains a limitation or exclusion of coverage for treatment of mental or nervous disorders. Insurance companies must be required to look beyond the undifferentiated diagnosis to determine the origin of the illness. If the cause is insurable, the resulting condition should also be indemnified. Nonetheless, it is incumbent upon the doctors and nurses who work in this field to refrain from simple diagnoses. Terminology must be clarified both with respect to the *Diagnostic and Statistical Manual of Mental Disorders* and the International Classification of Diseases so that postpartum psychiatric illness is recognized as a discrete organic disorder related to the physiology of pregnancy and childbirth. Until that day comes, though, documentation of the cause of the illness along with supportive medical journal articles should be provided to the insurers so that if payment of the claims is denied, it can be established that the refusal to pay benefits was wrongful. And because of the possibility of review under the arbitrary and capricious standard, it should be emphasized to the insurer that denial of coverage would be irrational and would go against the weight of medical authority.

Since most people are covered by insurance provided by employers, it should always be anticipated that the federal ERISA statute would govern the claim and its administration, and therefore, it is important to document as much as possible the basis for organicity. Also, in the event ERISA would not apply, a finding that denial of benefits was arbitrary and capricious would almost certainly support a "bad faith" claim and entitle the insured not only to recovery of the medical and hospital charges but would also compensate for the mental anguish caused by wrongful denial of coverage.

Insurance coverage for postpartum psychiatric illness is an issue that is often overlooked in the concern to treat the patient. Yet long after the patient has recovered, the legacy of unpaid bills could be as calamitous as the initial illness. Avoidance of claim denials by insurance carriers should be the goal, and with thought and careful documentation, insurance coverage should be provided.

References

American Psychiatric Association (1980, 1987). *Diagnostic and Statistical Manual of Mental Disorders, DSM-III, DSM-III-R.* Washington, DC: American Psychiatric Association.

Arkansas Blue Cross and Blue Shield v. Doe, 733 S.W. 2d 429 (Ark.App. 1977).

Employee Retirement Income Security Act (ERISA), 29 U.S.C. §1002 (1).

Firestone Tire and Rubber Co. v. Bruch, 109 S.Ct.948 (1989) 57 U.S.L.W. 4194 (2/21/89).

Gareis v. Benefit Association of Railroad Employees Insurance Co., 169 N.W. 2d 730 (1969).

Hayden v. Guardian Life Insurance Co. of America, 500 So. 2d 811 (La.App. 1986).

Malerbi v. Central Reserve Life of North America Insurance Co., 225 Neb. 543, 407 N.W. 2d 157 (1987).

Metropolitan Life Insurance Co. v. Massachusetts, 471 U.S. 724 (1985).

Metropolitan Life Insurance Co. v. Taylor, 481 U.S. 58, 95 L. Ed. 2d 55 (1987).

Pilot Life Insurance Co. v. Dedeaux, 481 U.S. 41, 95 L. Ed. 2d 39 (1987).

Prince v. United States Life Insurance Co. in the City of New York, 42 Misc. 2d 410, 248 N.Y.S. 2d 336 (1964); affirmed 23 A.D. 2d 723, 257 N.Y.S. 2d 891 (1965); affirmed 17 N.Y. 2d 742, 270 N.Y.S. 2d 891 (1966).

Sachs v. Commercial Insurance Co. of Newark N.J., 119 N.J. Super. 226, 290 A. 2d 760 (1972).

Chapter 24
Husband Support: A Neglected Aspect of Postpartum Psychiatric Illness

Robert Hickman

Psychiatric illness occurring after childbirth can be conceptualized as a spectrum of disorders that ranges from mild to severe depression and postpartum psychosis (Inwood 1985). Although the illness manifests itself within the new mother, it should be construed in a larger context, since the husband, the family and friends are all affected by the illness. Moreover, those close to the patient can play important roles supporting her treatment and influencing the outcome. The role of the husband is of critical importance. As the new mother's ability to fulfill important functions is diminished, he is expected to step in and compensate for his wife's disability. The demands on his time, energy, and patience can reach overwhelming proportions, yet he is needed to provide positive support to his wife throughout the illness.

The author of this chapter is a marriage and family therapist, and along with his wife heads a clinic specializing in treating postpartum disorders. Group therapy is remarkably effective in this area, since postpartum patients derive great benefit from meeting others who have had similar illnesses. Learning of their experiences first-hand and witnessing favorable therapeutic outcomes are very beneficial.

In the course of dealing with postpartum patients, I had occasion to talk with many husbands who accompanied their wives to the clinic. It has been apparent to me that much anxiety and fear, and sometimes anger, was exhibited or frequently concealed by these husbands. Seeing several of them in professional consultation confirmed my suspicion that postpartum illness generated many real problems among husbands of patients.

Since the sharing of experiences was so effective with new mother patients in support groups, it occurred to me that a group of husbands of postpartum patients would be an effective therapeutic innovation. This proved to be the case, a great deal was learned, and the participants affirmed that this approach was quite helpful. A second group of husbands has been organized and is in operation. This chapter presents a brief summary of the five principal problems and problem areas husbands presented, and some of the solutions that developed. Solutions often evolved from or were reinforced by the experiences of others in the group.

One of the first to document the reality of marital stress in postpartum psychiatric illness was Bruce Pitt (1968). He noted that marital problems that appeared to have been induced by postpartum illness often persisted long after most symptoms had abated. The importance of social support in expediting recovery, especially support by the husband, was stressed by Paykel and coworkers (1980). O'Hara and associates (1982) found evidence of a correlation between women's reports of earlier poor marital relationships and postpartum depression. J. Hamilton (1985), anxious to increase the participation of husbands and other family members in the diagnostic, therapeutic, and follow-up process, routinely initiated a family conference with the psychiatrist at the beginning of hospital treatment. Arizmendi and Affonso (1987) found that interpersonal stresses had an adverse effect on postpartum depression.

The first direct study of husbands' responses to postpartum illness was made by J. Harvey and G. McGrath (1988). These authors found that anxiety and depression were the principal reactions to a wife's postpartum illness. The present report, without quantification or control, seeks only to describe the nature of stresses, problems, and complaints that emerge in semidirected discussions with husbands, together with some answers that have developed.

The configuration of a husband group may vary greatly. With husbands' time under severe limitations, monthly meetings appear to be the most feasible. We were able to arrange meetings concurrent with patients' meetings. Among the leader's functions are an explanation of the illness (where an organic interpretation meets a very favorable reception), reassurance that postpartum illness is not a sign of other mental illness, and reassurance that postpartum illness, sometimes with a tedious course, has an excellent prognosis.

With husband groups, a number and variety of problems emerge rapidly. The areas of most concern and importance are described below, together with a few generalizations and/or solutions pertaining to each one.

The Predominant Problems

Family Relationships

All family relationships, and especially the marriage, can become severely strained. If the wives are severely incapacitated or hospitalized, the husbands may become the primary caregiver of the infant. If older children are present, the process of meeting their needs becomes very complex. Many husbands expressed exasperation because of the enormity of parenting demands. Husbands feel anxious because of the increased responsibilities and resentful as a result of the problems created by the illness, especially if it is protracted.

One aspect of postpartum illness is that the severe phase of illness may last a few weeks and then be replaced by a mild to moderate depression which may last for several months. Patients may be home on medication, and this can contribute to dullness and unresponsiveness. Husbands may note the marked improvement and then interpret the unresponsiveness of the later phase as personal rejection.

Solutions

The sharing of experiences in a husbands' group can be very beneficial. Reactions of the patient that can be interpreted as rejection or change of personality can be reinterpreted by other participants or the informed group leader. Sometimes husbands urge premature discontinuation of medications, and this can be interpreted as counterproductive, even dangerous. Husbands may also become overprotective of children and retard the gradual relinquishing of the mothering role to the recovering patient. Parents of the wife or husband may perform an invaluable service during the illness and then overprotect the child as the mother recovers. These parents can become a destructive influence because they misunderstand the etiology of the illness. Sometimes simplistic or judgmental explanations for the illness are inferred. The wife may be accused of malingering if the illness persists. The parents of one husband in the group were extremely critical of the wife because of the persistent depression she experienced. An informed husband can sense and rectify such misunderstandings.

Medical Concerns

The postpartum psychiatric illnesses are largely underrecognized. Since the manifestations are largely psychiatric in nature, treatment by a psychiatrist who is familiar with postpartum illness, or at least interest, is essential. Many husbands in the group reported frustration trying to to find a knowledgeable psychiatrist. One husband was told by a psychiatrist that he would not accept his wife as a patient if the couple believed that the illness was caused by a hormonal imbalance.

A nonmedical group leader can be put in a difficult position if asked directly about the qualifications of a physician. Often, if this is thrown out to the group, husbands may have some useful opinions. The leader can run no risk by indicating the physicians he knows are capable.

The couple who are dissatisfied with their psychiatric care have one resource that can be explained to them. Quite within the range of medical propriety and ethics, they can request a consultation, and a group leader can recommend a psychiatrist known to be capable.

One phenomenon has been observed in several husbands and may threaten the outcome of treatment. If an illness lasts longer than expected, husbands may begin to deny the severity of the illness. They may begin to suspect their wives of malingering and that they would be better off reducing the dosage of medication. Husbands may view reduction of the need for medication as the point where true progress is made. One husband in the group adamantly adhered to this belief, despite the caution he was urged to take by the leader. His need to put the illness behind him caused him to exert pressure on his wife to reduce the dosage of her medication. This could lead a wife to hide her distress from her husband. In cases involving psychosis, this situation could result in suicide or infanticide. It is incumbent on the leader to point out risks of relapse or recurrence following changes from recommended dosage without prior medical approval.

In many cases of postpartum illness, the husband or another family member will be asked to monitor medication. This requires great care. In cases of psychosis, patients may stop taking medicine because they have a delusion that it is poison. Problems of this kind or any unnatural behavior should be reported promptly to the physician.

Couples planning on attempting to have subsequent pregnancies should be warned of the substantial increase in the risk of recurrence, once one has had a postpartum illness. It is said that, while the risk of a severe postpartum illness is of the order of one in one thousand, this risk increases to one in three or four with a subsequent pregnancy. Many couples have been led to believe by well-meaning but uninformed individuals that such an increased risk does not exist. In one tragic case, an infanticide occurred after a couple was reassured by a licensed nurse-midwife that it was unlikely that the wife would become psychotic after a subsequent pregnancy (Japenga 1987). Couples need to know of this risk but also that there are prophylactic treatments which may reduce the risk substantially. (See Chapter 17.)

Financial Concerns

The financial concerns of husbands are often very great. The cost of psychiatric hospitalization is very high, yet psychiatric controls may be necessary to care for a patient safely.

One of the functions of a group leader is to provide advice on the procurement of adequate medical and hospital services within the financial capability of the patient or family. The most welcome advice is that a well-crafted diagnosis and skilled legal representation may result in the discovery that patients do, indeed, have good insurance coverage. The usual coverage for all kinds of special obstetrical problems is likely to cover postpartum illness, although this is a closely held secret. (See Chapter 23.)

The availability of public mental hospital facilities varies widely from one location to another. In some areas, physicians are very well informed about treatment of postpartum disorders. The leader of a husbands' support group can readily determine the facilities available with a few calls to social agencies. If a well-informed psychiatrist or physician advises that psychiatric hospital controls are necessary for the safety of the patient and funds are not available, husbands should be urged to make use of public facilities. Round-the-clock care and surveillance at home is an enormous and hazardous undertaking.

Family Activities and Plans

When a new mother becomes incapacitated by postpartum psychiatric illness, the family curtails many activities and plans, especially as symptoms are developing. When the symptoms are severe, curtailment is also severe and longlasting.

The husband's activities related to leisure and personal enrichment become limited out of necessity because of the burden of family management chores and patient care. Relaxation associated with these activities becomes a luxury and is replaced by worry and preoccupation. Many husbands in the group appeared weary as a result of the ongoing demands of their situation.

Social Relationships

As with other mental disorders, families of patients often experience social isolation. Many people still attach a stigma to mental illness.

Those who do not understand the condition may perceive it as a threat to their well-being and status within the community and distance themselves from it. An ill-defined dread of mental illness may be a motivating factor.

While couples with newborns tend to form relationships with other new parents, severe postpartum illness can obstruct this important pattern of friendship and support. One husband in the group and his wife felt extremely isolated socially after the birth of their first child. They attempted to get involved with other parents but felt that the others could not relate with the experiences associated with the illness. Consequently, this couple chose to help other new parents in this situation by forming a support group for wives and husbands.

The Long Road to Recovery

For husbands and families, the impact of postpartum psychiatric illness often increases with the duration of illness. The following reports by husbands provide some appreciation of the burden they carry.

For husbands, postpartum illness is an experience of loss, uncertainty, and concern. They may fear for the health and safety of their family without knowing what course of action may be useful. At the same time that a husband wants to be helpful, he may also feel alone and unsupported. All of his feelings are valid. In fact, he has lost the home he knew, the woman he loves, and the immediate future that he came to expect. These reactions, in addition to other common feelings of anger, frustration, sadness, and embarrassment, can make the course of this illness an emotional roller coaster for the husband. These are some of the reasons why it may be difficult for a husband to respond consistently in an effective and caring way.

A report to the Post- and Ante-Natal Depression Association (PANDA), the Australian organization of postpartum support groups, states by their permission:

My wife is not the only person in the family who went through this illness. I was a casualty, as were our older children, our family and friends. Meals were always a problem. I had a credit rating at every local take-away food venue. The housework just wasn't done. There was so much yelling, I got to the stage where I dreaded going home. I didn't know what the yelling was about. It was just happening. Then there were the silences.

Sex and affection were absent during that time. Not tonight—not tomorrow night—not next week—not ever!*

*Lack of sexual responsiveness is a common component of postpartum psychiatric illness. Many years ago, J. A. Hamilton (1962) reported that patients who received thyroid as a part of their treatment for depressions after childbirth experienced a recovery of sexual interest and responsiveness more rapidly than patients who did not receive thyroid.

Another husband states:

It was just three months after her second child that Paula started feeling "funny." It seemed as though it was directly related to her stopping breast-feeding. She began to become very emotional and started losing sleep. Complicating this problem was her slowly being unable to define reality from fantasy, or waking from sleep states.

Now I could not believe that any of this could be possible. How could someone I loved and knew intimately for ten years change so drastically, so quickly. I now had no one to share my problems with, much less to help with everyday household chores. At this time Paula had completely deteriorated as a functioning human being. It just seemed to be too much. I felt used up, defeated. My talks with Paula became senseless. Not only did I want to just "slap it out of her," but I felt that she wasn't trying to overcome her own feelings of depression and helplessness. Our conversations were incomplete, open-ended, with loss of topic. We were unable to communicate with each other—something that our relationship was based on. She could not hear me, she became paranoid. All I wanted was out! I quit! It seemed like my only hope of keeping my own sanity. My denial, my ignorance of the problem could have sent me on my own path. Fortunately, she was able to find help, and I did support her in her search for help. Now, thanks to many sources of help, our faith now is stronger than ever and our communication is better than ever.

Conclusion

All who have studied postpartum illness are agreed that women with this illness are particularly responsive to social support, encouragement, and the provision of an optimal psychological milieu. The husband is a critical person to provide these benefits. Many patients report that marital stress is an important aspect of their illness. Nevertheless, in the usual patient-oriented and sometimes child-oriented regimes of treatment, the husband receives scant attention.

This chapter describes an innovation: a support group for husbands. It appears that husbands do find themselves exposed to a great deal of stress incidental to postpartum illness. The major stresses, as developed in support groups, are outlined. The support group format with interaction of several husbands provides vitality and the sharing of experiences which is its unique asset. Because of the stringency of husbands' time and the recurrence of questions about postpartum illness itself, monthly meetings with an informed professional appear to be an optimal structure for the program.

References

Arizmendi, T. G., and Affonso, D. D. (1987). Stressful events related to pregnancy and postpartum. *J. Psychosom. Res.* 31:15–36.
Hamilton, J. A. (1962). *Postpartum Psychiatric Problems.* St. Louis: C. V. Mosby.

Hamilton, J. A. (1985). Guidelines for therapeutic management of postpartum disorders. In D. G. Inwood (Ed.), *Recent Advances in Postpartum Psychiatric Disorders*. Washington, DC: American Psychiatric Press.

Harvey, J., and McGrath, G. (1988). Psychiatric morbidity in spouses of women admitted to a mother and baby unit. *Br. J. Psychiatry*, 152:506–10.

Inwood, D. G. (1985). The spectrum of postpartum disorders. In D. G. Inwood (Ed.), *Recent Advances in Postpartum Psychiatric Disorders*. Washington, DC: American Psychiatric Press.

Japenga, A. (1987). The tragic ordeal of postpartum psychosis. *Los Angeles Times* Part IV, February 1, 1987.

O'Hara, M. W. (1985). Psychological factors in the development of postpartum depression. In D. G. Inwood (Ed.), *Recent Advances in Postpartum Psychiatric Disorders*. Washington, DC: American Psychiatric Press.

O'Hara, M. W., Rehm, L. P., and Campbell, S. B. (1982). Predicting depressive symptomatology: Cognitive-behavioral models and postpartum depression. *J. Abn. Psych.*, 91(6):457–61.

Paykel, E. S., Emms, E. M., et al. (1980). Life events and social support in puerperal depression. *Br. J. Psychiatry* 136:339–46.

Pitt, B. M. N. (1968). "Atypical" depression following childbirth. *Br. J. Psychiatry*, 114:1325–35.

Chapter 25
Information and Its Applications

James Alexander Hamilton, Patricia Neel
Harberger, and Robert M. Atkins

This book has compiled information pertaining to postpartum psychiatric illness from many sources. Certain parts of the information are well accepted and are becoming widely known: Severe postpartum illness can be a devastating catastrophe. Lesser degrees of postpartum illness are distressing and may impel profound changes in life patterns. If patients are cared for with knowledgeable use of the tools and facilities of modern psychiatry, most recover eventually. The severity of symptoms may be great and the duration long.

The improvement in treatment over the last decade is compounded by early recognition, awareness of the unique stresses and hazards of these illnesses, judicious selection and use of presently available therapeutic measures, and patients' acceptance of what may be several months of treatment. The 1980s saw real advances in public recognition and medical management of these illnesses. However, complacency with these advances could postpone further progress that could achieve two important goals: to reduce the severity of symptoms, and to reduce the duration of illness, perhaps very substantially.

This chapter examines a broad outline of the information that has come together and then suggests how the information can be extended, verified, and possibly applied effectively to patient care. Some of the information dates back a long time. It was in the fifteenth century that the first detailed clinical history of a postpartum case emerged, an autobiography dictated by the patient herself, one Margery Kempe of Lynn, England (Drucker 1972).

This dynamic lady was married to a wealthy former member of parliament, gave birth to a child, and became psychotic a few days later. The psychosis took the form of hallucinations, delusions, and violent emotional expression around a religious theme. After a few weeks she improved. She exhibited a strong urge to visit religious centers and ceremonies, in which she was indulged by her husband. In such places she was often seized by disruptive bursts of crying and screaming. Recurrences followed several pregnancies, with a similar pattern of explosive outbursts of religious fervor during the late phase of the illness. Early sexual precocity was followed by aversion to sex. She made a pact of celibacy with her husband and cared for him well in his old age. Her life story was dictated to two clerics. She could neither read nor write.

The fourteenth century was also the time of William of Occam, Franciscan monk, philosopher, and logician. Occam developed a rule of thinking which might illuminate the path from information about postpartum illness to its application. The fourteenth century was a time when political leaders and theologians found themselves in constant warfare over minutiae of doctrine, dogma, and ritual. William of Occam pleaded for a reduction of the controversies and a substitution of some simple interpretations of the works of God, man, and nature. He advanced the logical principle, later known as "Occam's razor," which held that if many causes are adduced to explain a phenomenon, the one most likely to be correct is the simple one. The irrelevant details were "cut away" by Occam's razor. Occam refused to support some of the doctrines advocated by his superior Pope John XXII, and was confined to the dungeon under the papal palace at Avignon. After four years he escaped and came under the protection of Holy Roman Emperor Louis IV of Bavaria, where he spent the rest of his life teaching and writing.

Following Occam, if one stands back and looks at the broad picture of postpartum psychiatric illness, a rather simple pattern becomes apparent. There are two severe disorders that appear after childbirth. The first is an agitated, volatile, changeable psychosis that appears after three days and has a peak incidence of onset on the sixth day. The psychosis may end abruptly or extend into months of a confused or depressed state, a state sometimes interrupted by a violent episode of psychotic thinking and behavior. The second severe disorder develops insidiously after the second or third week, has predominant depressive features, and often is associated with physical complaints, sometimes signs that are similar to those seen in thyroid deficit.

Mixtures of the two patterns occur frequently. Most cases recover after many months. A few deteriorate to a chronic mental state which has characteristics of dementia. These cases often have physical stigmata resembling known disorders of hormone deficit.

Postpartum psychiatric illness appears and runs its course rather precisely in the timetable of rapidly changing physiological events of the puerperium. Again, following Occam, one can stand back and look at the broad pattern of these events. During pregnancy, under the command of a very active pituitary, other glands respond with accelerated activity and hormone production. The pituitary's acceleration is pushed by large amounts of estrogen from the placenta. With the loss of the placenta, the pituitary moves from high activity to deceleration. Other glands follow, so that serum hormone levels move downward toward normal and perhaps into occasional deficit.

Hormonal substances do not act in isolation. Complex interrelationships and feedback mechanisms between hormones and target glands are present, so that the phenomenon has the quality of an equilibrium among many substances and activities. In general, the trend of hormonal production and activity after childbirth is a marked decrease from the acceleration of pregnancy. Hormone levels fall, but they fall at different rates, because of their different chemical characteristics and rates of synthesis, metabolism, and excretion. A temporary exception to postpartum hormonal fall occurs when autoimmune thyroiditis may cause a postpartum peak in serum thyroxine.

As these major transitions in hormonal levels and equilibria occur, it is to be expected that some levels would fall into a temporary deficit which could produce symptoms. A parallel possibility is that the phenomenon of kindling could alter the symptom-producing threshold of a hormone (see Chapter 16). Finally, the falling hormone pattern could reach a new equilibrium that was balanced but less than optimal.

Which hormone deficits are likely offenders? Marked thyroid deficits were relatively easy to associate with severe depression after childbirth because they are often associated with physical signs (e.g., myxedema). As Stössner saw in 1910, and as many others have seen, the physical signs and the depression disappear simultaneously as thyroxine is administered.

It was not so easy to find a known hormonal deficit associated with the symptoms of the early mercurial postpartum psychosis. Finally, the great laboratory of iatrogenic medicine produced an acute deficit of cortisol in the 1950s, when a great many people were given large doses of cortisone, suffered depression of their own adrenals, and became toxic. Their cortisone was stopped, and they became psychotic. The perceptive Ione Railton (1984) saw a similarity to postpartum illness, but few believed her.

One reason why it is difficult to fit the concept of a cortisol deficit into the simple picture of early postpartum psychosis is that there is no familiar model of a physical disorder of acute cortisol deficit today, as hypothyroidism is a physical disorder of thyroid deficit. However,

Sheehan's syndrome provides a model of both acute and chronic deficits of cortisol and thyroxine, and its psychiatric symptoms respond very quickly and favorably to cortisone and thyroxine.

Stripped of its embellishments by Occam's razor, the clinical and organic picture of postpartum illness appears plausible. What is to hinder its application? Erroneous interpretation of laboratory data often clouds the understanding of cases. Tests should be ordered and interpreted with knowledge of the changing values of the puerperium. Interpretation should take account the direction of changing values.

The serum level of thyroxine increases during pregnancy then falls during the first three weeks postpartum. The level may spike with autoimmune thyroiditis during the first few weeks. The level may plateau at a value well below the prepregnancy level, and yet remain within an arbitrary low-normal range set for the general population. A physical work-up may be made while serum thyroxine is falling, but before it has reached its nadir. Serial thyroid studies are needed for these assessments.

Detection of a significant cortisol deficit is more elusive. The total serum cortisol remains high during the time postpartum psychosis is most florid. But most of the cortisol is bound tightly to a large protein molecule (transcortin) and is physiologically inactive. It is the small percent of free cortisol that could be low and symptom-producing early in the puerperium, yet it is total cortisol that is measured commonly in the clinical laboratory. Measurement of free serum cortisol is an expensive, research laboratory procedure. Free urinary cortisol is a possible alternative.

Lacking conclusive laboratory evidence of a deficit of free cortisol as a cause of psychotic symptoms, clinicians are highly reticent to explore the possibility of a free cortisol deficit by administering a cortisol analogue. Part of this is due to lack of familiarity with the cortisol analogues. Another part may be attributable to a firm belief that drugs should not be used unless their efficacy in a given syndrome is "proved." Proof is equated with "experimental proof." There is no indication that criticism-free experimental evidence on this problem will be available in the foreseeable future. It may be that progress—or the alleviation of symptoms—is halted by a semantic problem. Perhaps the concept of "proof" should be examined.

Proof is the conclusive establishment of an assertion or a proposition. In modern medicine, proof is most acceptably accomplished by means of an experiment or a series of experiments. In its simplest form, an experiment begins with a defined population of subjects. From this population, two groups are selected at random, a control group and an experimental group. All conditions are held constant but one, which is manipulated in the experimental group. Proof consists of statistically valid differences that emerge between the two groups. Some kinds of proof require many experiments. The model for the introduction of a new drug approved by the Food and Drug Administration is a series of experiments. The cost of bringing a new drug to market may reach $100 million and take many years.

The foregoing model is not feasible in postpartum illness. Cases develop singly and in the United States are treated as individuals by individuals. To sequester a group of very sick new mothers without a physician's best effort is unthinkable. Pure experimentation with real patients is always a compromise. Even a compromise would cost many times the amount of money that has ever been available for study in this field.

A large experimental model involving many sick patients is inappropriate for another reason. The goal here is not the approval of a new drug. The goal is to establish the plausibility of a possible diagnosis. In the instance of postpartum illness, the first step is to establish the rationale for entertaining a given diagnosis, a rather simple hypothesis of organic etiology. A next step is to establish if it is reasonable to apply this diagnosis to a specific patient. A final step, one that is taken individually, is to apply risk-benefit analysis to a specific patient and to determine the risks versus the benefits involved in the trial of a specific medication.

Much information currently available and presented in this book supports or facilitates the first two steps. In addition, there are some very simple experiments that could illuminate, extend, or weaken the hypothesis of organic etiology in general or for a specific patient. Some of them are outlined below. (The risk-benefit analysis for individual patients favors the organic hypothesis; the specific medications are relatively safe in trial application, while many of the drugs in common use today have occasional severe side effects.)

The following are several areas wherein a small to moderate investment in research could extend knowledge in critical areas that are germane to advance in knowledge and to the treatment of postpartum psychiatric illness:

1. In 1956, R. R. Hughes and V. K. Summers reported that in patients with postpartum hypopituitarism the normal alpha waves on an electroencephalogram (EEG) were often replaced by slow theta waves, and occasionally, by very slow delta waves, particularly in the occipital region. Sheehan and Davis (1982) reported that these abnormal EEG waves disappear along with psychiatric symptoms, almost immediately after the introduction of cortisone, or cortisone and thyroxine therapy. With the exception of one patient described in another

context later in this chapter, there is no record of EEG studies on postpartum psychiatric patients. While not every patient is an appropriate candidate for EEG studies, it would be useful to look for EEG abnormalities in suitable patients.

2. Maternity blues bears considerable resemblance to the symptoms and timing of the early agitated psychosis in postpartum illness. The first trial of estrogen for prophylaxis was based on the observations that this substance, administered for lactation suppression, also appeared to prevent maternity blues. (See Chapter 7.) Does Diana Riley's recommended pyridoxine for prophylaxis also prevent maternity blues (Riley 1984)?

3. H. L. Sheehan and J. C. Davis (1982), after many pathological studies of the pituitary after postpartum hypopituitarism, conclude that the tissue necrosis is the result not only of a fall in blood pressure but also of several hours of concurrent constriction of small arteries which support the portal system of the pituitary. (See Chapter 15.) George Stein and coworkers (1976), and later Handley and associates (1977), found low tryptophan associated with severe maternity blues. An important cause of pituitary vasoconstriction could be a shortage of serotonin in vasodilator neurons of the pituitary arteries. Both pyridoxine and tryptophan are on the metabolic pathways leading to serotonin synthesis. Does pyridoxine protect against diminished postpartum tryptophan?

4. As relationships between maternity blues and severe postpartum illness become identified, it would be reasonable to follow Jan Campbell's suggestion in Chapter 7 and consider that maternity blues might be considered a model for the early psychosis, postpartum psychotic depression. (See also Chapter 18.) A reasonable expedient would be to give a small dose of an analogue of cortisol to a case of the blues and literally *watch* its effect. Note that for such a test, the dose and total amount of the cortisol might be less than is often given for an attack of hay fever. If this test is seen to abort maternity blues, a small series of low-dose trials, with double-blind controls, should outline the parameters of the response.

5. Pharmacological agents in current use for postpartum psychiatric illness include neuroleptics, antidepressants, antianxiety agents, and thyroxine. Anticonvulsants are not likely to be considered. However, an experience of one of us (R.M.A.) with an anticonvulsant drug raises this possibility.

A 26-year-old primipara, without prior psychiatric history, was admitted to a psychiatric facility eighteen days after delivery. For the preceding seven to ten days she had exhibited increasing confusion, agitation, bizarre thinking and speech, and increasingly threatening behavior toward her child. In the hospital, physical studies were negative except for an abnormal EEG. She had hallucinations as well as persecutory and grandiose delusions. The violence of her behavior required body constraints. Haloperidol (120 mg daily) and then chlorpromazine (550 mg daily) failed to relieve her agitation and disturbance of consciousness. Medication was reduced gradually, and lithium carbonate (1,800 mg daily) was started. Within a few days she experienced vomiting that lasted for many hours. All medication was discontinued, and a few days later she became asymptomatic. After about ten days she was discharged on no medication.

Two days after discharge, the patient suffered a relapse and was readmitted. Lithium was begun with small doses, gradually working up to 1,800 mg daily. Her response reached a plateau, with behavior that could be described as infantile, with pressurized speech, and occasional aggressive disruptive behavior. This was interrupted occasionally with brief periods of lucidity and insight. This continued for 4½ months.

Review of the case took note of the periodic nature of the patient's behavior, the persisting EEG abnormality, and the poor response to neuroleptics. The hypothesis was adduced that the patient could have a syndrome of episodic dyscontrol. This is a seizurelike phenomenon described by Russell R. Monroe (1959 and 1974) as a "third psychosis." On the basis of this, the patient was treated with carbamazepine (Tegretol), 500 mg twice a day. Complete remission occurred within thirty-six hours. The dose was tapered and symptoms began to recur. Resumption of the full dose was followed by complete remission. She returned to her home and normal activities. After several months the carbamazepine was reduced gradually and discontinued without a problem. She was followed for five years by her psychiatrist and remained asymptomatic. A second pregnancy and delivery were without complications and without psychopharmacologic intervention. She has had no subsequent psychiatric problems requiring treatment.

This case is of interest for several reasons: The onset is typical in timing and behavior to that of a severe postpartum psychotic depression (or postpartum psychosis). There was a variety of presentations, with interspersed periods of lucidity. The syndrome was refractory to haloperidol and chlorpromazine and only partly responsive to lithium. The EEG, characterized by prominent theta waves, is usually associated with abnormal activity of the diencephalon. Also, these abnormalities are characteristic of Sheehan's syndrome. (We have no prior account of abnormal brain waves in postpartum psychiatric illness, although EEG study was suggested by H. L. Sheehan in 1960.) The striking apparent effectiveness of an anticonvulsant, Tegretol (carbamazepine), would weigh in favor of an organic syndrome. Also, Tegretol could be a valuable resource when other medications fail. While lithium is a very effective drug, its unfortunate side effect of frequent injury to the thyroid makes it a candidate for replacement, if a satisfactory substitute were available. This would be particularly true in postpartum psychiatric illness, where the thyroid gland could be under other adverse influences as well.

The foregoing case history recounts a single incident, the epitome of the much maligned anecdotal method. It is true that nothing is proved by a single case. However, this case could provide two valuable clues for further study of EEG patterns and the use of carbamazepine. Had someone acted on the 1910 anecdote of Stössner regarding the curious association of postpartum depression and myxedema, the dismal history of the twentieth-century research in postpartum illness might have been averted.

6. Chapter 2 described an attempt to treat late postpartum depression with the rapidly acting analogue of thyroxine, triiodothyronine (Ballachey et al. 1958). The effort was abandoned as an experiment because, after marked elevation of mood by triiodothyronine, the sudden letdown with placebo control appeared to introduce a serious suicidal risk. Another experimental design, with different instructions and with in-hospital supervision could develop as an effective predictor of thyroxine appropriateness.

7. As noted in Chapter 17, measurement of the serum level of thyroxine may fail to diagnose a deficit as reflected in clinical signs and in the response to administration of thyroxine. This phenomenon is observed not only in postpartum syndromes but also in conditions related to childbearing. While the reason or reasons for this may not be known, it is apparent that a need exists for measurement of tissue activity of thyroxine to supplement the quantitative determination of its presence in the serum.

The oldest index of thyroid function, the "basal metabolic rate," was such a measure. It was a determination of the rate of oxygen consumption under relaxed and resting conditions but not sleep. The variable element of agitation and restlessness would probably preclude the use of this measure for patients with postpartum psychiatric disorders. Other functions which may vary with tissue availability of thyroxine are: (1) the reflex relaxation time of striated muscle, as measured most conveniently with the Achilles tendon reflex, (2) the rate at which a flickering light of standard intensity fuses, the "flicker fusion test," (3) basal body temperature and peripheral skin temperature, and (4) serum cholesterol.

Two or more of these measures could be combined. A first useful step would be to measure, for example, the Achilles tendon reflex and the rate of flicker fusion on an unselected obstetrical population at three months pregnancy, during the third trimester, and six weeks postpartum. With average levels and variability established, studies of patients with identified hypothyroidism and with postpartum psychiatric illness could be studied.

8. Data presented in Chapter 14 suggest that a ratio of two fractions of urinary 17-ketosteroids may reflect thyroid function. The 17-ketosteroids are produced in the liver as a stage in the metabolism of estrogen, androgen, and other steroids. One fraction, androsterone, is normally somewhat larger than the other, etiocholanolone, so that the ratio (the A/E ratio) in health is 1.5 to 3.00 or more. It was discovered that patients with periodic psychoses in an active phase often had ratios of 1.0 or well below 1.0 (Nomura et al. 1979). Later it was found that postpartum patients had low A/E ratios. Administration of desiccated thyroid to patients with severe postpartum depression resulted in alleviation of depression and a striking concurrent rise in the A/E ratio (Nomura et al. 1983). The separation of the two fractions of the 17-ketosteroids is described by T. Wakoh (1959).

The apparent wide span of the A/E ratio, from 0.5 to 3.0 or above, suggests that this could be a very valuable supplement to the measurement of serum thyroxine. It might be particularly useful for lesser degrees of depression severity, or for cases where serum studies yield equivocal or negative results.

9. Living models afford exceptional opportunities for the accumulation of information. When the Swiss physician V. S. Bürgi (1954) decided to study cases of postpartum illness that had become chronic, he found plenty of subjects in the back wards of public psychiatric hospitals. Similar patients could be found today, studied with modern diagnostic tools, perhaps treated rationally and humanely.

10. Estrogen prophylaxis for high-risk patients is in a holding pattern while alternatives to injection of estrogen in oil are explored. One alternative could be introduction of estrogen by way of transdermal patches for the critical first forty-eight hours.

The foregoing research opportunities are, for the most part, examples of work that could extend current information regarding postpartum illness into some of the areas where the picture puzzle is still incomplete. The central objective is to expand detailed knowledge of important organic features that make postpartum disorders unique entities.

At this time, it is neither feasible nor necessary to create a mammoth study to explore postpartum psychiatric illness. The funds are not available, and clinical applications may be reached more quickly by a series of less elaborate, prudently selected studies. A first step toward clinical application is the absorption of the mass of information that points toward organic mechanisms, and specifically hormonal deficits and imbalances, in these illnesses. This book has assembled much information toward this end.

The final decision is a diagnostic one which applies to the individual case. Specifically, does current general information and information about the single patient justify a trial of the hormone-deficit hypothesis? For an individual patient this is a risk-benefit decision, a decision which balances the probability that the patient does have a hormonal deficit that may be correctable, against the hope that the patient may be helped sufficiently by use of an array of nonspecific psychoactive drugs, each with its own hazards and claims.

The route from information to clinical application is opening for thyroxine in late depressive reactions. The route toward the application of a cortisol analogue in postpartum psychosis of early onset is virtually blocked. One reason for this is that much existing information has not been disseminated. Another reason is that the use of total serum cortisol determination has led to the erroneous conclusion that serum cortisol is normal. This conclusion cannot be made correctly without knowledge regarding *unbound* cortisol.

The existing information, together with the inferences of H. L. Sheehan (1960) and the observations of Ione Railton (1984), may be insufficient to convince clinicians to favor a trial of cortisol analogue for these early disorders. The investigations suggested in this chapter may facilitate their decisions.

A final barrier that may block the trial of a cortisol analogue in early postpartum psychosis is the reticence of physicians to prescribe drugs that are outside their usual armamentarium, particularly those that are known to cause severe reaction when used in excess or for too long a time. The solution to this, a solution which Ione Railton used thirty years ago, is to associate oneself with a trusted endocrinologist.

The pathway from research and information to application can be traversed. A large number of women and their families are waiting for this to happen.

References

Ballachey, E. L., et al. (1958). Response of postpartum psychiatric symptoms to 1-triiodothyronine. *Jour. Clin. & Exper. Psychopathol.* 19:170.

Bürgi, V. S. (1954). Puerperalpsychose oder Diencephalosis puerperalis? *Schweiz. Med. Wochenschr.*, 84:1222–25.

Drucker, T. (1972). Malaise of Margery Kempe. *New York State Jour. Med.* 72:2911–17.

Esquirol, J.E.D. (1838). *Des maladies mentales considérées sous les rapports medical, hygiénique et médico-légal*, Vol. 1. Paris: J.B. Baillière.

Handley, S. L., et al. (1977). Mood changes in the puerperium and plasma tryptophan and cortisol concentrations. *Brit. Med. Jour.* 2:18–22.

Hughes, R. R., and Summers, V. K. (1956). Changes in the electroencephalogram associated with hypopituitarism due to postpartum necrosis. *Electroencephalogr. Clin. Neurophysiol.* 8:87–96.

Monroe, R. R. (1959). Episodic behavior disorders: Schizophrenia or epilepsy. *Arch. Gen. Psychiat.* 1:205–14.

———. (1974). Episodic behavior disorder: an unclassified syndrome. Ch. 11 in S. Arieti, *American Handbook of Psychiatry*. 2 Ed. Vol. 3.

Nomura, J., et al. (1979). Role of the central nervous system in hepatic steroid and ammonia metabolism. *Psychoneuroendocrinology* 4:47–56.

Nomura, J., et al. (1983). Studies on the cerebrohepatic relationship with reference to the pathogenesis of acute psychoses. In N. Hatotani and J. Nomura (Eds.), *Neurobiology of Periodic Psychoses*. Tokyo: Igaku Shoin.

Post, R. M., Trimble, M. R., and Pippenger, C. E. (1989). *Clinical Use of Anticonvulsants in Psychiatric Disorders*. New York: Demos.

Railton, I. (1984). The use of prednisolone for postpartum psychiatric symptoms. San Francisco: Scientific Program of The Biennial Meeting of the Marcé Society.

Riley, D. (1984). Pyridoxine prophylaxis. San Francisco: Scientific Program of The Marcé Society.

Sheehan, H. L. (1960). Personal communication with James Hamilton.

Sheehan, H. L., and Davis, J. C. (1982). *Post-Partum Hypopituitarism*. Springfield: C. C. Thomas.

Stein, G. S., et al. (1976). Relationship between mood disturbance and free plasma tryptophan in post partum women. *Brit. Med. Jour.* 2:457.

Stössner, K. (1910). Ein Fall von Myxödem im Anschluss an Gravidität. *München Med. Wochenschr.*, 57:2531–33.

Wakoh, T. (1959). Endocrinological studies on periodic psychosis. *Mie Med. Jour.* 9:351–96.

Appendix: The Words of Marcé

In the history of medicine, few have observed so carefully, inferred so wisely, and written so clearly as Louis Victor Marcé. Probably no physician, and certainly no specialist in mental disorders, has been misquoted so systematically and with such disastrous consequences.

This Appendix provides sample pages of Marcé's writing about psychiatric illness after childbearing. They are taken from his 1858 treatise on peripartum illness and his 1862 textbook on the entire field of mental illness. A short biographical note precedes the comments on the facsimile pages.

Louis Victor Marcé was born in 1828. He had a brilliant record in the medical school at Nantes. After graduation, he was offered a position at the mental hospital at Ivry-sur-Seine, near Paris. The hospital had been founded by France's first leader in postpartum illness, J.E.D. Esquirol, and it had an excellent reputation for treatment of psychiatric cases associated with childbearing. Concurrently, Marcé became affiliated with the University of Paris, where he received a gold medal prize in 1853 (Ritti and Limas 1865).

Continuing the tradition at Ivry-sur-Seine, Marcé familiarized himself with the extensive literature about postpartum illness and began to work with patients. By 1858 he had studied seventy-nine postpartum cases. Reviewing them and hundreds of other cases studied by other physicians at hospitals such as the Salpêtrière, he published *Traité de la folie des femmes enceintes, des nouvelles accouchées et des nourrices,* in 1858. He was 30 years old at the time and was listed as *ancien interne* [senior resident], *lauréat des hôpitaux et de la Faculté de médecine.* Four years later, in 1862, he published his textbook, *Traité pratique des maladies mentales.* At that time he was listed as *Professeur agrégé* [clinical professor] *à la faculté de médecine de Paris.* He died in 1864 at the age of 36.

Marcé's position on postpartum illness was that it displayed many and varied symptoms, and that these symptoms bore some similarity to symptoms that may be observed in cases unrelated to childbearing.

However, he made it very clear that the combinations of symptoms, the syndromes of postpartum illness, the way one syndrome moves to another, and the consistent association between the changes in psychiatric syndromes and the changes in the generative organs, all of these were unique to postpartum illness.

Marcé was particularly impressed by the tandem march of the physical changes that follow childbearing and the changes which he observed in his patients as their illnesses evolved. He was convinced that there was a *connexion* between the generative organs and the mind that could not be accounted for by known structures of the nervous system, which he called *une sympathie morbide*. His inferences may have foreseen the discovery of the endocrine system by about one-third of a century.

Plates I to V are the title page and table of contents of Marcé's "Treatise on the 'Folie' [Madness] of Pregnant Women, the Newly Delivered, and Nursing Mothers." Plates VI and VII introduce the various forms of the "folie" of the newly delivered together with comments on the unusual characteristic of these illnesses to change from one form to another.

Plates VIII and IX discuss the depressive reactions which Marcé believed to be a variety of the disorder of the newly delivered. Some of these develop during the first fortnight, while others appear after several weeks. Marcé describes and discusses a quality of these depressions that he and others believed to be unique to the postpartum state and that appeared frequently: *délire triste*, or "sad delirium."

The four pages of Marcé's first book, Plates VI through IX, include a large variety of symptoms and syndromes, together with a notation of the striking tendency for syndromes to change from one to another, or to periods of apparent lucidity. It was with this range of expression in mind that the authors of Chapter 3 advanced the suggestion that the category of postpartum disorder which corresponded generally to the "madness" of the newly delivered be designated as postpartum psychotic depression.

Plates X and XI discuss the characteristics of the postpartum illness of late onset, the "madness" of nursing mothers, with its prominence of depressive symptoms. The appearance of a variety of physical symptoms and signs is described. Marcé makes a comment that the "disorders of health" almost always precede the "disorders of the mind," in this condition. The authors of Chapter 3 believe that this illness of late onset, an illness with depression rather than psychosis as the dominant feature, should be called major postpartum depression.

Plate XII is the title page of Marcé's general textbook of mental illness. Chapter 2 is titled *Des causes de la folie*. In this chapter Marcé indicates unequivocally how the etiology of postpartum illnesses should be classified: in the section on "physical causes," the subsection on "physiological causes," or in modern terminology, among the organic mental disorders.

Plates XIII through XV are part of Marcé's discussion of "physiological causes." Plate XIII describes the major disorders. The first paragraph of Plate XIV suggests that he believes that the general cause is a hereditary predisposition. He then begins a list of secondary causes. Of particular interest is item *e* (Plate XV): hemorrhage after delivery. This observation is very close to a prediction that postpartum psychiatric illness is related to Sheehan's syndrome, or postpartum necrosis of the pituitary following hemorrhage. This relationship was predicted more specifically by Professor H. L. Sheehan in 1961. (See Chapter 2.) It is explored exhaustively by Doctors Collin Davis and Mohammed T. Abou-Saleh in Chapter 15. Most of the psychiatric reactions of postpartum necrosis of the pituitary respond within days to cortisone with thyroxine medication. If this is tried and is effective for postpartum psychotic depression, this will indeed be an affirmation of Marcé's prescience.

References

Marcé, L. V. (1858). *Traité de la folie des femmes enceintes, des nouvelles accouchées et des nourrices.* Paris: J. B. Baillière et Fils.
———. (1862). *Traité pratique des maladies mentales.* Paris: J. B. Baillière et Fils.
Ritti, M., and Limas, M. (1865). Éloge de Marcé. *Ann. Med.-psychol.,* 86:133–43.

TRAITÉ DE LA FOLIE

DES

FEMMES ENCEINTES

DES

NOUVELLES ACCOUCHÉES ET DES NOURRICES

ET

CONSIDÉRATIONS MÉDICO-LÉGALES QUI SE RATTACHENT A CE SUJET,

PAR

LE Dr L. V. MARCÉ

Ancien interne, lauréat des hôpitaux et de la Faculté de médecine;
membre titulaire de la Société anatomique.

PARIS

J. B. BAILLIÈRE et FILS,

LIBRAIRES DE L'ACADÉMIE IMPÉRIALE DE MÉDECINE,

Rue Hautefeuille, 19.

LONDRES	NEW-YORK
H. BAILLIÈRE, 219, REGENT-STREET.	H. BAILLIÈRE, 290, BROADWAY.

MADRID, C. BAILLY – BAILLIÈRE, CALLE DEL PRINCIPE, 11.

1858

Plate I

TABLE DES MATIÈRES.

Plate II

TROISIÈME SECTION.

De la folie transitoire au moment de l'accouchement............ 134

QUATRIÈME SECTION.

CHAP. Ier. — **Des causes de folie des nouvelles accouchées et de la folie des nourrices** 147

CHAP. II. — **De la folie des nouvelles accouchées**.......... 190

Plate III

26

Plate IV

CORBEIL, imprimerie et stéréotypie de CRÉTÉ.

Plate V

CHAPITRE II.

La folie des nouvelles accouchées est la plus fréquente de toutes les variétés de folie puerpérale ; déjà nous avons eu occasion de le prouver par des chiffres ; qu'il nous suffise de répéter ici que sur un total de 79 faits, nous en avons trouvé 44, c'est-à-dire un peu plus de la moitié, qui appartiennent à cette catégorie.

Les formes de folie que nous avons observées, sont la manie ; la mélancolie ; les lésions partielles de l'intelligence, hallucinations, monomanies intellectuelles ou instinctives ; enfin une variété toute spéciale d'affaiblissement mental, qui semble causé par d'abondantes pertes de sang, et peut facilement guérir par un traitement approprié.

En traçant une démarcation aussi nette entre les diverses formes d'aliénation mentale qui se présentent après l'accouchement, je dois faire quelques réserves peu importantes. Peut-être observe-t-on dans l'état puerpéral un moins grand nombre de ces formes mixtes, impossibles à classer et à définir nettement dans la pratique; mais on rencontre, ici comme

Plate VI

partout, ces transformations morbides qui ne sont pas un des phénomènes les moins curieux de la pathologie mentale : nous avons vu la manie avoir pour prodromes plusieurs journées de langueur, de faiblesse et d'abattement. Chez une de nos malades (observ. 55), il y eut, six semaines après l'accouchement, un accès de délire maniaque qui disparut au bout de peu de jours laissant après lui des hallucinations, des conceptions délirantes isolées qui, deux années après, persistaient avec la même intensité. Dans un autre cas (observ. 44), la folie avait débuté par des conceptions délirantes partielles qui, au bout de deux mois seulement, se compliquèrent de la dépression mélancolique la plus complète. Ainsi, manie, mélancolie et monomanie ont des connexions intimes et n'existent pas d'emblée avec tout leur appareil symptomatique.

Ces formes diverses d'aliénation mentale sont loin d'être également fréquentes. Sur 44 malades, j'ai trouvé 29 cas de manie, 10 cas de mélancolie, 5 cas de folie partielle, et deux cas seulement d'affaiblissement intellectuel passager. La prédominance de la manie chez les nouvelles accouchées est un fait qu'il n'est pas sans intérêt de noter, car chez les nourrices la forme mélancolique est au moins aussi commune que la manie ; le nombre des monomanies est à peine égal au cinquième des cas de manie.

Chacune de ces variétés a sa marche et son pro-

Plate VII

l'affligent vivement. Enfin, nous rencontrons parmi les antécédents de la plupart des malades un état intellectuel déjà modifié profondément et ayant reçu, à un moment plus ou moins éloigné du début de la maladie, des atteintes sérieuses qui le rendent apte à subir l'action de toutes les causes morbides.

Cette particularité est la seule qui nous ait paru exercer une influence spéciale sur le développement de la mélancolie. Sans doute, l'idiosyncrasie du sujet, ses habitudes morales, sans doute aussi les causes débilitantes peuvent être ici spécialement invoquées, mais à part ces données générales, nous ignorons en vertu de quelle cause spéciale la mélancolie se développe chez certains sujets plutôt que la manie ou toute autre forme d'aliénation mentale.

§ 3. La mélancolie débute, comme la manie, soit dans les premiers jours qui suivent l'accouchement, soit vers la sixième semaine; elle se développe d'emblée avec tout son appareil symptomatique, ou parfois ce sont des idées isolées de nature triste qui précèdent l'invasion du délire et l'apparition de la dépression mélancolique. Enfin dans certains cas on observe pendant quelques jours, dans les actes et dans le langage, une excitation générale qui se rapproche de l'excitation maniaque, et plus tard seulement le délire se systématise.

Les deux éléments principaux qui caractérisent

Plate VIII

la mélancolie, la dépression d'un côté, et de l'autre, le délire triste, se sont rencontrés associés entre eux à des degrés différents chez toutes les malades dont nous avons recueilli l'histoire. La dépression a offert les nuances les plus variées, depuis l'inertie, le manque d'activité et d'entrain, le sentiment d'impuissance que l'on retrouvait surtout chez une de nos malades, jusqu'à la stupeur la plus profonde, qui masque sous une immobilité complète la nature des fausses conceptions ; la figure un peu bouffie, pâle, contractée, stupide, participe alors à la fois du facies des mélancoliques et de l'aspect spécial des nouvelles accouchées ; la voix dolente, mal articulée, est aussi lente que la pensée ; la démarche pénible et incertaine, les mouvements rares et peu étendus, la lenteur des digestions, la constipation constante, indiquent que la dépression porte autant sur le système musculaire que sur l'état intellectuel. Le délire a été, comme il l'est toujours dans la mélancolie, de nature triste, et souvent même peu varié dans son expression : les idées de persécution, la crainte de la mort, du déshonneur, d'une expiation à subir, puis, par une conséquence logique, les idées de suicide ont constitué le fond des conceptions délirantes (obs. 20), tout ce que voient les malades est interprété dans un sens défavorable ; tous les objets sont envisagés à un point de vue funèbre.

Les hallucinations de l'ouïe, de la vue et du

Plate IX

Il résulte pour nous, de quelques faits cliniques, que, chez des femmes bien portantes ayant supporté la lactation avec une aisance parfaite, la suspension d'une sécrétion abondante qui s'est prolongée quelquefois pendant plus d'une année, et est devenue pour l'économie une habitude, détermine un état de pléthore qui peut devenir le point de départ des accidents. Ceci est tout à fait remarquable dans une observation de manie hystérique intermittente survenue trois semaines après le sevrage, dont l'histoire se retrouvera plus loin; tous les accidents s'exaspérèrent sous l'influence du fer et des toniques; les saignées seules pratiquées un peu avant l'époque menstruelle, et plus tard la diète lactée, amenèrent la guérison des accidents. (Observ. 64.)

En résumé, dans l'immense majorité des cas, la folie, à la suite de l'allaitement ou du sevrage, survient chez les femmes profondément épuisées, que la moindre perturbation fonctionnelle jette dans un trouble nerveux complet; dans quelques cas assez rares, elle est liée à un état de pléthore déterminé par la suspension d'une sécrétion abondante.

Nous dirons plus tard comment distinguer ces deux cas; qu'il nous suffise d'appeler ici l'attention des praticiens sur une distinction qui n'avait pas encore été faite et dont l'importance, au point de vue pratique, est réellement considérable.

§ 7. Quelle que soit l'époque à laquelle elle se

Plate X

développe, la maladie *débute* de deux manières : ou brusquement, à la suite d'une cause occasionnelle, comme un refroidissement, une vive émotion morale; ou lentement et par gradation insensible. Les désordres de la santé physique précèdent presque toujours les désordres intellectuels; les femmes maigrissent, deviennent pâles et languissantes; des bruits de souffle se font entendre dans les gros vaisseaux, et il y a des palpitations; en même temps, les digestions deviennent difficiles et s'accompagnent de rapports acides et de flatuosités ; chaque fois que la nourrice a allaité, elle éprouve un sentiment de faiblesse et de vide à l'épigastre ; quelquefois la sécrétion lactée s'amoindrit, d'autres fois elle reste intacte, et la femme n'en maigrit que davantage ; des accès fébriles, à forme irrégulièrement intermittente, véritables accès de fièvre hectique, viennent se surajouter à cet état morbide.

Les troubles intellectuels ne tardent pas à survenir, souvent même ils remontent à une époque très-éloignée ; il arrive en effet parfois que, pendant toute la durée de l'allaitement depuis la délivrance, les malades éprouvent de l'affaiblissement de la mémoire; les idées sont moins nettes; le caractère offre des bizarreries inexplicables, et les femmes ont souvent même conscience de leur état maladif. Tous ces symptômes ne font que grandir, à mesure que la lactation continue; les excitants, comme le

Plate XI

TRAITÉ PRATIQUE

DES

MALADIES MENTALES

PAR

LE DR L.-V. MARCÉ

PROFESSEUR AGRÉGÉ A LA FACULTÉ DE MÉDECINE DE PARIS,
MÉDECIN DES ALIÉNÉS DE L'HOSPICE DE BICÊTRE.

PARIS

J.-B. BAILLIÈRE et FILS

LIBRAIRES DE L'ACADÉMIE IMPÉRIALE DE MÉDECINE
Rue Hautefeuille, 19.

<table>
<tr><td>**Londres**</td><td>**New-York**</td></tr>
<tr><td>Hipp. Baillière, 219, Regent street.</td><td>Baillière brothers, 440, Broadway.</td></tr>
</table>

MADRID, C. BAILLY-BAILLIÈRE, PLAZA DEL PRINCIPE ALFONSO, 16

1862

Plate XII

nombre des nourrices étant moins considérable que celui des nouvelles accouchées, cette proportion ne saurait être prise dans un sens absolu. Enfin, les cas de folie survenant pendant la grossesse égalent tout au plus le tiers de ceux qui se développent pendant la lactation.

Les nouvelles accouchées offrent principalement la forme maniaque : chez elles, la folie se développe à deux époques distinctes, tantôt dans les huit ou dix premiers jours qui suivent la délivrance, et alors son origine peut être légitimement rapportée à la fièvre de lait et à l'ébranlement nerveux qui accompagne l'accouchement ; tantôt vers la cinquième ou sixième semaine, c'est-à-dire au moment de la première époque menstruelle ; chez les nourrices, la mélancolie est aussi fréquente que la manie : Esquirol, qui rencontrait un plus grand nombre de cas de folie à la suite de la lactation chez les femmes de la classe pauvre que chez les femmes aisées, l'attribuait à l'insuffisance de leur alimentation, et les faits que nous avons observés viennent presque tous à l'appui de cette opinion : la plupart de nos malades présentaient de l'anémie, de l'amaigrissement, des vertiges et divers accidents nerveux ayant précédé l'invasion des troubles intellectuels. Quant au sevrage, son influence sur la production de la folie est incontestable, mais plus difficile à expliquer, puisqu'il met fin à une sécrétion dont l'abondance épuisait les malades. Cependant il n'est pas rare de voir l'organisme épuisé s'habituer pendant quelque temps sans secousse et sans malaise à des pertes qui l'énervent d'une manière quotidienne et régulière ; mais que ces flux se suppriment brusquement, il peut arriver, comme chez les hémorrhoïdaires ou chez des sujets habitués à une longue suppuration, qu'il se produise dans l'économie une réaction d'autant plus vive et plus dangereuse que le sujet est plus enclin aux accidents nerveux.

L'état puerpéral n'exerce pas chez tous les sujets une

Plate XIII

égale influence au point de vue de la production des troubles intellectuels; dans l'appréciation des causes de la folie puerpérale, il faut toujours tenir le plus grand compte, non-seulement de la prédisposition et surtout de l'hérédité, sur laquelle nous n'avons pas à revenir, mais encore de certaines conditions d'un ordre secondaire dont l'action est bien démontrée. Ainsi :

a. L'âge des nouvelles accouchées : plus les femmes s'éloignent de cette période de la vie dans laquelle les fonctions génératrices jouissent de toute leur énergie, plus elles se trouvent exposées à la folie lorsqu'elles deviennent enceintes. J'ai prouvé ce fait autre part à l'aide de statistiques irrécusables.

b. Le nombre des grossesses augmente la prédisposition à la folie, à cause de la profonde débilitation amenée par des parturitions nombreuses et très rapprochées. Cette cause et la précédente s'enchaînent l'une l'autre et se trouvent naturellement juxtaposées; on les retrouve non-seulement pour la folie des nouvelles accouchées, mais encore pour la folie des femmes enceintes.

c. Un accès antérieur d'aliénation mentale prédispose à la folie puerpérale, il en est de même d'un état mental fâcheux pendant la durée de la grossesse.

d. Le sexe de l'enfant que la femme a porté ou allaité devient quelquefois cause de folie. On a vu des malades devenir aliénées après avoir mis au monde un enfant mâle, et rester exemptes d'accidents après l'accouchement d'une fille. Ces faits au premier abord semblent inexplicables : on comprend cependant qu'un enfant mâle, fort, développé, et plus tard, lorsqu'on l'allaite, exerçant des efforts de succion énergiques, arrive à épuiser plus promptement sa mère et à déterminer des accidents que la gestation et l'allaitement d'une fille auraient pu éviter.

MARCÉ. — MAL. MENT.   10

Plate XIV

e. L'hémorrhagie pendant ou après l'accouchement hâte le développement des accidents nerveux.

f. La folie peut survenir chez les nouvelles accouchées, à la suite de convulsions éclamptiques. Tantôt elle succède immédiatement au coma qui accompagne les convulsions; tantôt elle n'éclate que plusieurs heures ou plusieurs jours avant la fin complète de l'état convulsif, alors que l'on semblait pouvoir compter sur la cessation de tous les accidents cérébraux.

g. La première menstruation qui suit l'accouchement exerce sur le développement de la folie puerpérale une influence que M. Baillarger a signalée le premier, et que nos propres observations confirment d'une manière non douteuse : sur 44 malades atteintes de folie après l'accouchement et qui n'avaient pas allaité, j'en ai trouvé 11 qui sont tombées malades vers la sixième semaine, c'est-à-dire précisément au moment du retour des règles. Quelquefois le délire précède de cinq à six jours l'apparition des règles, mais dans le plus grand nombre des cas, la folie débute avec l'écoulement menstruel ou pendant sa durée. Enfin, j'ai vu la menstruation faire complétement défaut et le délire éclater précisément au moment où les règles devaient apparaître. Chez les nourrices, l'invasion du délire a lieu fréquemment de la quatrième à la sixième semaine qui suit l'accouchement; et chez les femmes qui, ayant allaité pendant un certain nombre de mois, deviennent malades après le sevrage, le délire éclate très souvent au moment même où les règles reparaissent après une longue interruption.

h. Dans quelques cas, les difficultés de la parturition, un phlegmon du sein passé à suppuration, un refroidissement, paraissent être devenus le point de départ d'un accès de folie chez des femmes prédisposées. Je ne citerai que pour mémoire les inhalations de chloroforme signalées comme

Plate XV

Contributors

M. T. Abou-Saleh, M.B.Ch.B., M.Phil., Ph.D., M.R.C.Psych., is a staff member of the Department of Psychiatry, University of Liverpool, Royal Liverpool Hospital, Liverpool, England.

Robert M. Atkins, M.D., M.P.H., is Coordinator of Mental Health Services and Director of Education in the Department of Psychiatry, York Hospital, York, Pennsylvania.

Nancy Gleason Berchtold, B.S., is founder of the Depression After Delivery Support Network. She is a member of the founders' group of Postpartum Support, International and a lecturer in the field of postpartum disorders.

Ian Brockington, M.D. F.R.C.P., is Professor of Psychiatry at the University of Birmingham, Queen Elizabeth Hospital, Birmingham, England. He is a founding member of The Marcé Society and co-editor of *Motherhood and Mental Illness* (1982, 1988).

Jan L. Campbell, M.D., is Assistant Professor of Psychiatry at the University of Kansas and serves as staff physician at the Veterans Administration Medical Center, Kansas City, Missouri.

J. C. Davis, M.D., F.R.C.Path., is a staff member in the Department of Endocrine Pathology at the University of Liverpool, Alder Hey Hospital, Liverpool, England. He is the co-author of *Postpartum Hypopituitarism* (1982).

Mark D. DeBofsky, Attorney-at-Law, is a specialist in medical insurance matters. His practice is based in Chicago, Illinois.

Jeanne Watson Driscoll, M.S., R.N., C.S., is a psychotherapist in private practice. She is Vice-President of Life Cycle Productions, Inc., Waltham, Massachusetts.

Ricardo J. Fernandez, M.D., is Clinical Assistant Professor in the Department of Psychiatry, Robert Wood Johnson/Rutgers Medical School. Based in Princeton, New Jersey, Dr. Fernandez acts as advisor to the Depression After Delivery Support Network, and his area of special interest centers on postpartum psychiatric problems.

Robert B. Filer, M.D., is based in the Division of Reproductive Endocrinology, Department of Obstetrics and Gynecology, York Hospital, York, Pennsylvania.

Galina M. Gorodetsky, M.D., earned her Certificate for Specialization in Obstetrics and Gynecology (Endocrinology) at the First Leningrad Institute. She served as Chief Consultant in Gynecology/Endocrinology at the Kalinin Medical Center and Hospital of Leningrad. Dr. Gorodetsky is currently Assistant Clinical Professor of Psychiatry at the University of California, San Francisco, where she served her psychiatric residency from 1981 to 1985.

James Alexander Hamilton, Ph.D., M.D., is Associate Clinical Professor of Psychiatry (Emeritus) at Stanford University and former Psychiatry Chief of Staff at Saint Francis Memorial Hospital, San Francisco, California. Dr. Hamilton is the author of *Postpartum Psychiatric Problems* (1962) and a founding member of The Marcé Society.

Patricia Neel Harberger, M.S., C.F.N.P., A.C.C.E., is Director of Primary Prevention and Counseling Services, Family and Community Health Associates, York, Pennsylvania, and former coordinator of Behavioral Sciences and Family Dynamics for the Family Medicine Residency Program, York Hospital, York, Pennsylvania. She is a founding member of Postpartum Support, International.

Elizabeth K. Herz, M.D., is Associate Professor in the Department of Obstetrics and Gynecology and Psychiatry at the George Washington University School of Medicine. Dr. Herz also serves as director of the Program of Psychosomatic Obstetrics and Gynecology at George Washington University Hospital in Washington, D.C.

Robert Hickman, Ph.D., M.F.C.C., is a licensed marriage and family therapist. Dr. Hickman is co-director of the Postpartum Mood Disorder Clinic and facilitator for the Postpartum Husbands' Support Group, San Diego, California.

Susan A. Hickman, Ph.D., M.F.C.C., is a licensed psychotherapist and certified childbirth educator. Dr. Hickman has served as an expert witness, and she is a member of the California State Task Force on Postpartum Psychosis, San Diego, California. Her special area of interest focuses on problems relating to birth and parenting.

Jane Israel Honikman, B.A., formerly directed the Santa Barbara Birth Resource Center. She is a founding member and chairperson of Postpartum Support, International, and co-founder of Postpartum Education for Parents (PEP), Santa Barbara, California.

Daniel Maier Katkin, J.D., is professor and head of the Department of Administration of Justice, Pennsylvania State University, State College, Pennsylvania. He is the author of *The Nature of Criminal Law* (1981).

Laurence Dean Kruckman, Ph.D., is Associate Professor of Anthropology in the Department of Sociology/Anthropology, Indiana University of Pennsylvania, Indiana, Pennsylvania. He is co-author of *Postpartum Depression—A Research Guide and International Bibliography* (1986).

R. Kumar, M.D., Ph.D., F.R.C.Psych., is Reader in Psychosomatic Medicine at the Institute of Psychiatry and Consulting Psychiatrist at Bethlem Royal and Maudsley Hospitals, London. He is co-editor of *Motherhood and Mental Illness* (1982, 1988) and a founding member of The Marcé Society.

Donald L. LeVine, Attorney-at-Law, specializes in criminal defense. His practice is based in San Diego, California.

Maureen Marks, D.Phil., is a research psychologist in perinatal psychiatry at the Institute of Psychiatry, De Crespiguy Park, London.

Junichi Nomura, M.D., is Professor and Head of the Department of Psychiatry, Mie University School of Medicine, Tsu, Mie, Japan. Dr. Nomura specializes in psychoneuroendocrinology.

Tadaharu Okano, M.D., is Assistant Professor in the Department of Psychiatry, Mie University School of Medicine, Tsu, Mie, Japan. Dr. Okano specializes in psychiatric problems related to childbirth.

Barbara L. Parry, M.D., is Assistant Professor of Psychiatry at the University of California at San Diego. She edited and contributed to the journal *Psychiatric Clinics of North America* (March 1989), in an issue entitled "Women's Disorders."

Bernhard Pauliekhoff, M.D., Ph.D., is a professor at the Universitäts Nervenklinik, University of Münster, Germany. He is the author of *Seleische Störungen der Schwangerschaft und nach der Geburt* (1964) and *Endogene Psychosen als Zeitstörungen* (1986).

Deborah A. Sichel, M.D., is an instructor in psychiatry at Harvard Medical School and director of the Postpartum Mood Disorder Program at Newton Wellesley Hospital, Newton, Massachusetts.

Bruce Singh, M.D., is Professor of Psychological Medicine, Monash University Medical School, Melbourne, Australia.

Roger Smith, M.B., B.S., Ph.D., F.R.A.C.P., is Associate Professor of Medicine at the University of Newcastle Medical School, Newcastle, New South Wales, Australia, and serves on the staff of Misericordiae Hospital, Woratah, New South Wales. Dr. Smith's primary area of research focuses on the hypothalamic-pituitary-adrenal axis and the endocrinology of the placenta.

Joan Sneddon, M.D., was formerly Senior Lecturer in Psychiatry at the University of Sheffield, England.

Richard H. Trapnell, M.D., is Chairman of the Professional Advisory Committee Mental Health Association in San Francisco, California, and formerly served as Psychiatry Chief of Staff at Saint Francis Memorial Hospital, San Francisco, California.

Index

This book was set in Baskerville and Eras typefaces. Baskerville was designed by John Baskerville at his private press in Birmingham, England, in the eighteenth century. The first typeface to depart from oldstyle typeface design, Baskerville has more variation between thick and thin strokes. In an effort to insure that the thick and thin strokes of his typeface reproduced well on paper, John Baskerville developed the first wove paper, the surface of which was much smoother than the laid paper of the time. The development of wove paper was partly responsible for the introduction of typefaces classified as modern, which have even more contrast between thick and thin strokes.

Eras was designed in 1969 by Studio Hollenstein in Paris for the Wagner Typefoundry. A contemporary script-like version of a sans-serif typeface, the letters of Eras have a monotone stroke and are slightly inclined.

Printed on acid-free paper.

More Praise for *The Circle Way*

"In this beautifully written book, Christina Baldwin and Ann Linnea share the simple elegance of their PeerSpirit circle process and how it can be used in organizational and community settings with powerful impact. We have learned a great deal from the way of the circle as a call to remember our collective capacities to design and host catalytic conversations around the questions that most matter to our common future."

——Juanita Brown and David Isaacs,
cofounders, The World Café

"*The Circle Way* offers over twenty years of experience by the authors, who share how sitting in a circle allows for optimum self-governance, facilitates quality conversations that make a difference both personally and professionally, and encourages leaders to become more effective within their organizations and communities. Relevant, accessible, practical, and invaluable for all generations."

——Angeles Arrien, PhD, cultural anthropologist and
author of *The Second Half of Life*

"Christina and Ann take us through the anatomy of the circle process with poetic clarity and simplicity, demystifying elements of the circle process while, at the same time, showing us the indescribable mystery of what can happen in circle. *The Circle Way* is one of those rare books that can truly be called a transmission."

——Jack Zimmerman, coauthor of *The Way of Council*
and *Flesh and Spirit*, and Elder, Ojai Foundation

"We learn circle best by doing it and letting the circle teach us, letting it reveal itself as we embrace it. Or we can learn circle by immersing ourselves into the deep and profound stories that Christina and Ann recount for us. They lay the bones of circle and then weave colorful threads of countless stories that create the tapestry of our understanding."

——Pamela Austin Thompson, CEO, American
Organization of Nurse Executives

"The definitive work on circle process. Rich with stories and detailed instructions, this book will inspire hope and a vision of exciting possibilities in anyone who has ever wondered how to breathe life and love into unproductive or conflict-laden meetings."

— Roger Harrison, PhD, organization development consultant

"Christina and Ann bring the magic and discipline of circle fully to life in *The Circle Way*. They have opened the door for circle to enter our boardrooms, corporate meetings, community gatherings, and living rooms. I can hear them cheering us on, 'Now it's your turn.' I'll gladly take the wisdom of *The Circle Way* with me. It's like walking with Ann and Christina by my side."

— Teresa Posakony, Board Chair, The Berkana Institute, and practitioner, Art of Hosting

"Christina and Ann present us with the gifts that working the circular way offers us at this time of great shifting in our world. Their writing is a piece of art in itself from two masters who through diligent practice have stayed the constant apprentices of this fine art. I am grateful for its clarity and practicality."

— Toke Paludan Møller, cofounder and CEO, InterChange; cofounder and practitioner in the Art of Hosting network; cofounder and designer of the Flow Game and the Warrior of the Heart dojo

"I often wonder how the world would be if we remembered one thing: to practice meeting together in circle whenever we gather. This book is our 'MapQuest' back to our authentic selves."

— Phil Cass, PhD, CEO, Columbus Medical Association and CMA Foundation

"Somewhere along the way we humans forgot how to come together to have conversations that matter. Masterfully written, *The Circle Way* provides practical, nuanced insights on how to convene gatherings that foster clarity and inclusiveness. If you are a leader who values true collaboration, this is a book to read."

— Larry Dressler, author of *Consensus Through Conversation* and *Standing in the Fire*

The Circle Way

A LEADER IN EVERY CHAIR

Christina Baldwin & Ann Linnea

Foreword by Margaret J. Wheatley

BK

Berrett–Koehler Publishers, Inc.
San Francisco
a BK Business book

Berrett-Koehler Publishers, Inc.
235 Montgomery Street, Suite 650
San Francisco, CA 94104-2916
Tel: (415) 288-0260   Fax: (415) 362-2512   www.bkconnection.com

Ordering Information

Quantity sales. Special discounts are available on quantity purchases by corporations, associations, and others. For details, contact the "Special Sales Department" at the Berrett-Koehler address above.

Individual sales. Berrett-Koehler publications are available through most bookstores. They can also be ordered directly from Berrett-Koehler: Tel: (800) 929-2929; Fax: (802) 864-7626; www.bkconnection.com

Orders for college textbook/course adoption use. Please contact Berrett-Koehler: Tel: (800) 929-2929; Fax: (802) 864-7626.

Orders by U.S. trade bookstores and wholesalers. Please contact Ingram Publisher Services, Tel: (800) 509-4887; Fax: (800) 838-1149; E-mail: customer.service@ingrampublisherservices.com; or visit www.ingrampublisherservices.com/Ordering for details about electronic ordering.

Berrett-Koehler and the BK logo are registered trademarks of Berrett-Koehler Publishers, Inc.

Printed in the United States of America

Berrett-Koehler books are printed on long-lasting acid-free paper. When it is available, we choose paper that has been manufactured by environmentally responsible processes. These may include using trees grown in sustainable forests, incorporating recycled paper, minimizing chlorine in bleaching, or recycling the energy produced at the paper mill.

Library of Congress Cataloging-in-Publication Data
Baldwin, Christina.
The circle way : a leader in every chair / Christina Baldwin & Ann Linnea ; foreword by Margaret J. Wheatley.
   p. cm.
"A BK Business book."
Includes bibliographical references and index.
ISBN 978-1-60509-256-0 (softcover : alk. paper)
1. Ritual--Psychology. 2. Circle--Psychological aspects. 3. Communication in small groups. 4. Group decision-making--Psychological aspects. 5. Leadership--Psychological aspects.
I. Linnea, Ann, 1949- II. Title.
BL604.C5B35 2010
302.3'4--dc22   2010000532

First Edition
15 14 13 12 11 10   10 9 8 7 6 5 4 3 2

Interior design and project management by Jonathan Peck, Dovetail Publishing Services..
Cover design by Gopa&Ted2, Books and Design; Cover photograph by Margaret J. Wheatley
Back cover author photograph by Debbie Dix:Interior author photograph by Bonnie Marsh

To the dear people who leaned into the circle
and who have been our peer spirits
along the path of remembering and application.
Thank you.

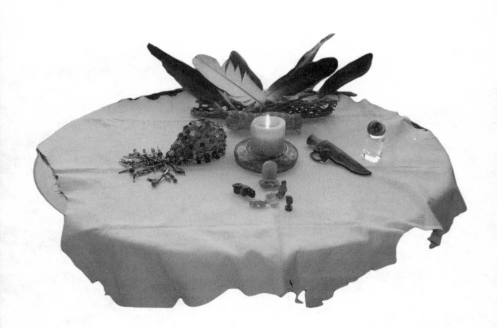

If we change the chairs,
we can change the world.

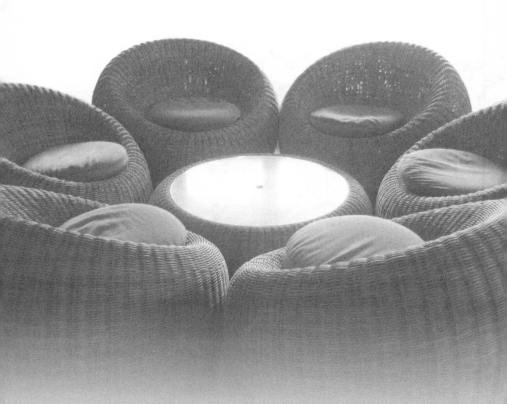

CONTENTS

The Stories and People in This Book

Sometimes people and situations are identified by full name, position, and organization. In such cases, these individuals have granted us permission to use their experiences as teaching tales for circle practice.

Other people are identified by first name only or merely by gender or profession. In these cases, their identities have been disguised so that their story could be told without divulging details of the actual situation. We include these stories to illustrate important lessons we have learned and have altered the contexts to honor the promise of confidentiality that governs many circle settings.

We give thanks for all these stories. We share them in great respect for the tender, difficult, and profound moments of circle that illuminate those of us who sit at the rim.

Story is the sweet nectar of language. Story is the crystallizing of thought, turning it into something digestible, sweet on the heart, even when the details are hard to bear. Story is the way we dribble sweetness over the often harsh realities of life's everyday grind... rolling what happens on the tongue until we discover the nugget of meaning, humor, heartbreak, and insight.

Christina Baldwin, *Storycatcher*, pp. 10–11

When Did We Forget This?

Margaret J. Wheatley

I first discovered the power of the circle way in 1998 working with Christina and Ann. But that's not an accurate statement—we don't "discover" circle practice so much as remember it. As humans, our species' memory is filled with circles, not just those we painted on pots and cave walls long, long ago but also the physical formations in which we arranged ourselves as we got to know one another. The extraordinary Chilean biologist Humberto Maturana writes in "The Biology of Love" that humans first developed language when we moved into familial groups.[1] The closer we got to one another, the more curious and expressive we became. As soon as fire was discovered, some early version of us formed a circle around the fire, experimenting with new forms of expression. Circle is the way humans have always sat together and gotten to know one another.

It's important to remember this long, loving lineage as we now daily sit in rows in classrooms, auditoriums, buses, and airplanes, looking at the back of each other's heads. Or as we sit along the straight edges of tables and desks struggling to find a way to communicate and reach one another. After all these centuries of separation and isolation, circle welcomes us back into a shape where we can listen, be heard, and be respected, where we can think and create together. Circle is the means to draw us away from the dramatic and angry public exchanges that now are not just commonplace but seemingly the only option available for discourse. Sitting together as equals, slowed down, held by the shape, drawing on ancient familiarity—just what we need at this time!

In today's world, dozens, if not hundreds, of group processes are available. In the midst of so much choice, it's important to remember the long lineage of circle and its role in human community. Circle process is not a technique; it's a heritage. It is a way to be together that is familiar to people everywhere on the planet. In indigenous communities, it's easy to notice the presence of circle—as people sit in fields resting from their work, in homes and public places, even in airports as they travel. But generally, circle has been suppressed and forgotten. Cultures of hierarchy and control long ago abolished circle, because circle serves democracy. Those seeking to dominate and rule over others know instinctively that circle is dangerous to their desire for power. By its simple shape, circle includes everyone without distinction, welcomes and invites all to participate, and creates equality among those gathered.

So it is that this most ancient of forms becomes revolutionary in today's world. And also most welcome. Welcomed by those who are excluded, by those who never speak to power, by those who don't believe they have anything to say. In this way, it opens up the creativity and contribution of all who sat silent for far too many years. Circle ends our collective and individual silence.

The shape itself offers many benefits. Circle is the form of endlessness, continuation, calming down, pacifying. In a circle, there's no beginning or end—once you're in the circle, you're there, participating in wholeness. Nobody is superior; no one is better than anyone else. We sit together in our differences in one nice, round shape.

We don't pay nearly enough attention to shape, to the form of the meeting. We spend a great deal of time preparing content and agendas and dealing with politics but then barely notice the shape of the room in which we're doing the work. We accept whatever's in the room—the tables, the chairs, the disarray from the last meeting. We just want to get on with the work (and get out of there as quickly as possible). If we do start to rearrange the room, often colleagues ask us what we're doing, why we're bothering. Or they try to embarrass us and accuse us of becoming "touchy-feely." But if we don't work on the shape of the meeting, it's predictable what will happen. Rectangular tables promote difficult discussions based on opposition; public forums with microphones at the front promote drama and anger; stages and speakers create critical observers; circles create coequal participants and reflective thinking.

As in architecture, form should follow function. Once we define what we want to accomplish in the meeting, it becomes important to determine the shape in which we'll meet. No one form is good for every circumstance—every form has its uses.

Please let's start paying attention to this! If you want to maintain power and control, keep using the forms that support that. If you need to convey information but not conversation, set the room for a lecture or teaching. If you want to include diverse colleagues and think well together, use the circle. But don't assume for a single minute that you can mix up or ignore the form. It's the most essential element to consider, predictive of the outcome of the meeting.

In this beautiful book, under the wise and loving guidance of Christina and Ann, you'll travel into the ancient lineage of circle and learn how it has been brought forward into our modern organizations. You'll see how deeply embedded this pattern of circle is, how it's a true archetype of the human spirit, one that summons people everywhere to step into the conversation. As you read the stories and understand the practices, I hope that you will feel the stirrings of memory in you, that you will be taken to a place of recall of a time when we were sitting together, drawing on each other's presence and perspectives.

Then and now, no matter what's happening in the external world, human beings can get through anything as long as we're together. May we take these practices to heart as our path going forward, out of the darkness of isolation into the clear seeing that circle makes possible.

The Origin of the Peerspirit Circle Process

This is a book about remembering something basic to human nature—the desire to cooperate and participate in conversations in which we can speak and listen fully. This book reintroduces the use of circle process so that anyone, anywhere, can have a meaningful conversation and rise with support to do what needs to be done.

This body of work arose out of the meeting of two midlife, Middle American women in July 1991 during a five-day summer institute writing seminar that Christina Baldwin was teaching at the University of Minnesota, Duluth. The classroom looked out over great lawns and low brick buildings with a view of Lake Superior, the world's largest lake, an inland, freshwater sea. Sixteen adult learners clustered around the topic of memoir. Ann Linnea came to write about the death of her best friend and to prepare herself to carry a story line through her anticipated adventure kayaking along the perimeter of Lake Superior the following summer.

Ann was a professor's wife with a bachelor's degree in botany and a master's degree in education. She had taught both primary and high school classes and worked as a Forest Service naturalist before she and her husband adopted two children. She was currently dedicated to her parenting and to teaching environmental education to parents, teachers, and students. She was an accomplished amateur athlete who had run and skied in marathons, backpacked in the mountain West, and taken her children for months-long travels in the desert wilderness, a version of home schooling on the road. Her first book, *Teaching Kids to Love the Earth*, cowritten with several educational colleagues, documented her lifelong devotion to sharing the wonder of nature.

Though she lived with her family in a modest home a few blocks up the hill from the university campus, wilderness was not far from her door. Ann hiked or skied every ravine in town and headed up the North Shore, the Gunflint Trail, the Boundary Waters, and out onto the wild and unpredictable waters of the Great Lake, training for her upcoming rite of passage.

Christina was a freelance writer with a bachelor's degree in English literature and a master's in educational psychology who had pioneered the field of journal writing and women's leadership. When her first book, *One to One: Self-Understanding Through Journal Writing*, was published in 1977, the Library of Congress had to create a new category for it: "personal writing, therapeutic uses thereof." Her second book on journal writing, *Life's Companion: Journal Writing as a Spiritual Quest*, had just been published that January, and Baldwin was taking a leadership role in what had become a renaissance in private writing and a burgeoning literary genre of diaries, memoir, and autobiography.

She lived at the suburban edge of Minneapolis, walked her dog and rode her bicycle on paved trails, taught at the Loft Literary Center, hung out with writerly friends, and was seeking her next steps forward. The writing of *Life's Companion* had opened something in her—a sense of calling that did not yet have a name.

Midforties, midcareers, each with new books out in our fields: we were at a crossroad. Ann had noticed how burned out and overextended her participants often were and was seeking ways to introduce reflection and spirituality that could help sustain parents and activists for the long-haul challenges. Christina wanted to encourage the women and men who had been writing their way to personal healing to connect this inward journey to informed action and engagement with social issues. Our first seminar, offered that fall, combined these skills and interests and drew participants from both our mailing lists. We sat down in the circle.

It was not unusual for us to teach this way. Christina had walked into her first journal-writing class in 1975 and immediately recognized the need to change the chairs so that writers could face each other as they talked about the topics they were putting on the page. Ann had been leading wilderness adventures since age sixteen, integrating campfire councils into her time with younger children, and then adapting the love of speaking around the fire into all her outdoor work. What we had not yet understood was that our use of the circle itself was creating a different kind of experience for us as collaborative teachers and for participants as empowered learners.

Throughout the following year, 1992, we noticed that putting our adult education seminars into a ring of chairs and teaching from within the rim had a profound impact on the depth of learning. We came to the conclusion that there was something about the use of the circle that transformed groups of people into participatory learners and leaders. We noticed that when the circle was called, it elicited a depth of speaking and listening that seemed to emerge from within the form itself.

People participated in ways that surprised them. They heard themselves speak wisdom, make commitments, and understand ideas or issues at a synergistic level. From these early circle experiences on, participants have felt empowered, connected to a community of practice, and have credited the circle with giving them the ability to change aspects of their lives. They eagerly asked us to codify what we were doing so that they could replicate circle process. In response, we entered the next level of our exploration: to define and name the essential elements that sustain the circle. Christina began writing her first version of *Calling the Circle: The First and Future Culture.*

Ann circumnavigated Lake Superior in the summer of 1992. She was the first woman to kayak the lake with the largest surface area on the planet: the equivalent of paddling from Duluth, Minnesota, to Miami, Florida, in a 17-foot plastic banana—an Aquaterra Sea Lion, the state-of-the-art kayak at the time. The trip took sixty-five days in what turned out to be the coldest, stormiest summer in a hundred years. It was a profound midlife rite of passage, and she returned to her home, marriage, and children ready to make equally profound changes in the course of her life. That fall, while sorting the impact of what had happened to her in the wilderness, she began transcribing her journal and making notes on her experiences that eventually became her second book, *Deep Water Passage: A Spiritual Journey at Midlife.*

It was a terribly rough autumn. Ann was going through major challenges incorporating her posttrip self into her pretrip life; Christina was separating from a seventeen-year partnership. We were teaching together occasionally and each trying to figure out new directions for our lives. We continued to explore the potency of circle and tried to research whatever we could find about it. In the pre-Internet, pre-Google days, this was a difficult task. The book was due at Bantam in early 1993. Christina worked hard to meet the deadline and sent the manuscript off on time. Silence from the editor, silence that went on for several months.

Circle was such a new topic, we felt like Helen Keller's teacher, Annie Sullivan, hand-spelling the word into society's palm. C-I-R-C-L-E: it means something; it is a way to get somewhere else than where we are. Civil War was raging in the former Yugoslavia, with ethnic cleansing and factions everywhere. Best Picture in the Academy Awards went to *Schindler's List.* In April, there was a terrorist attack on New York's World Trade Center: a truck bomb blew up in the lower-level garage and damaged the building. The city was in a state of shock. C-I-R-C-L-E means something; it is a way to get somewhere else than where we are.

Christina called her editor and after an amicable conversation bought the manuscript back. The publisher didn't know what to do with the concept and couldn't imagine who would read the book. So we found ourselves with an unfinished manuscript, no editor, and no publisher. We continued our explorations. That spring, we were teaching at Hollyhock Retreat Centre on Cortes Island, British Columbia, when we met David Kyle, who owned a very small press in Oregon called Swan, Raven & Company. We handed him the manuscript and a few days later he joined us for tea on the deck of the lodge. "I think I can help you," he said. "I'm intrigued."

In March 1994, Ann and her two children and Christina and her dog all relocated to Whidbey Island, just north of Seattle, Washington. Christina was at work on the next reiteration of the book. Ann was getting her children settled into their new lives. Her memoir about her kayak trip sold, and she bought a house. One step at a time, we were figuring out what we were doing. C-I-R-C-L-E: it means something; it is a way to get somewhere else than where we are. Nelson Mandela was elected president of South Africa with 60 percent of the vote. The Chunnel opened between France and England. The Internet was not yet a household word or phenomenon, although the technology was growing behind the scenes in Silicon Valley.

We knew we were not inventing the circle. We were trying to understand its power and how to frame this ancient social lineage in modern language and application. The *circle*, we were learning, *is essentially a gathering of equals, people who set aside external, hierarchical positions that categorize and separate them and sit down in a ring of chairs with a clearly defined intention or purpose symbolically represented in the middle.* With the rim and the center in place, each person contributes as a peer to the process of reflection, speaking, consideration, and action. The *circle*, we were experiencing, *is an energetic social container capable of helping a group draw on wellsprings of insight, information, and story that inspire collective wisdom and action.* The form itself invites *spirit* to participate in people's interactions. Thus the PeerSpirit Circle Process was born and named.

We formed a small educational company, PeerSpirit, Inc., to carry forward our belief that the circle was needed in mainstream culture. The first edition of Christina's book, in print from 1995 to 1998, sold fifteen thousand copies and connected us to a circle of colleagues with whom we are still in touch. We began training these colleagues in circle process—and learning together many of the deeper insights and practices that appear throughout *this* book.

In 1997, Christina got a call from an agent who wanted to represent the book to larger presses. He sold it back to the same Bantam editor who reissued the edition of *Calling the Circle,* which has been available since 1998. Unfortunately, the circle concept was still so edgy that the book was categorized as "ritual/psychology" and most often shelved in the occult section of the bookstore—not exactly mainstream! Meanwhile, we kept doing our work, expanding our outreach, and through training other facilitators, consultants, and leaders in many fields, kept working to normalize circle as an alternative group process. As Amazon and the Internet came along, the book could be more easily found without people even knowing of its relegation to the back room, and the title took on a second surge.

C-I-R-C-L-E: it means something; it is a way to get somewhere else than where we are. In 1998, we entered the e-mail world and built the first PeerSpirit Web site, reluctantly entering cyberspace as a medium to try to explain the importance of retaining face-to-face communication. Google was founded; the dot-com boom was in full force.

Other books were coming out based on similar explorations of circle. We met Joan Halifax, who had brought the circle process to the Ojai Foundation, and Jack Zimmerman and Gigi Coyle, who worked with Joan and cowrote the book *The Way of Council* in 1996. We met Sedonia Cahill, coauthor of *The Ceremonial Circle* (1992), and Charles Garfield and Cindy Spring, who along with Sedonia wrote *Wisdom Circles* in 1998. One night in a howling rainstorm, we drove to the top of a peak in the Santa Cruz Mountains and met the founders of the Ehama Institute, WindEagle and RainbowHawk (*Heart Seeds: A Message from the Ancestors,* 2003), who are carriers of a circle lineage traceable back three thousand years. Angeles Arrien had contributed *The Fourfold Way* (1993). Jean Shinoda Bolen wrote *The Millionth Circle* (1999), and all these movements were growing in from the edges in attempts to bring circle back to common practice.

We began to feel that we belonged to a "tribe" of people who had been called in different ways to reinstate the circle in modern culture. We at PeerSpirit kept focusing on getting the circle from the edge to the center, wanting it out of the "occult" and into the office. Our training as consultants is experiential; we come from arts, service, and educational backgrounds rather than from business backgrounds; yet we felt compelled to bring the circle into the organizational heart of Middle America because we believe that's where it is most needed and where social change will arise.

In 2000, through our association with the societal and organizational visionary Margaret Wheatley, PeerSpirit Circle Process started going global in the From the Four Directions network and later in the Berkana Learning Centers and Art of Hosting networks. In 2001, especially in life-affirming reactions to the 9/11 attacks, we found ourselves in an expansive, self-organizing movement to create a "culture of conversation." With escalating political, social, and environmental challenges all around us, talking and listening to each other seemed an increasingly vital first step toward sustainable futures. Margaret Wheatley wrote about circles and conversations in *Turning to One Another* (2002). Kay Pranis, Barry Stuart, and Mark Wedge were taking circle into the court system (*Peacemaking Circles: From Crime to Community*, 2003) and training facilitators across North America. Juanita Brown and David Isaacs released their model, The World Café, through a book with that title in 2005. After years of practice and training, the third edition of Harrison Owen's *Open Space Technology: A User's Guide* came out in 2008. And in 2007, Peggy Holman, Tom Devane, and Steven Cady compiled a 700-page resource, *The Change Handbook*, that showcased more than sixty methodologies, many of them using some form of circle process to provide dialogue and feedback for systemic change. We had another "tribe." As old and new colleagues and consulting associations began calling on us, we jumped eagerly into the learning curve that is reflected here in this entirely new book on PeerSpirit Circle Process. The infrastructure has stood the test of time and application. The level of practice has deepened, and the breadth of people with an openness to try circle as a way to get somewhere else than where they are in their lives and work has greatly expanded.

Now Berrett-Koehler, a publisher specializing in books on business best practices, leadership, and organizational development, has recognized circle practice as mainstream enough to add *The Circle Way* to its business group process list. When we pause to reflect on this journey, we are amazed at the rapidity of social and technological change and are deeply gratified to be part of this work and conversation. And now we invite you into the circle—to join this amazing cadre of people who sit at the rim and lead from within the group, who believe that the wisdom we need is in the room and that talking our way forward leads to informed and wise action. Welcome.

Christina Baldwin
Ann Linnea

Whidbey Island, Washington
November 2009

The Circle Way

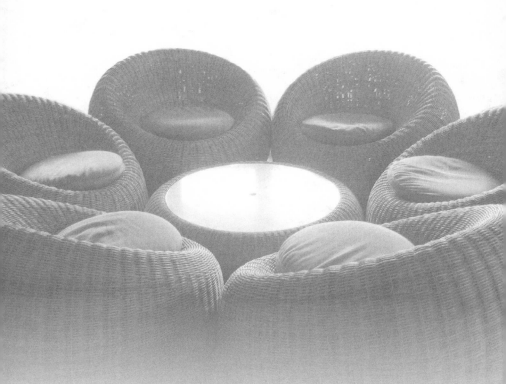

1

Where Circle Comes From and Where It Can Take Us

The room sizzles with tension. Emotions are high, opinions are formed, polarities harden, and alliances and divisions are drawn. Twelve women and men dressed in the current armor of business are about to engage one another on the battlefield of a contentious meeting. In the next two hours, they will decide things that shape their organization's future. The agenda is overfull, and there will be insufficient time for discussion or consideration of consequences. Perhaps this doesn't matter, as the decisions have essentially been made through background e-mails, late and early cell phone calls, text messages, and side conversations in the catacomb of cubicles and corner offices. The players wander in: the CEO, the guy from accounting, department managers, and supervisors. The boss's assistant sets up coffee, flip charts, and related papers and gets ready to take notes.

These are good people.

These are the people who keep business running—in the United States, Canada, Europe, India, China, Australia and the Pacific nations, Latin and South America, and Africa. Wherever there is enough stability in society to hold together commerce and community, some variation of these people gather, around the clock, around the world. They have spouses and partners and children they love whom they send off to school in the mornings and cheer at soccer games. They walk the dog, pet the cat, read the paper, watch television, and enjoy a good meal and perhaps a glass of wine or a cup of tea to draw a line through the end of the day. They put the kids to bed and often head back to their laptops or hand-helds to tend to correspondence they have no time for in the rush of their workday.

"Two to three hundred e-mails a day," they tell us, "and we're required to have our BlackBerrys on 24/7." Another one says, "I get up every night at two A.M. to see if the early meetings have been changed—sometimes we have to be here by six A.M., and I have an hour commute. Then I have to wake my husband and negotiate how we're doing the kids if I'm gone by five—surprising how many other road warriors are on the freeway that time of day." A man laughs sardonically: "I sometimes think of myself as a six-figure lemming rushing toward the cliff. I was going to transition out, but my financial parachute burned up back in 2009. Now I'm just grateful to have made it through the layoffs."

Underneath their resignation is tremendous frustration at what it takes to run the world this way—and to be run by the world. And the place that much of this underlying discontent shows up is in how we run our meetings—how we greet and treat each other and how we wield interpersonal power in the attempt to hold on to some sphere of influence that satisfies our desires to make a difference. This world, however, the world of human interaction and participation, is *our* world to mold and change to fit our needs. What is about to happen here in this room is not predestined; we can redesign it. There is another way: the circle way.

Where Circle Comes From

When humanity's ancestors began to control the use of fire and to carry the embers of warmth and cooking and light along with them from site to site, fire brought a new experience into being: the need for social organization. We speak of this imagined scene many times in circle, awakening our connections to the dreamtime of human origin.

> The man is wet to the skin and shivers. The lifeless body of a rabbit bounces against his shoulder as he hurries through the twilight. The woman trotting at his side pauses in the fading light to gather a few leaves, scratch a surface root free with her toe, and deposit it in the skin pouch at her waist. They move in this fashion along a trail they hope will lead to welcome, warmth, and company for the night. They smell smoke before they can see it, and then hear voices. Finally, they round a bend and there it is—fire glow on a cave wall. Other travelers have already gathered. Not wanting to be mistaken for prey or foe, the man grunts loudly, making the sound for "man-friend." The people at the fire are alerted now and

shush each other, listening cautiously. There is chatter; then one among them grunts back, "Man-friend, man-friend." The woman opens her throat and ululates the haunting cry of female welcome. The women at the fire call back to her. They have two things to offer: food and story.[1]

With flame, hominid scavengers could provide one another with increased safety, warmth, and food. These elements allowed hominids to cluster in larger groups, and larger groups required an increased capacity for complex social behavior. Evidence of the controlled use of fire dates back to the Lower Paleolithic, some 200,000 to 400,000 years ago, when *Homo erectus*, a now extinct hominid, was first exploring its way out of Africa. The skilled use of fire seems to have been passed along to *Homo sapiens sapiens*—us—who arrived about 165,000 years ago. Solid archaeological evidence of hearth rings has been excavated in South Africa and dated back 125,000 years.

What makes this interesting in a book about collaborative conversation is the supposition that language as a social tool developed alongside the use of fire and the sophistication of hand tools. Just as archaeologists and anthropologists can verify the progressive development of tools, neurolinguists such as Stephen Pinker, in his book *The Language Instinct*, can verify the brain pattern of a developed language center faintly etched in the frontal lobe on the inside of fossilized *Homo sapiens* crania. Based on this evidence, Pinker states, "All *Homo sapiens* talk, and all *Homo sapiens* use language as the way they interpret and filter the world around them."[2] This combination—*fire*, which provided the capacity for extending physical gathering; *tools*, which supported hunting and gathering and eventually agriculture and architecture; and *language*, which provided a way to organize experience, transmit knowledge, and process human thought and feeling—has proved to be an unbeatable combination.

Once upon a time, fire led our ancestors into the circle. It made sense to put the fire in the center and to gather around it. A circle defined physical space by creating a rim with a common source of sustenance lighting up the center. These ancestors needed the circle for survival—food, warmth, defense—and they discovered that the circle could help design social order.

This may seem like quite a leap of imagination, but it seems less so when we notice how strongly the impulse toward circle remains active, almost instinctual, in human beings today. When people are engaged in dialogue and relationships, we generally arrange ourselves in a circular formation. This automatic behavior is based on the need to be able to see and hear each other and to communicate our intentions through body language and facial expressions as well as through words. The dialogue may be heated, with emotions roused, or it may be comforting, with emotions relaxed; nevertheless, we still stand where we can keep an eye on each other and on what we and they are saying. This social patterning comes from somewhere and has obviously been of service since it has been maintained in the psychosocial lineage of how we behave together. The seminal researcher who articulated the sources of psychosocial lineage was the twentieth-century Swiss psychiatrist and philosopher Carl Gustav Jung, the founder of analytical psychology, who lived from 1875 to 1961.

Jung hypothesized that all human beings share a number of images that seem to spring from a common imagination deep within the human psyche. Jung called this source *the collective unconscious* and noted that it was filled with recurring and universal mythic symbols he named *archetypes.* Archetypes are expressed culturally but are deeper than culture. For example, the archetypal image that arises when you read the words *wise old man* is influenced by race, religion, and cultural origin—you may imagine Merlin, the Dalai Lama, James Earl Jones, or Black Elk; the point is that calling up an image is universal. Speak an archetypal phrase to a group, and everybody will imagine something. Jung studied the power of circle by examining anthropological evidence and making psychological corollaries; we discovered the power of circle by noticing what happens when people sit in a circular shape.

To understand the power of circle as a collaborative conversation model and the kinds of insights that can pour into this group process, it is helpful to understand that when we circle up in a ring of chairs, we are activating an archetype. Archetypal energy tends to make our experiences seem bigger, brighter or darker; our words become imbued with shades of meaning, and our dialogue, decisions, and actions take on a sense of significance. This is part of the attraction to circle process: the archetypal energy can magnify issues among the group and help transform them.

People who have experienced circle often refer to this archetypal energy as the "magic of circle" that occurs when the best (or sometimes the worst) comes out of us and we find ourselves capable of responding with a level of creativity, innovation, problem solving, and visioning that astound us. Others talk about circle as an experience of synergy, as being able to tap into something they didn't know was in them and could not have predicted as a possible outcome at the start of a circle meeting.

In Germany a few years ago, we were offering a four-day training to sixteen sophisticated consultants from five countries. One of our participants was a leading scholar and academician who wrote and edited journals on political theory and the legacy of Carl Jung in European pedagogy. He pressed us constantly for cognitive information. It was a very helpful interaction for all of us, especially working cross-culturally and choosing English words we hoped would translate meaningfully into German.

The second day into our conversation, something happened that sparked the group and took our learning into insight—we don't remember the particulars of the moment but do remember how urgently this man leaned forward and said, "Stop. Stop—right now, what is happening? What is this energy?" He gestured into the space between us, eighteen people sitting in a room at the back of a little retreat center outside Frankfurt on a sunny spring day. He looked at Ann on one side of the room and across the circle at Christina on the other side. "You, what are the two of you doing? How does this happen?"

"It's not the two of us," we told him. "It's all of us and the circle itself." Synergy is the experience of interaction between elements or people that when combined produces a total effect greater than the sum of the individual parts. The man's question led us into a rousing discussion on synergy, with clarifications being offered in several languages. After a while, satisfied with their explorations, the participants moved on. Later that evening, with a mischievous smile on his face, our colleague brought a pitcher of beer and a bowl of pretzels to our dinner table and popped the next question: "OK, now I want to discuss from where comes synergy?"

Circle as an Archetype of Group Process

Even though the wheel as a *tool* wasn't invented until about 5,500 years ago, the circle as a *symbol* appears in cave paintings and carvings dating back 35,000 years to the Late Paleolithic era. In his research, Jung discovered that the circle, often in the form of the sun wheel (a pie cut into eight equal pieces), is represented in cultures that developed in complete isolation from each other. The circle shows up around the world as the medicine wheel, the wheel of law, the wheel of the year, the Catherine wheel, the dharma wheel, the Kabbalah wheel or tree of life, the mandala, the zodiac, the Uroboros, the triad cross, the Celtic cross, and many other variations. When we pull the chairs away from the table and out of the rows and into a ring where we face each other, we are turning ourselves into a sun wheel. We assume the shape of the symbol itself—and synergy comes with us.

Since the 1990s, when PeerSpirit began offering circle process in an increasing variety of mainstream settings, experimenting with the circle's ability to hold conversation in social settings that range from North America to Europe to South Africa, we have remained consistently aware that the ancient, ever-present circle archetype is evident in the modern methodology. We have repeatedly seen people surprised by their own capacities to access insights and come to decisions no one had imagined when their meeting started. They have asked, "How did we just do that? We didn't get into power struggles. We came up with a course of action no one had seen as possible before." Or they comment, "The director came into this room with 'my mind is made up' written all over his face. Twenty minutes later, he's at the flip chart diagramming options." And people begin to wonder, just as we do, "Is there something about the circle itself that encourages us to newness? Could this process work where folks are really stuck? Could slowing down and talking together really make us more productive? Could circle make our work lives more sustainable?"

Not everyone in the room needs to be interested in or thinking about synergy, archetypes, or social evolution for circle to work. However, group process is strengthened when a few thoughtful participants understand that we are playing with the fires that made us who we are. These fire tenders can then help a group remain steady through the kinds of experiences circle elicits, many of which are shared in stories throughout this book.

Circle may start as one small shift that turns out to be a tipping point. Often we suggest that people introduce a bit of circle process by offering a round of *check-in,* using the first ten or fifteen minutes of a meeting to invite each participant to share a short relevant story that relates to the group's purpose—essentially, to let the group members know how they appear to each other. Sometimes people worry that the exercise is taking time away from the agenda, and yet this simple routine gathers people's attention and focuses everyone on the purpose of the meeting. And sometimes the power and wisdom of the archetype shows up.

In the late 1990s, when PeerSpirit worked with the Center for Nursing Leadership (CNL), we had an experience of archetype streaming through and changing check-in. Founded in 1996 by members of the American Organization of Nurse Executives and funded by a grant from the Hill-Rom Company, CNL developed a one-year educational and midcareer renewal program called Journey Toward Mastery. Founding members had read Christina's book *Calling the Circle* and were incorporating PeerSpirit methodology into their meetings. We were invited to join them to strengthen their understanding of circle practice. In the first few minutes, we offered the following check-in suggestion: "Tell us the story of how you came to enter the profession of nursing."

We watched in amazement how the power of the right question can open a group's synergy. The two of us, coming in as sensitively as we could yet outside the profession we were serving, expected people to check in fairly succinctly. We expected participants to offer a brief anecdote that would better inform us of the motivation behind their career choice and lead into our teaching design for the morning session.

Instead, we witnessed stories of great heart. One person explained that she was the first girl in her large family to go to college; others grew up in small towns and rural areas where their grandmothers had delivered most of the babies. One knew as a child that she had healing abilities that she couldn't talk about; another had a sense of being called at an early age to serve humanity; another's father had died when she was fourteen, and her experience of caring nurses during that time made her determined to become such a caregiver. People listened with rapt attention and without interrupting as one by one they reached into their personal histories and brought forward the memory of the moment they had chosen their path. They laughed with one another and cried with one another, and by the time we had finished check-in, the morning was over.

The experience of circle that morning was a far more powerful lesson than we could have provided talking about circle methodology. And after lunch, when we began a more cognitive conversation about how circle process could influence learning within the cohort group and among the nurse leaders in their organizations, everyone had a profound reference point. This is another aspect of circle that constantly informs us: that the process can hold great depth, that it can survive and resolve long-standing conflicts, provide a space for healing, and then shape-shift into an efficient, peer-led, agenda-based meeting. All this happened at CNL in the course of a few hours.

Three archetypes were activated in this experience: the *healer* that shaped the participants' life journeys, the *circle* that provided a learning ground different from any they had previously experienced, and the *leader* that guided them into the fullness of their careers.

Years later, we still meet these women and men in the places where their work has called them. They are CEOs, chief nursing officers, vice presidents in large and small health care systems, directors of education, professors at nursing schools, and consultants to their profession. Cathy Michaels, currently on the faculty of the University of Arizona College of Nursing, remembers, "It was a profound shift to be invited into story. The question sent us into reflecting on how we had come to live this life.... And when that chord was struck, we became a community that wanted to listen. The serendipitous nature of the question met a waiting readiness in people to let go of everything else and speak from the heart."

Today, Cathy and other nurse leaders tell us stories of the times since that day when they have pulled chairs into a ring and used such a question to check in with staff and team members. They understand how to help teams become grounded in their foundational stories and to stand together on that shared foundation while using circle to manage their work relationships and tasks.

Triangle as an Archetype of Group Process

"Change the chairs and change the world" is a snappy slogan that contains a deeper truth. Whether or not we realize it, social design is always influencing us. Over time, the arrangement of things in our environment becomes such an ingrained norm that we assume that our way of being together is the only way of being together. We do not see that the arrangement itself sets the ways we interact and that if we shift the arrangement, we can shift the interaction. As we bring the circle back into places where the form of arrangement has become codified by organizational charts and chairs bolted into rows facing lecterns, we are greeting the archetype that has become the modern norm: the triangle activated as hierarchy.

The triangle is a universal symbol as old as the circle, one that similarly appeared in the Late Paleolithic. The triangle is chiseled and painted on cave walls as a representation of the Great Mother and continues down through time, showing up as the Great Pyramid, the Star of David, and the Trinity. We mentally relate to the number three and the three-pointed configuration represented by the triangle. The triangle is the basic unit of family (father/mother/child); the triangle divides how we see ourselves (body/mind/spirit); the triangle shapes how we view society (church/state/individual). Looking at the triangle through a psychological lens, we understand Abraham Maslow's hierarchy of needs, with survival at the base and self-actualization at the top. Looking at the triangle as a system of socialization, we get powerful leaders located at the top and followers, employees, and ordinary citizens located at the bottom, with gradations of authority assigned and maintained in a status-based worldview.

As powerful archetypes manifesting in human affairs, the triangle and the circle have probably always coexisted in the organization of human society. One way to look at the world today is to think about the triangle, representing hierarchical power, as having overtaken its partnership with the circle and, as is the nature of power, decidedly come out on top. Hierarchy as a model offers an efficient means for charting systems and for carrying out specific and repetitive tasks when coordinated effort is required. Hierarchy is useful for passing on information, giving directions, establishing chains of command, developing armies, developing work-forces, organizing data, programming computer software, and mass-producing goods. Yet it lacks a holistic understanding of networked systems and biological interdependence and connectivity.

Within a hierarchical worldview, people look for their place. They can either accept their place as an unchangeable fact or strive ever upward toward greater perceived stability and privilege. That is our heroic story: the rise to power and the escape to greater freedom. The closer people are to the top, the more they tend to accept and defend hierarchy, and the closer people are to the bottom, the more they tend to acquiesce to or resist hierarchy. Every time people enter a meeting that plays out the scene that opened this chapter, we activate the triangle archetype and struggle to find our place within the implied power grid.

For the past five thousand years, the increasing valuation of triangle over circle, of hierarchy over collaboration, has gone through many evolutionary changes until what is a mutable imbalance of power is accepted as innate human nature: that's the arrangement. What started off as a concept of partnership in the deepest recesses of the human mind has become a distorted and destructive worldview in which collaborative ways of social organization are denigrated as child's play, relegated to the past, and discounted as utopian, naïve, or "new-age." And yet this world, the world of human interaction and participation, is our world to mold and change to fit our needs. We can rearrange who leads, how we lead, and what happens to all participants in a system. When we understand the archetypal shift, we can rearrange the chairs in ways that rearrange our world.

Where Circle Can Take Us

The circle way is a practice of reestablishing social partnerships and creating a world in which the best of collaboration informs and inspires the best of hierarchical leadership. The chief needs a council that brings the voices of the village to his or her ear. The president needs a cabinet. The coach needs a team. The teacher needs students. The elders need children. And the meetings need to change.

The ancient ways of circle are waiting for us to remember and activate a true experience of collaboration. So if the opening scene of this chapter is how most of the world currently gathers, we have the opportunity to change that scene by changing the meeting into circle process. The room buzzes with creative tension, emotions are optimistic, diverse opinions have been welcomed into the conversation, and the past several days of background e-mails, phone calls, text messages, and side conversations in the cubicles and corner offices have all supported the development of an agenda that is focused, with time allotted to each item and premeeting information shared among all participants. Twelve women and men are about to engage each other in the dynamic interactions of a meeting held in circle process. In the next two hours, they will decide things that shape their organization's future. They have scheduled time for sufficient dialogue and consideration of consequences. They are ready to vote on some issues and to gather information and survey the wisdom in the room on other issues.

The leaders come in and take their places at a round table. The CEO has one agenda item prepared for presentation; the guy from accounting has another. One of the department managers will serve as *host* today, assuring that the process moves smoothly along; one of the supervisors will serve as *guardian,* watching over timeliness and helping the host maintain orderly momentum. The boss's assistant sets up coffee, flip charts, and related papers and prepares to serve as *scribe,* to note the essential insights, decisions, and action items.

Here the triangle of leadership is embedded within the collaborative circle. The host is not the boss; the guardian is not the enforcer; the scribe is not the historian: these roles are loose, rotating, voluntary, assumed and released as the sessions of a circle-based group advance toward fulfilling their intention. The triangle of leadership stabilizes group process so that the ideas, stories, wisdom, and synergy that emerge can stream through the conversation and be preserved in helpful ways. With this understanding in place, and the reestablishment of the ancient partnership, these good people can change the chairs *and* change their world.

The group can learn new ways of distributing leadership and responsibility. Participants can set agreements for respectful interaction before speaking and define what material is confidential and what can be shared. They can mark the moment between casual socializing or multitasking and paying full attention to one another. They can blend the dynamism of collaborative conversation with voting, achieve consensus, and acknowledge the authority of informed hierarchy within their roles in the circle.

Creating a Renewed Culture of Conversation

Recognition that we can talk and listen ourselves into the changes we need is simultaneously occurring to people in a number of environments. PeerSpirit Circle Process, the infrastructure of circle we have designed to serve in modern settings, travels in the company of other circle carriers and ways of calling forward this heritage—the Way of Council, the Ehama teachings, Peacemaking Circles, the Millionth Circle, and other interpretations of lineages continue to elucidate circle process and capacity. In addition to the various circle processes, we find ourselves connected to a growing number of conversational modalities that have circle at their base: Open Space technology, World Café, Conversation Cafés, Art of Hosting, Appreciative Inquiry, restorative justice circles, Bohmian dialogue. Variations of collaborative group process are constantly being designed and offered as contributions to our social exploration.

We are in big trouble, so we need big help. We have inherited and created many problems, so we need many solutions. These collaborative conversational modalities are replicating, adaptive, global, democratic forces through which ordinary people are rediscovering their abilities to connect with each other's hearts and minds and make things happen as a result. These emergent conversations are not, at their essence, policy discussions or strategic planning; they are spontaneous eruptions of empowerment based on the release of energy that occurs while speaking to and listening to each other within the container of the archetypes.

What is generated by this emerging culture of conversation is a social paradigm shift that can occur anywhere, at any time, within any group of people. It operates through an intelligence that integrates the heart and mind. It seeks to restore principles of belonging and to find meaningful ways for everyone to contribute. Perhaps this culture of conversation is occurring now because science has given us a much more complete story of our origins and history: we have come to truly understand that we are one people, literacy among the populace is greater than ever before, and we live in a technologically as well as biologically interconnected world.

In symbolism, the circle and triangle are often found together. A triangle within a circle appears on the back of the U.S. dollar bill and on the front of the Alcoholics Anonymous medallion and is recognized as an international peace symbol. The partnership of archetypes is the willingness to combine the best attributes of both social structures and to know when to call on each of their strengths and to experience their balance. It is the nature of circle to invite in, to provide both access and boundaries, to provide a participatory process, to set social expectations, and to absorb diverse, even opposing, views through the alchemy of a symbolic central "fire."

Circle functions best in an environment where people feel socially safe and have the time to make authentic, thoughtful contributions to the process. How to foster that social safety is a major purpose of this book. Circle invites contribution—particularly for problem solving or insights from unexpected sources (the janitor who solves a managerial issue, the child whose comment shifts a situation for teachers and staff). Circle provides a social container in which all voices may speak and be heard.

By contrast, *hierarchy* functions best in an environment where tasks need to be clearly delineated and carried out quickly with little or no debate, where authority requires clear boundaries, and where leaders have the time, space, and education to make good judgment calls and set directions for people who have different responsibilities (the paramedic handling triage, the skipper directing a crew through wind-whipped seas, the platoon leader on military reconnaissance). Triangle provides a social container in which safety depends on each person doing his or her part.

In the mid-1990s, Christina was editing pages for *Calling the Circle* while seated next to an airplane pilot who was flying home in economy class. He read over her shoulder for a while and then announced in a tone of friendly challenge, "From what I see on your pages, you and I are diametrically opposed human beings in how we see the world." A spirited conversation ensued, and our civility as temporary companions led us to listen to one another.

After expounding on the need for "one pilot, one decision," and the sense of responsibility he felt flying these magnificent machines, he mentioned that the research on plane crashes and other in-flight disasters had caused the Federal Aviation Administration to mandate communications training between the cockpit and the cabin crews so that they would better understand each other's skills and roles in moments of crisis. "Oh," Christina smiled, "like being able to call a circle in the air?" The two of them came to agree that he led with hierarchy and accepted circle, while she led with circle and accepted hierarchy. It was a five-mile-high dialogue of balance and partnership.

So here we are. We are facing new terrain and a plethora of challenges and disasters we can hardly imagine. No one has come this way before, yet we stand at the front edge of the long and winding path of our human heritage. The greater the number of people who understand where the application and experience of circle can take us, who have the confidence to put a candle or photo or mission statement in the middle of a shouting match and suggest a return to listening, the more empowered we will be to create the kind of world for which we long and on which our ultimate survival depends.

CHAPTER

The Components of Circle

Every conversation has an infrastructure, an understood pattern of participation. The conversational structure of PeerSpirit Circle Process is outlined here through a map known as the Components of Circle. The entire process is first presented here as a reference within the longer narrative, explicated in Chapters 3 through 6, and placed in the context of circle as a social art form in the remaining chapters of the book.

This chapter serves as the operator's manual to actual circle practice. The information here is like that little booklet in the box that says "Some assembly required" in seven languages. To assemble the circle you will need the following skills: interest in other people, a good question, and a supply of trust, tenacity, and time. Once assembled, you will have the following tools: a ring of chairs, a center, a bell, and a talking piece. With these skills and tools you'll be ready to engage your family, friends, and colleagues in an amazing collective experience. Step one in the assembly of circle: understanding that all forms of conversation are based on social infrastructure.

Social infrastructure is the pattern of exchange that allows us to interact with a sense of confidence that we are being appropriate to the moment. ("Hi, how are you?" is a social infrastructure, and so is the nearly automatic response, "Fine." We don't even need to think about it: one sentence signals the next.) There is social infrastructure in a lecture (unless you're the speaker, be quiet and listen; taking notes is a sign of respect), in a debate (timing is everything, get your points in, look bold, interrupt if possible)—and in circle.

In circle, we interact in a slightly more formal pattern than casual conversation. Circle's potential for depth and insight is ever present, and it requires that we pay increased attention. The actual content of what we say may be the same, but the patterns of engagement—who speaks when and how we listen, how we interact, and what is expected of us after the circle conversation is finished—are influenced greatly by circle structure.

A Structure for Conversation

Everything has structure: a shape or form that defines what it is. The human body, for example, is defined by the internal structure of our bones. The flesh of our physical bodies comes in nearly seven billion variations of size, shape, age, skin tone, and hair. Yet from as far off as we can see someone coming, we recognize and name that moving shape "human" based on how our skeletons hold us up and allow us to move.

Even as a two-year-old walking into a day care center in Los Angeles, Ann's grandson was not confused by an array of toddlers of all colors. "Baby, baby, baby . . . ," he would call out, practicing a favorite word. His friends all looked up: an array of little Asian, Hispanic, African American, and Caucasian faces, each different in appearance but similar in structure. We are recognizable by our bones.

We also know the circle by its "bones"—a definable structure that fleshes out in different articulations of the same form. As PeerSpirit moved into the twenty-first century, we were increasingly called on to make circle process accessible to more diverse and international audiences. Aware of our white, middle-class, American backgrounds, we went looking for a way to talk about circle that would translate cross-culturally. We began to think of the structural elements of circle as having a skeletal quality, a basic infrastructure that could flesh out with great diversity and still retain its integral form. As long as those "bones" were in place, people would recognize circle as the underlying pattern. This articulation of the conversational infrastructure as "bones of circle" first occurred to us in December 2000, when we were part of a facilitation team offering circle process to an international group of young and middle-aged community organizers.

We met at Hazelwood House, a genteel Victorian retreat center in Devonshire, England, as part of a teaching team in a movement then called From the Four Directions (F4D). F4D had been founded by Margaret J. Wheatley to introduce living systems theory and circle process in support of cross-cultural community leadership development. Having arrived from countries as different as Zimbabwe and Croatia, thirty people squeezed into a circle of chairs in a rectangular room. The conversation occurred in English, though for many this was a second or third language. In preparing for this event, the two questions PeerSpirit had been considering were *How could we most readily present the universality of circle?* and *How could we talk about the invisible elements of conversational structure in such a way that everyone could identify how circle was already present in the cultures they came from?*

By the time everyone gathered, England was in the midst of a hundred days of winter rain. The house was drafty, and many participants had arrived from warmer climates with inadequate clothes. To warm up, the young people put on music and the whole group rose to dance—arms and legs akimbo until we found a common rhythm. In that rhythm, suddenly it was obvious: we saw social interaction as a kind of dance with shape and form that defines what it is. We saw interaction as a skeletal system, in which the understood rules of engagement shape our meetings and *allow* us to move in certain ways and *restrain* us from moving in other ways.

In that room in Devon, we handed out the Components of Circle illustration (see Figure 2.1) and referred to it as the "bones of circle process." The metaphor translated well, and we have introduced it this way ever since.

The Components of Circle in the PeerSpirit model are also skeletonlike in that they connect to each other, move each other, and work best when all are active. This chapter presents the entire skeleton so that you can think about the model as a whole and can talk it through with others.

Circle can be introduced using a few pieces of structure or using the entire structure. It can work without activating all components at once—much as we shake hands without using the whole body. Yet our handshake conveys the structural strength of the whole body. Both parties know they can engage more deeply as needed—as when a handshake turns into a hug or a casual greeting turns into a heartfelt exchange. When circle interaction is gentle, we sit relaxed. When interaction is strenuous, we lean in to avail ourselves of the strength of the full structure. For purposes of simplicity, we are going to assume that *you* are calling the circle. You are getting ready to invite circle practice into a new setting or into an ongoing group that you hope will be willing to adopt circle as the process for its meetings or conversational time.

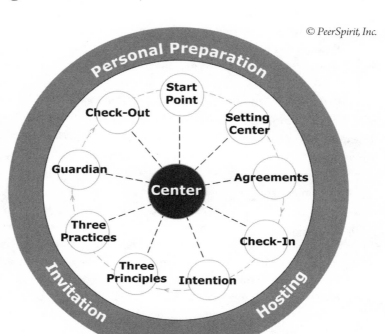

FIGURE 2.1
The Components of Circle

On the Rim

Circle structure begins at the rim with three components: *personal preparation, invitation,* and *hosting.* There is prep work to do in calling a circle. It starts with personal readiness, then invites others into the process, and finally asks you to take the initial leadership role as the circle's first host.

All processes have their own jargon. It is our intent to provide a common vocabulary of understanding about what goes on in circle and then to demonstrate how circle allows people to adapt the process to their own environments and purposes so that they might integrate circle jargon in meaningful ways.

Personal Preparation

Circle requires an intensified sense of showing up. While this intensified and intentional presence fosters rewarding conversations, it's not casual: every person's engagement or lack of engagement is noticeable. There is literally no space to hide out, to multitask, text-message, read unrelated materials, or nap. We will be leading from every chair, sitting as peers, taking risks that call on the capacities of participation and leadership from everyone in the room. Everyone is accountable to everyone else and to the purpose of the meeting.

This is often not the kind of space we are entering as people rush down hallways finishing phone calls and tossing drive-by comments to those they pass: "Joe, Tuesday, lunch. We'll talk about that staffing issue." One of the gifts of circle is to slow us down and provide a place to stop and listen, to take a breath and consider the fullness of what we want to say to each other. Personal preparation is, essentially, the practice of shifting from whizzing to attending. When we turn off the phones, the beepers, whatever little pieces of equipment keep us attached to the multitasking world, it is an invitation to take a few breaths, look around, get nourished and comfortable, focus on the people actually in the room, and take a place so that the meeting can begin.

If you are acting as host, there is additional preparation you need to have done. The host prepares the ambiance of the meeting space and has done whatever prep work may be needed. He or she has carefully considered who needs to be present and invited them. The host comes prepared to open the meeting with a start-point and check-in and has made sure people have what they need to participate.

When a friend of ours decided to host her book group in circle, she reminded everyone of the time and place and put some thought into refreshments and ambience. She finished reading the book early so that she could come up with several good questions. On the day of the meeting, she took time for a walk through the park after work and arrived ten minutes early at the library community room to make sure the space was inviting, warm, and ready. She had taken care with her own sense of groundedness and readiness and approached the evening with relaxed preparedness.

Invitation

People appreciate clarity. A verbal or written invitation addresses the questions *For what reasons are we coming together? Who will be or needs to be present? What kinds of contributions are expected of me?* (And if circle process is being introduced for the first time, *Why are we using this approach, and what does it look like?*)

Invitation is understood in both work and informal settings. When Ann's parents turned seventy-five, nearly the entire family gathered for a shared summer vacation. The invitation announced that Saturday evening would include a "talking piece council" to honor these parents and grandparents and invited everyone to think of a favorite story that illustrated the values these two elders brought to the family. The invitation prepared family members for participating in something slightly different than the usual barbecue.

In a work setting, a new board chair decided to ask the board to try using circle process for three meetings to see how it might affect their communication and decision making. He e-mailed board members this invitation:

At our next meeting, we will be addressing the need to update our mission and vision statements. I would like us to try an approach known as "circle process." It will follow the structure outlined in the attached "Basic Circle Guidelines." Please read this document before the meeting and come with an open mind. Please also bring an item that you feel represents the contribution our organization is making to its constituency. These objects will help us focus our discussion. In both the family and the board situation, hosting is happening: someone has taken the leadership role to say, "Please come," "Let's do things this way," "Let's talk about this."

Hosting

Hosting is part of our ingrained sense of social order. A host prepares and holds the space for a conversation to occur and then participates in the conversation as it occurs. At a dinner party, the host prepares the menu, sets the table, creates the ambience, puts thought into people's comfort—and *joins in* when the party begins. Things usually start off as expected, surprises happen, the event takes on a life of its own, and most of the time it all works out. Someone says, "Oh, let's do this again—next time I'll host."

In an ongoing group, it is helpful if different people host over time so that leadership rotates and everyone has the opportunity to practice. In a management leadership circle, one manager at a time hosts the conversations. The next month, the hosting shifts. In this case, hosting involves reserving a comfortable and private room, reminding the group of agreed topics of conversation, and taking leadership at the end of the gathering to ensure that topics are set for the next meeting—for which a new host steps forward.

The host can be responsible for the invitation and for introducing the components of circle—especially at the first few meetings as others learn circle process. The role of a host is more integrated than that of a facilitator. Facilitation is usually conducted by someone who stays outside the process, who attempts to take an overview, may introduce the process and the agenda and perhaps even the outcome, and devises the way the group will get to its goal. A host sits within the process. Like everyone in the circle, the host notes what topics arise, invites participation, and calls the group to shared accountability for how it will reach its goal.

Internal Components of Circle Structure

The first thing to do in calling a meeting into circle process is to literally form a circle shape. Perfect roundness is not required. Circle shape can accommodate living room furniture, square walls, or, when necessary, a boardroom or dining room table. In a recent meeting in a very oblong room dominated by a rectangular table that didn't seat the entire staff, we invited everyone who was at the table to push back their chairs and everyone who was stuck in the corners to roll their chairs forward and join the rim. This made a shape more like a big egg than a circle, but it accomplished what was needed: the people in the room became one group. We then enjoyed a meaningful round of conversation. The purpose of sitting in a circle is to allow people to notice all who are present, to see who is talking, to hear one another better, and to interact fully with the other participants.

However, walking in and finding the chairs arranged in a circle can be a bit discomfiting at first. Circle signals a much higher degree of participation and a greater sense of physical exposure. Ideally, if your invitation was effectively crafted and issued, people will come to this experience assured that their time and energy will be well used and their participation valued.

It's OK to be creative about the question of gathering around a table versus using a circle of chairs with no table or a low coffee table at the center. We have helped hosts work the issue out in a number of ways. One committee we've watched over the years developed a pattern of opening the meeting by sitting in a circle of comfortable chairs around a small coffee table that held symbols of the meeting's purpose. Because people appreciate having a table for writing and spreading out documents, they then switch to a nearby table for an agenda-based circle. At the end of the meeting, the group returns to the circle of chairs for closure. In another group, where there are often forty to fifty participants, everyone gathers in a large circle of chairs with an elaborate center that helps fill the space, and all conversations of the whole are held there. From this space, the participants periodically adjourn to clusters of small circles in an adjoining room. As people grow accustomed to the use of circle process, they often find that gathering around a table inhibits their sense of engaged interaction. They want to sit fully in the simplicity of a circle shape—gathered around a center with a full-bodied presence.

Center

The conscious placement and use of the center is one of the primary contributions of circle to conversational methodologies. If we think of the circle as a body, the center is the heart. If we think of the circle as a wheel, the center is the hub. If we think of the circle as a campfire, the center is the fire itself.

Because circle was originally held around a fire, the center always produced warmth and light. Fire requires tending: adding logs to refresh the flames, cooking food in hanging pots or wrapped and placed on the coals, banking embers for the night. The center of the circle also requires tending. We put something in the middle that is meaningful—a symbolic representation of a group's intention, purpose, or goal—and these objects allow people to visualize their reason for gathering.

In business, this might be a display of placards of company values or project goals; in education, it might be student photos and the school logo; in an informal group, the center might consist of a candle, some flowers, or a few natural objects. One simple object can make an unobtrusive and yet powerful center. Think of a circle called during a crisis and in the center of the carpet is a smooth gray rock the size of a brick into which the word IMAGINE has been laser-etched. Think of a circle gathered around a table with a small spiral of pens and Post-it notes in the middle and the invitation to take note of each other's essential contributions. People tend to rest their gaze on whatever is placed in the center, to use it as a focal point.

A tangible center creates an intangible third point between people, a sort of common ground. In customary dialogue, person A speaks, person B listens and responds, person A signals that he or she is listening, and the words go back and forth like a verbal game of table tennis. In circle, person A speaks and verbally places his or her comment in the common ground of the center, then person B speaks and places his or her response in the common ground. The sense of placing a comment or story in the center can be done by gesture, body language, voice tone, or statement ("I put this story to the center"). The center provides a neutral space where diversity of thought, stories of sorrow and outrage and heartfulness, can be held and considered by all participants.

What most often causes us to shut down and stop listening to each other is the sense that we are being barraged by another person's intensity: the person won't stop talking until we either agree or disagree. However, in circle, people can agree and disagree and keep on listening as long as each person's intensity is laid down in the center instead of against another's chest. Use of the center becomes like working together on a jigsaw puzzle, piecing our knowledge, wisdom, and passion into a coherent sense of what is going on and how we can respond. As people talk, ideas link up and synergy builds.

Start-Point

A meeting in circle has a beginning, middle, and end. We shift from social space into circle space, do the process, and then shift back out into social space. The host or other volunteer offers a simple ritual to signal these shifts. It may be ringing a chime that beckons silence, lighting a candle or setting out the center objects, or reading a quote or short inspirational reading. Any of these actions elicits the reflective attention of those who are gathering. The circle is beginning: the infrastructure is now called into play.

A friend of ours, a community college president, always begins her staff and faculty meetings, and even college assemblies, by reading a poem. "Poetry, recited aloud in settings where that is no longer common," she says, "calls people to a kind of listening I find useful. The cadence of poetry offers a sense of calm, prepares people to interact differently, and often inspires a metaphor that shows up later in the day."

People use start-points whenever they want to initiate a contained conversation. In Alcoholics Anonymous, participants recite the Twelve Steps. At school, students recite the Pledge of Allegiance or sing a school song. In organizational settings, people may read their intention statements and group agreements.

Circle Agreements

Like all social processes, the success of circle rests on the ability of participants to understand, contribute to, and abide by rules of respectful engagement. Agreements provide an interpersonal safety net for participating in the conversations that are about to occur. In a circle, where people rotate leadership and share responsibility, agreements remain constant while leadership changes and task or intention evolves. Agreements are the circle's self-governance, and they create a way for each member to hold both self and others accountable for the quality of interaction.

In an ongoing circle, we recommend that people take time to generate agreements specifically suited to their purpose and articulated in their own vernacular.

Since the circle has gathered around an intention, and in response to an invitation, the host may ask, "What agreements do we need to have in place to be able to fulfill our intent?"

When hosting a new circle or in a brief or onetime meeting, we offer the following generic agreements:

○ *Personal material shared in the circle is confidential.* It is worth spending time considering the applicable parameters of confidentiality in order to ensure that all participants share a definition of what is meant and expected of them regarding this issue.

○ *We listen to each other with curiosity and compassion, withholding judgment.* Curiosity allows people to listen and speak without having to be in total agreement: curiosity invites discernment rather than judgment.

○ *We ask for what we need and offer what we can.* This agreement is a form of self-correction in direction. Generally, if a request fits the task and orientation of the group, someone in the circle will volunteer to help carry it forward. If a request doesn't fit task and orientation, no one is likely to volunteer.

○ *From time to time we pause to regather our thoughts or focus.* To create these pauses, one member of the circle volunteers to serve as the guardian, who employs a bell or other nonverbal aural signal to introduce a moment of silence into whatever is taking place.

Sometimes negotiating agreements is a fairly quick and easy process; sometimes it is slow and complex. Negotiating agreements is a strong indicator of the level of trust and confidence, or of tension and concern, that already exists in the social field. A group will learn a lot about itself in this process, and sometimes much confusion will be cleared away. It's not always comfortable. A wise young Englishwoman once announced in the middle of our negotiations, "People, these are not frivolous phrases—we're making a life raft here! Our agreements are what carries us through stormy seas." In response to her charge, the group made strong and thoughtful agreements—and she was right: we needed them.

Check-In

As circle starts, the first time everyone has an opportunity to speak is called *check-in*—a chance for all participants to introduce themselves, respond to the invitation, or share stories about what brings them to the circle. Check-in is often framed as a specific question or direction offered by the host:

> "Please share a brief story of what drew you to participate in this circle."

> "What excites you about being here, and what concerns do you have?"

> "What has happened in the past few days that inspires you about this organization?"

The use of the talking piece greatly helps the check-in process. A talking piece is any object passed from hand to hand that signals who has the right to speak. When a person is holding the talking piece, he or she is talking and everyone else is listening without interruption or commentary. (The use of a talking piece controls the impulse to pick up on what a person is saying, to interrupt with jokes or commentary, or to ask diverting questions. It is a powerful experience to listen to one another in this way. The talking piece has served this purpose in circle since ancient times.) Circle protocol always respects the choice of someone who wishes to pass along the talking piece without speaking and remain in listening mode. At the conclusion of the round, the host usually asks if those who passed up the first opportunity are now ready to speak and offers them a chance to talk without any implication that speaking is required.

The talking piece is a great equalizer among those who differ in age, ethnicity, gender, or status. The piece assures that everyone at the rim has a voice. In modern settings, where clock time is always a factor, it is helpful to suggest a time frame for a round of the talking piece. Do "time math" for the group: "We are *X* number of people. If we each speak for two minutes, that means . . ." In the first round of a new circle, check-in may take longer than at later meetings. Typically, people become quite skilled at checking in with both meaning and brevity.

In smaller circles or among long-standing groups, the talking piece is sometimes placed in the center and people reach for it when they are ready to contribute. Although circle process does not require constant use of a talking piece, its use is suggested for check-in, for check-out (to be discussed shortly), and whenever it would be helpful for people to slow down and hear everyone's contribution.

Intention

Rotating around the Components of Circle diagram, we come to intention. Intention is the understood agreement of why people are present, what they intend to have happen, and what they commit to doing and experiencing together. The invitation articulates the host's intention. Sometimes intention is concrete: we are gathered to vote on finalizing this year's budget. Sometimes intention combines the concrete and visionary: we are gathered to vote on a budget that will enable us to focus on meeting the changing environmental needs of our community. Sometimes intention is ideological: we're here to have a conversation about how to improve community relations.

Defining intention is a process of self-examination for both the individual and for the group as a whole. Intention gets us in the room with each other, usually glad that someone took the initiative to host the conversation, and starts us toward action—and then, once we all contribute, intention evolves. For example, if the intention for a meeting is to generate ideas to improve customer service, each person arrives with a slightly different personal intent. One person's intention may be influenced by the fact that she is in charge of customer service and needs to present herself as being "on top of things." Another person's intention may be influenced by the fact that he is tired of customer service "getting all the attention" and wants to move through the agenda item quickly and into his area of expertise. Ultimately, the group intention is shaped by all these individual tensions and, hopefully, draws forth a synergy of creativity that becomes a collective vision.

Intention requires a conscious balancing between personal and collective needs. There is something each person wants to have happen: there is something the group wants to create. When these two energies emerge and coexist, the circle really steps into a sense of itself.

It is as important to the long-term success of a circle to spend as much time honing the intention as it is spending time crafting the agreements. Intentions can be made clearer by including a time frame. For example, in gathering to save trees and create a park, the group may agree to meet for six months and work toward that goal and then revisit their progress. Softer, more loosely defined intentions also benefit from a time frame: "Let's have a monthly breakfast meeting to talk about neighborliness and then check if we are being personally nourished by the conversation and want to continue it." The clearer the intent of the people in circle, the more focused the dynamic of the circle will be. Reworking intention can save a circle that's floundering or help a group understand how to set itself back on track.

Three Principles of Circle

Circle process functions under three principles of participation: rotating leadership, sharing responsibility, and relying on wholeness.

Rotating leadership means that every person helps the circle function by assuming increments of leadership. This is evidenced in the roles of host and guardian (and scribe, when that function is needed), and every person is invited to interact in circle with a sense of self-determination, volunteerism, and tending to common needs. "I could do that, let me take that on." Rotating leadership trusts that the resources to accomplish the circle's purpose exist within the group. If no one is interested, that lack of interest becomes the next topic of conversation, an exploration without blame or judgment.

Sharing responsibility means that every person watches for what needs doing or saying next and makes a contribution. Sharing responsibility breaks old patterns of dominance and passivity and calls people to safeguard the quality of their experience, to jointly manage the allocation of time, and to notice how decisions arise out of group synergy. "Guardian, could you ring the bell? We've veered off topic here, and I want us either to get back or to make a clear decision to digress."

Reliance on wholeness means that through the act of making individual contributions, people in circle generate a social field of synergistic magnitude. Reliance on wholeness reminds people that the circle consists of all who are present *and* the presence of the circle itself. Wholeness is an animation of circle process beyond methodology; it acknowledges the archetypal energy of circle lineage. Things happen that we do not expect, and we discover in ourselves the capacity to respond brilliantly.

Many of the stories throughout this book illustrate the principle of reliance on wholeness; these are the memorable moments that people ponder, are moved by, and look back on as turning points. Whatever skills and talents we bring to a circle meeting, whatever hesitancy and doubt accompany us into an issue we fear is irresolvable, this principle invites us to remain present and attentive to our interactions on the rim and to attach our energies to the center, like spokes on a bicycle wheel, so that the synergism of wholeness may hold us and spin us.

Three Practices of Council

The practices of council invite circle participants to speak, listen, and act from within the infrastructure in place.

Attentive listening is the practice of focusing clearly on what is being said by someone else. In circle, listening is a contribution we offer one another. There is too little actual listening in the world; too often we are waiting for our turn to insert our own thoughts and stories. Listening through the center of the circle allows us to receive people's thoughts, feelings, and stories and stay separate from them, stay curious, look for the essence, seek a place to connect even when there is surface disagreement. Attentive listening is a kind of spiritual practice that shifts us out of reactivity and into deep inquiry.

Intentional speaking is the practice of contributing stories and information that have heart and meaning or relevance to the situation. It comes from the patience of waiting for the moment when we each really understand what to contribute and when receptivity is alive in the group. Intentional speaking does not mean agreement; it means noticing when the piece of the truth that is ours to say may be received and then to say it, avoiding blame and judgment—to speak in neutral language. It means that attentive listening is in place and that each person is able to make a contribution while still tending to the well-being of the group.

Attending to the well-being of the group is the practice of considering the impact of our words and actions before, during, and after we speak. It is important to take time before speaking to inquire of ourselves what it is we want to contribute. Typical questions to the self might include the following:

- What is my motivation or hope for sharing this?

- What is my body telling me about tension or excitement?

- How do I offer my contribution in a way that will benefit what we're doing?

- How do I need to consider what I say, before I say it, and still speak my "truth?"

These practices are profound gifts of circle process: that we can speak the fullness of what we have to say and listen to the fullness of what others have to say and do so in ways that sustain relationship.

Guardian

While all participants hold the infrastructure of circle, the role of mindful watching falls to the guardian. We adapted this role to circle process after attending a lecture in the early 1990s by the gentle Buddhist monk Thich Nhat Hanh. He sat on a simple meditation cushion on a raised dais so that the thousand people in the hall of the hotel conference center could listen attentively as he spoke softly into a microphone. Several times in the middle of his speech, his traveling companion rang a small, resonant bell from somewhere in the middle of the audience. Thich Nhat Hanh ceased speaking and entered a thoughtful silence—and so did the thousand listeners. After a while, Thich Nhat Hanh would announce quietly, "The bell calls me back to myself," and resume speaking while we resumed attentive listening.

The guardian observes both practical and spiritual needs and tries to be extraordinarily aware of how group process is functioning. To employ guardianship, the circle needs to supply itself with a small brass bell, chime, or other object that makes a pleasant sound loud enough to be heard during conversation (a rattle, rain stick, or small drum might be appropriate, depending on the setting). Usually rotating on a meeting-by-meeting basis, one person volunteers to serve in the guardian role. The guardian has the group's permission to intercede in group process for the purpose of calling the circle back to center, to slow down conversation that has speeded up, to focus on the group's intention or task, or to return to respectful practices as outlined in the agreements. The guardian also works with the host to stick to the time frame of the meeting or agenda and to call for breaks when necessary.

The use of a chime or bell as part of group process is becoming increasingly common. A pair of Tibetan cymbals, called *tingsha,* will resonate in human ears for fifteen seconds—time to take an elongated breath. *Tingsha* has its own Wikipedia entry, along with Tibetan singing bowls. Tone bars or bar chimes, consisting of a horizontal silver tube suspended on a wood base, are available at mainstream music stores.

When the guardian rings the bell, conversation and interaction stop. Everyone takes a breath and waits for the guardian to signal the return to action by a second ring of the bell: *ring, pause, ring, resume.* Often the guardian, or the person who asked the guardian to ring, will speak a few words about why—"I thought we had speeded up and stopped listening" or "I needed to take a breath."

Over and over again in the years since *Calling the Circle* was first released, we have found the guardian to be central to the PeerSpirit process, particularly in those inevitable times when tension arises. *Anyone may ask the guardian to ring the bell at any time.* This is one of the ways that leadership rotates in a circle. One person holds the responsibility of guardian, and others help. The bell becomes a voice in the circle that honors the process.

Scribe

Not every circle requires a record of its process, but when such a record is wanted, the role of scribe can be activated to help gather these insights. There are many creative ways to keep such a record: participants can work collectively with journals on their laps or individually on laptop computers, on chart pages spread out on table or floor, on a flip chart stand placed along the rim of the circle, or even on a wall on which papers can be pinned.

Like the guardian, the scribe sits in a more observational mode and listens for essence statements, new insights, and decisions rising to the fore. In the energy of heightened conversation, there is often a collective awareness that something significant has just been said. "Whoa, did we capture that? Who's scribing?" is a common comment at these moments. We like to use the word _harvest_, rather than _report_, for recording these insights. At the conclusion of circle time, a collective harvest may be part of check-out: "What did you hear today that you take away as your primary learning?" is a harvest question. And if no scribe has been writing earlier, the host may ask someone to take on that role during closure.

The role of scribe is not the same as that of a minute-taker. If minutes are required in an organizational context, circle members need to discuss how to handle this because the intensity of minute-taking and the required detail and accuracy greatly limit the ability of the person to participate fully in the gathering, thus making it an unsuitable role for the scribe to fulfill.

Forms of Council

There are basically three forms of council: talking piece council, conversation council, and silence. The principles, practices, agreements, guardian, and center are _essential_ in each form.

Talking piece council is a more formal pattern of speaking and listening. When engaging a talking piece, permission to speak passes from person to person. One person speaks; the group listens. The purpose of talking piece council is to hear each voice, to garner insight and show respect for each person's presence, to seek collective wisdom, and to create consensus. These are the ancient practices of circle process. As the talking piece passes around the rim, the commentary often takes on a spiraling quality, gathering depth and calling people one by one to increased clarity.

Talking piece council is often used during check-in so that every person has a way to participate verbally and to signal the shift from socializing to circle. In talking piece councils, people have a chance to witness the stories each member of the circle wishes to share. When used to elicit responses to a specific question, each person speaks without necessarily making reference to what others have said.

Conversation council is employed when people desire a more informal structure or a quickened pace of contribution and response. In conversation council, as in ordinary conversation, people pick up on what others are saying. They react, interact, brainstorm, disagree, persuade, and interject new ideas, thoughts, and opinions. The energy of open dialogue stimulates the free flow of ideas. There are times when conversation is essential to circle process and times when circle will work better if it's slowed down a bit, allowed a calmer pacing and more contemplation.

The two forms of verbal council shift back and forth according to need and may hybridize such as when tossing a Koosh ball from speaker to speaker.

Silence has not usually been considered a form of meeting except in meditation settings. However, silence in circle is an important way to support deepened thoughtfulness. Silence provides time for members to write in their journals together or respond in writing to a pertinent question. It can also be a time for inward centering that is shared collectively. A host might say, "This is an important moment for us as a group. Let's take a moment of silence to be thoughtful. Guardian, would you ring us in and out, tending to time?" A few minutes of silent council can be an incredibly effective centering tool before or after a longer talking piece council.

Silence in most social settings, especially in business, can convey many different things, and people may be uncomfortable unless a context is set. When silence occurs spontaneously in reaction to something that has happened, it is helpful to have it named and welcomed. The host might say, "It seems we don't know what to do or say next. We've fallen silent, so let's welcome this pause and hold our peace until the way forward is clear."

Consensus and Voting

People often ask us, "Can a circle make a decision? How does a circle make a decision?" *Consensus is a process in which all participants have come to agreement before a decision goes forward or action is taken.* Consensus is applied when a group wants or needs to take collective responsibility for actions. In a PeerSpirit group, there needs to be a sense that everyone supports what the circle is about to do. Consensus doesn't require that everyone have the same degree of enthusiasm for each action or decision, but it does require that each person approve the group action or is willing to support the action the group is about to take. Consensus provides a stable, unifying base. Once consensus is reached, the circle can speak of its actions as "we."

One way to signal consensus is to institute a thumb signal:

thumb up = "I'm for it."

thumb sideways = "I still have a question."

thumb down = "I don't think this is the right way for us to go."

Clarifying conversations occur, led by anyone with a sideways or downward thumb. Although the downward thumb indicates disapproval, it may not necessarily block action. With further conversation, the person may actually be willing to say, "I don't support this action, but I support the group." Keeping dialogue open in the middle of the thumb vote allows for continued insight and learning, and the decision made is stronger by including space for hesitancy or resistance.

Consensus can also hybridize according to a circle's needs. Some groups operate with a consensus-minus-one philosophy. Group members listen carefully to the dissenting voice, and if the group remains confident in its decision, they honor the principle to move ahead so that no single person can stop a decision.

Check-Out

Having opened the circle with respect, it is equally important to close in a way that signals the circle's completion. Because heightened attention is required to listen and speak carefully in circle, people want to know when to relax. Before closing, the host may invite the participants to revisit their insights, action items, or agreements, especially if there is need to clarify confidentiality..

A common circle closing invites a brief check-out so that every person has a chance to speak briefly what he or she has learned, heard, appreciated, or committed to doing. The circle may want to designate the host for the next meeting and pass along certain duties in order to maintain coherence. Final closing may then be offering a quote, poem, or brief silence, followed by the bell.

We'd like to return to the seventy-fifth birthday circle Ann organized for her parents, mentioned earlier in the chapter. After an hour of talking piece council and dozens of thoughtful, funny, and sometimes poignant stories, Ann closed the circle with a rousing rendition of "Happy Birthday." Immediately after the song ended, cacophony erupted in the room. The measured cadence of story sharing was over. It was time for chatting, refreshments, and release from careful listening. Bring on the cake!

It may not be anyone's birthday, but this sense of celebration at good process well done is often alive in the room. In the egg-shaped staff meeting circle, even though people had been vulnerable and the company had had to make some difficult decisions that affected people in the room, participants left the meeting in good spirits, able to get on with their day, knowing that they had been listened to and feeling pleased with their contribution to the conversation.

Coming Full Circle

Circle structure is intuitive. Once we begin these practices, we remember this way of being together. There is a fundamental familiarity with circle process from our long social history that is lying dormant, just waiting to be reactivated. Over the years, we have experimented with a number of ways to communicate this basic structure. The longest versions are book-length. The medium-length versions are this chapter and our self-published booklets. On our Web site, the two-page downloadable document, "Basic Circle Guidelines," is available in a growing number of languages. And we have fit the most essential elements onto one side of a business card. The chapters in Part II elucidate these components with further insights and stories. We will keep exploring how the circle's bones will hold you and hold the group—they are weight-bearing, and they are strong.

So now you have the operator's manual. You have assembled the knowledge needed to start hosting. Just try it. We can check in and check out with each other in almost any environment, and doing so will improve the quality of our connections. We can begin to shift our engagement at work, at home, and in community organizations from competition to collaboration simply by how we show up and contribute and the things we acknowledge about what's going on. We can live the agreements, principles, and practices—whether or not they have been introduced to the group we're in. When *we* show up differently, different things happen. People get curious.

Curiosity is an effective model of circle introduction. Several years ago, we offered a one-day circle training with a group of beleaguered managers who were not sure if they dared take this back to their departments—they feared resistance and were unsure of their skills to really hold to the form. The group came up with the idea that they should start by practicing with each other. They decided to host monthly manager meetings in circle in order to gain confidence in their hosting capacities, and they adopted an agreement that they could stop action and talk about the process while practicing it. The managers met in the education room near the reception area where there was space to make a circle of chairs. They experimented with how to blend needed topics of conversation with needed time to get to know each other better. Sometimes the tenor of the meeting was hushed with emotion or poignancy, and other times the inviting sounds of raucous laughter leaked under the door. Even though the janitor told the receptionist who told the departmental assistants that occasionally there was a lot of Kleenex in the waste bins, people noticed that their managers seemed happier and more focused after these meetings. People began to ask, "What are you doing in there?"

Pretty soon the managers were ready to say, "We're practicing circle. Want to join us?"

Practicing is the key. Circle is not a succeed-or-fail environment: it is a constantly shifting, imperfect, self-correcting learning field. "What if I mess up?" is a common concern. Well, the guardian is there to pause the process and invite the group to inquire with curiosity:

- What's not working here?

- Why isn't it working?

- What are we willing to do about it?

- What's our wisdom?

You, the host, are not succeeding or failing: we, the whole circle, are learning. This is the shift: the host is not like the driver of a car, steering all alone and responsible for whether or not the vehicle stays on the road or crashes into a tree. The whole group is steering. Everyone is connected to the hub of the wheel. And most of the time, most of the people want the process to work, want the host and guardian to offer the level of guidance needed in the moment, and want everyone's participation to be received and meaningful. Most people would rather learn from little readjustments of course than wait until problems become big swerves necessary to avoid impact.

In the fully participatory model of PeerSpirit Circle Process, everyone will eventually take a turn as host, guardian, and scribe; everyone will serve as leader of an agenda topic, holder of a question, and spinner of synergy. This inclusivity of risk taking creates a strong desire to support whoever is serving as leader at the moment. We are going to want similar support when our turn comes.

Circles at Work in the World

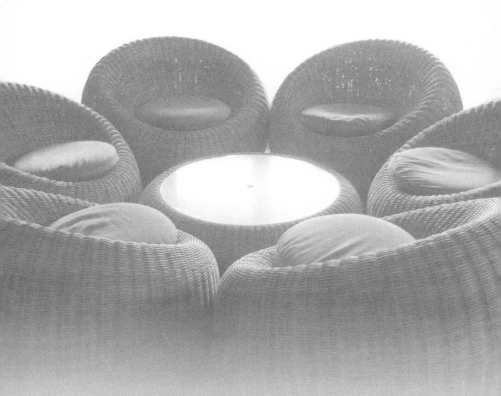

CHAPTER

The Power of Preparation, Invitation, Intention, and Center

Meetings of all kinds function better when the right people are in the room and they know why they have gathered and how they might contribute: this is the power of invitation and intention. Placing a visual representation of shared purpose in the center creates a focus for the group.

A leader in the human resources department, PJ, was enjoying circle process in her women's group and wanted to bring her experience of careful listening and cohesive purpose from her monthly gathering to her meetings at work. She entered the process of preparation. "I knew something good was happening in the rounds of check-in in the women's group that could translate to team building within the company," she said, "if I could just figure out how to do it. And I knew that if I described what was happening in a girlfriend's living room—half a dozen candles lit on her coffee table, Enya playing in the background, passing a conch shell from hand to hand and talking about our feelings—that I'd be up a creek and speaking Greek!" She laughed heartily imagining pandemonium. PJ's first act of preparation is to switch the vernacular of circle to a more business-oriented frame while still honoring the experience and infrastructure of circle. This is a fairly common need for translation: people learn of circle in business and want to take it home, or they learn of circle in a personal setting and want to take it to business.

37

PJ calls herself a "pacing thinker." She has worn a track in the carpeting around her desk that everyone agrees is a productive sign. "I knew the invitation had to sound businesslike and still remain somewhat holistic," she said, pacing by. "I mean, it was possible that an appropriate but perhaps a bit surprising level of truth and heartfulness would emerge because that is what circle does. However, I didn't want folks to feel ambushed, and I didn't want to doom the experiment by trying to design in emotional content rather than allowing the authentic feelings people already have to emerge from the structure of circle itself."

Whenever circle is called with invitation and intention, we need to be prepared—not necessarily for trouble but for a release of power. There are conversations eagerly waiting to occur that cannot happen until a strong interpersonal container is set out for them. In the midst of all the talking, e-mailing, and texting that goes on in our wired days, there is a corresponding silence around deeper conversations. Once people slow down, sit down, take a breath, and raise a question, these waiting topics come forth. It's not a policy of "don't ask, don't tell" so much as an unconscious omission of space that allows us to ask so that we may tell.

In a harried moment around the coffee pot, the question *So why did we become nurses?* is likely to elicit quick repartee—"I just like blood!" (said with a laugh) or "Me? I was twenty and wanted to stay up all night and make money. Now I'm fifty, and I can't get to sleep. Go figure." A patient light goes on, and everyone scatters to the next task. But as we saw in Chapter 1 in the story of the Center for Nursing Leaders, the same question offered in the rim of a circle allows people to tap into the wellspring of their life purpose and to learn some poignant history about one another. So PJ is wise to tend first to preparation—of herself and of the space in which to hold such conversation.

Levels of Preparation

This is often how preparation for circle in an organization begins: one person, who becomes the initial host, reads about circle process or has an experience of circle process that is transformative and wants to apply it meaningfully somewhere else in his or her life. These initiators want to take it into the places where relationships or processes need to be more collaborative, thoughtful, and creative. Like PJ, they begin to articulate their desire for something different to themselves and imagine changed outcomes..

There are three facets to preparation: getting one's own motivation clear, writing and extending the invitation, and literally finding time and space.

Exhibit 3.1

What I Have Enough Of	What I Have Too Much Of	What I Want More Of
Support from husband for doing this work; good friends who let me download and find humor in situations	Meetings that are ill-planned, more meetings that are ill-planned, and even more meetings that I have to plan; number of e-mails and calls per day	Weekends! Time when I am really not mentally at work; time to exercise; time to enjoy cooking for us—not just take-out
Fair compensation, good health, etc.	People thinking I have to know everything—they don't trust their own autonomy.	Mini-vacations that revive my spirit; time to have fun with family and friends.

PJ began her self-explorations by making a chart with three columns (see Exhibit 3.1). Then she asked herself, *What do I think circle has to do with this?* She opened a folder on her computer and began an informal journal in which to jot down more questions, thoughts, and ideas that came to her in the following weeks.

While attending to her inner preparation, PJ also began to explore what her workplace had in the way of tangibles for holding a circle—chairs, tables, meeting spaces. "We're talking major shift here," she noted in a conversation with a friend from the women's group. "People are used to sitting in rows, and I think they kind of like the time to check out, look like they're listening to what's coming down from admin, and take a little brain nap. And all our work teams sit around rectangular tables with the project leader at the head. The only place I could even find comfortable, movable chairs was in reception, and the only place I could find round tables was in the snack room. So this was going to take some thought."

As she searched for literal space, PJ wrote a vision statement—an image of the circle experience she wished to offer and participate in. It began, "I am sitting with my team in a ring of comfortable chairs, and we are ..."

These reflective activities of preparation can be refined to fit the personalities of any of us. They are useful tools in that they help us attach to a source of inner leadership that gives us courage to invite staff and colleagues to get behind a potentially huge shift in how business gets done. Leading from the rim, hosting as a peer, calling on the willingness of everyone in the room to participate fully—these are not easy requests to make. As we prepare to call the circle, we need to examine the "what I want more of" parts of our working days; we need to look for allies, other people who express a similar longing for improved relationships and uses of time. We need to think about what we will lean on for support while the group leans on us in its learning curve and early experiences.

Every morning on the way to work, PJ pulls into her favorite drive-through coffee stand and purchases a skinny tall latte. Sipping this as she moves her Toyota Matrix in and out of lanes of traffic en route to work, she attaches her iPod to the sound system and listens to music her husband has downloaded for her. "This routine calms me down and makes me ready for whatever happens when I enter the glass doors of our building. Call it a routine or ritual; all I know is, my day would not go well without it." We all have ways we tap into intuition or guidance, a sense that we are being assisted to make wise choices of word and deed. When preparing to host a circle, taking time to amplify our connectedness to these inner resources will serve us in the circle.

It has been our experience over the years that it is exactly this inner preparedness we most need as circle work takes its turns and shifts, deepens, and lights our way. When we who host launch a question and a talking piece in the circle, we do not control what happens next. We can set expectations about time and timeliness, we have the guardian ready to help us hold the space, we sometimes have a scribe ready to record the essence—and then we trust each other and the process.

There is an inner core of preparation that serves us in this work. The more we are each able to listen for a sense of guidance, rather than pulling our responses to situations out of our habitual thinking, the more readily we prepare to receive the wisdom that lies waiting in any gathering of people. Whether calling a circle for an HR staff meeting, a men's or women's group, or a community gathering, taking the time to attend to all levels of personal preparation steadies us to offer the methodology and to participate with the mystery.

This is the learning curve throughout this book: leading from the edge requires that we keep calling each other back to our core purpose and that we allow a certain amount of digression, confusion, excitement, and surprise to pour through the conversation so that our creativity is enlivened by being together.

Invitation and Intention

A major aspect of calling a group into circle is the art of issuing a clear invitation. This is a "Please join me" statement that allows people to say yes, no, or maybe, to understand why they are being invited, to know who else is coming, and what commitment is requested. When composing an invitation, the host may want to consider the following questions:

- What is the topic to be addressed or the experience into which people are invited?

- What will be the major focus, expectation, and activity?

- Who needs to be present, and why? (This personalizes the invitation to different essential participants and helps them determine if they wish to send an appropriate substitute if necessary.)

- What time commitment and potential follow-up commitment are required?

- What does each person need to know about circle process when considering the invitation?

To issue a clear invitation, the host needs to have a clear intention. The invitation gets the right people into the room so that they can respond to and influence the intention.

PJ's invitation for the first meeting of the year read as follows:

Subject: Happy New Year, Everyone!

When you enter the meeting room tomorrow, please gather first at the circle of chairs you will find there. You can place your papers on the rectangular table for our business meeting. We'll open with a brief opportunity for each person to respond to this request—"Share one story from the past week that demonstrates our new company initiatives at work." The initiative statements will be resting on a small table in the center of the circle of chairs. Our check-in will take about 15 minutes. The remainder of the meeting will take place at our usual table. The agenda is printed below. Let me know if you have any questions.

In her invitation, PJ clearly states her intention and invites participants to be prepared for something slightly different from the usual. Her plan is to introduce check-in and check-out, with the rest of the meeting proceeding in their usual pattern—at least for a while. At the end of the meeting, she intends to ask, "Would you be willing to add check-in and check-out to more of our meetings?" Even though she's convinced that circle would add to the quality of her staff's interactions, her cautious respect demonstrates one way of weaving circle into an organization over time.

Here are some other sample invitations for onetime gatherings:

> *Please come to my birthday party and know that at 4:00 P.M. we will hold a brief circle to share our experiences of turning 40, 50, or 60.*

> *From 12:00 to 2:00 P.M. next Thursday, you are invited to a complimentary lunch to celebrate Joe's contributions to our company. We'll eat first and then ask Joe to sit in the middle of the dining room while people offer appreciative comments regarding his service.*

> *I am calling a circle to respond to the opportunity to start a neighborhood garden in Kathy's yard. We need to work out the land use covenants and building costs for this project and develop a way to make collaborative decisions about what to grow, who does what, and how to manage the harvest. Imagine whirled peas! Come join this fun and fruitful way to build our community and eat well.*

A well-thought-out invitation allows people to begin to imagine their participation with some confidence about what will transpire and what is being asked of them. People come to the birthday party already thinking about their own decade birthdays. They come to Joe's lunch with an anecdote in mind, and those who don't wish to speak in public may write out their appreciation and slip it to him privately. Neighbors showing up at the garden meeting have been invited into an atmosphere of friendship as well as work and know they are making a long-term commitment, including a financial contribution.

All of us experience meetings and events that are not clearly called, held, or completed that work out fine. Sometimes, as in going to a friend's house for supper or out for pizza after the ball game, we want things to be loose, undefined, and spontaneous. However, when we are asked to attend meetings that are loose, undefined, and spontaneous, frustration rises. One of the major complaints about how our time is spent, particularly in business settings, is that there are too many meetings where nothing happens. Clarity of intention and invitation will radically change the spirit of efficiency and participation in circle meetings.

Evolving Intentions for Ongoing Circles

As intention moves beyond a single event, the complexity of what's being addressed may quickly change or expand and require additional thought from the caller of the circle and from the group.

Here is a private example of shifting intention. A few years ago, Christina was seeking a small monthly circle of local friends willing to join in a conversation deeper than after-dinner gatherings. She sent out an invitation that articulated her idea for the general framework. Three people responded, "Yes—let's try it together." As it turned out, all three are women who keep journals. After a couple of months, it became clear that the deepest need for each of them was to enjoy a few hours of quiet writing time, followed by reading their journal entries and a check-in. Almost without noticing, they shifted their intention from topical conversation to writing reflection. At the end of each year, they revisit the structure and choose whether or not to enter another cycle.

While this circle is ongoing, someday it is likely to come to a completion. The women honor the cyclical nature of circles by asking each other from time to time: Is this still nourishing us? Do any of our patterns need to change? Is there anything more or less we want of each other? These are not the kinds of questions we ask very often in business—and what a shift would occur if we did.

Here's an organizational example. Our colleague Bonnie Marsh provided a powerful template for bringing circle to her organization. At the time we first worked with Bonnie in the mid-1990s, she was corporate senior vice-president for strategic development at Fairview Health Services in Minneapolis, Minnesota. Bonnie had read a newspaper article about the first edition of Christina's book, *Calling the Circle*. She purchased a copy, was excited by the ideas, and approached her CEO, Rick Norling. "If I am going to do this huge work of bringing together departments that have not worked together before, I need to do it differently," she said to Rick. She handed him a copy of the book. "This is what I'd like to try. What do you think?"

A few days later, Rick strolled down the hall, put the book back on her desk, and said, "It could be a little soft as a management process. On the other hand, if it works, it could be exactly what you need." Bonnie promptly gave copies of the book to each of her eighteen managers, asked them to read it, and invited them to try staff meetings in circle. Most of the managers under her jurisdiction—organizational development, human resources, and strategic planning—had never met together before. People agreed to try the experiment, and we traveled out to offer three days of training. They didn't know it, but the team was our first big corporate client. Our time with them was truly a mutual learning experience.

Bonnie's attention to the importance of getting permission from her superior and then getting acceptance from her reporting colleagues set a tone of inclusivity and ownership that ultimately led to great success. She respected the triangle structure in place and used it as a foundation on which to introduce circle structure. In Fairview hierarchy, Bonnie was the boss: in the circle, she was a colleague holding her corporate rank in the background. Like so many creative leaders, she genuinely believed in gathering the wisdom of the whole, and she had to do it without pretending that the other structures didn't influence the circle.

When the circle comes into organizational settings, the triangle is always present. Circle process morphs back and forth between moments of freewheeling collegiality and recognition of authority. Bonnie deliberately avoided hosting as much as possible because she didn't want her status in the hierarchy to weigh heavily in the group. And yet there were times when the circle counted on her to carry issues and ideas to the CEO.

As the months progressed, the circle established itself as a "no guilt" zone where these incredibly busy department leaders could use the safety of their agreements and confidentiality to share their challenges and support one another. As Bonnie had hoped, the old mode of communicating only within departmental silos changed significantly.

Over the next four years, we made annual visits to consult with the management circle. "I believed thoroughly that we needed to bring more heart and spirit into our work, and I knew that it was absent in most of the forums I was in," explained Bonnie. "Circle provided a phenomenal shift for us." By the end of the second year, these managers talked about how to have maximum impact on their eighteen thousand–employee system. They even considered dropping all department titles and redesigning themselves into a single "strategic development department."

"For me, that was clearly the biggest marker that something different was happening," said Bonnie. "Another important moment was the day one of our members came to the circle asking for help in how to respond to a corporate memo that told her there was nothing to be done about employees' complaints in a unit that desperately needed resources and attention. She wanted the circle's assistance to formulate a position statement that would communicate to top management that this was an unacceptable response that was sure to create more problems. It was a delicate and complex situation where the manager felt responsible to the unit, which had worked to voice a coherent complaint and request help, and she understood the priorities and constraints at the upper-management level. The circle helped her to craft clear language. She took her intervention to corporate and worked toward a better resolution. I don't think corporate ever knew she stood with the circle at her back the way she did and that we were watching her progress."

In an ongoing group like Bonnie's managerial team, intention needs to be periodically revisited. She set an intention for meeting in a more inclusive, circular fashion, and both her boss and her team responded positively to the invitation as issued. Once they had experienced the impact of circle process for several months and claimed it as their own, they needed to revisit intention so that the words continued to serve their needs and reflect their evolution.

Over the next few years, as the group matured and shifted, added new members, and changed responsibilities, it required a number of conversations about the role and intention of the circle in the expanding corporation. They held on to their agreements and Fairview's core values; they held on to their time together for four years. Bonnie and others moved to positions outside Fairview, and slowly the circle dissipated as the remaining people ended up reporting to different vice-presidents and others were laid off. However, that circle seeded circles in other organizations that are evolutions from this pioneering experience.

Personal Intention in Group Process

Groups always consist of some people who are primarily focused on tangible accomplishment and want reflection afterward and other people who enjoy reflecting on the quality of process and relationship before diving into action. For those focused on tangible accomplishment, talking about group process is often frustrating because they don't perceive it as part of the "doing." For those who ground their work through understanding process, overlooking circle's potential for deepening relationship seems a misuse of the form: they want to "be" together before "doing" together. Circle requires members to constantly balance individual style and group intent. Remember, there is something each person wants to have happen; there is something the group wants to create. These two energies need to coexist and cooperate.

In Christina's personal circle, the original intention was to create a social container to explore specific questions. In Bonnie's managerial circle, the intention was to increase communication between different departments. Both of these intentions are quite broad compared to an intention among neighbors to start a shared vegetable garden. Whether circle intention is broad or specific, individuals arrive with their own motivations, desires, and agenda. The ability of people to hold their personal intentions within the collective intention is greatly helped by keeping these issues part of the ongoing conversation.

In a cooperative environment, personal intention (what *I* hope to contribute and gain) and group intention (what *we* can accomplish by being together) are held in balance. However, since we live in an atmosphere dominated by tition, people often come to circle carrying an internalized competitive edge, even if they don't mean to. We often speak of circle as a process of remembering how to behave differently—switching from acculturated competition to voluntary cooperation. One way to help this shift occur is to acknowledge that everyone has a personal intention and to name it as part of group process. Perhaps everyone completes statements such as these:

- I joined this group because . . .
- I most want to contribute . . .
- I most need to receive . . .
- I'd like to look back on this experience and see that I . . .

Each person then reads his or her statement to the group in a round of talking piece council followed by open conversation. Sometimes we invite people to write their statements on large sheets of paper and post them along one wall of a room or spread them out in the space between the rim and the center so that we can work with the patterns of commonality and diversity that show up.

Another possibility is to open a circle using the check-in question: *What intention do you offer circle today?* Individual intentions are then all clearly placed in the center—sometimes with people literally placing an object symbolic of their personal intention in the center. A rich conversation about how to combine them into a cohesive working intention can then emerge.

Center

Two things are immediately noticeable when participants walk into the room where circle is being held. First, the chairs are in a true circular shape, or as close to that shape as furniture allows, and second, the head of the table or front of the room has been replaced by a center.

The conscious placement and use of the center is one of the primary contributions PeerSpirit Circle Process offers modern conversational methodologies. Because circle was first held around a common fire, center is remembered as a place of warmth and light. Just as fire requires tending, the center of the circle also requires tending. Even when no fire is present, people will talk to a center point and understand that the energy of shared intention resides in the carefully chosen symbolic objects placed in the middle of the circle.

The Fairview circle conducted its twice-a-month business meetings sitting in a circle of chairs with a low coffee table in the center. At the first training, we inscribed four placards for the group,, that stated the four corporate core values: "Service," "Integrity," "Dignity," "Compassion." The placards were then placed on the coffee table along with a small vase of flowers. The group adapted and maintained this center and counted on the visual presence of the four values. Periodically, individuals also placed objects in the center in response to a check-in question.

Objects placed in the center allow people to visualize and remember their reason for gathering. Centers are as variable as circles themselves, for they reflect the highest intention for the group's gathering. At a school board meeting, the center might be a bowl of apples. In a gathering of nurses, a replica of the Florence Nightingale lamp might reside in the center. A group of wilderness guides will likely be gathered around a real campfire. A group of financial planners might place client portfolios and ethics statements in the center with an old-fashioned piggy bank.

Perhaps the most elaborate center we've experienced was in the middle of a gymnasium floor with forty-five Wheaton Franciscan sisters seated in padded chairs around it. The gymnasium was the only place in their motherhouse large enough to host a circle of so many women. The yellow pine floorboards with the black markings for basketball games seemed an unusual place to engage in a dialogue with religious women about the future of their province. Yet the highly visionary leadership team of Provincial Marge Zulaski and Gabriele Uhlein, Patricia Norton, and Alice Drewek, understood the introduction of circle process as the paradigm shift they sought for their community and the legacy of their leadership.

Sister Gabriele volunteered to design a strong visual center. The transformation of the gymnasium was amazing: rice paper screens encircled the backs of the chairs, creating an effect that the whole circle was being held and protected. The center itself was about twelve feet in diameter with candles, flowers, and cloths coordinated with the colors of the liturgical season (see Figure 3.1).

During the opening of each "wisdom circle" (two- or three-day gatherings held quarterly over an eighteen-month period), the sisters spoke into a hand-held microphone that served as their talking piece and each placed a personal object at the edge of this center—thus adding their individual intentions to their work together. Day after day, the women spoke into the reflected beauty of their lineage to voice thoughts, feelings, and opinions. During evening sessions, when the mood was set more for story and reflection, the center shimmered with candlelight to evoke heartfelt sharing.

Later one sister commented, "The center prepared the space, and bringing an object to the center prepared us. When I looked around to choose an object

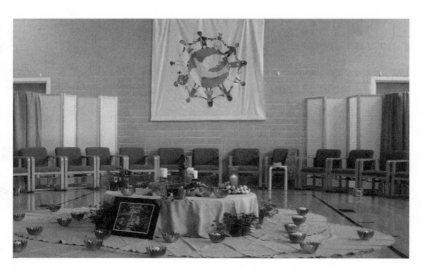

FIGURE 3.1

for the center, it required thinking about how I was coming to the meeting. Our center enabled a clearer quality of arrival in us."

Intention and _center_ are the most basic components of circle. Intention holds the rim and sets the parameter. Center holds the heart and the mindfulness of why we're gathered. If a circle stops feeling like a circle and slips into versions of triangle in the round, reviewing intention—both personal and collective—is a democratic way of reestablishing focus. And reactivating the center so that it has a pleasing aesthetic and meaning can provide a calming attachment to the archetype that supports us in these modern experiences of our ancient social patterning.

PJ is right to be thinking things through. The initial call to circle she made for the January meeting has immediate and long-range potential to change the ways she works with her team and how the team works with her. She needs to be ready, and so does the team. The power of preparation, invitation, intention, and center releases the ability of circle process to accommodate significant shift. Though the circle no longer meets at Fairview, this pioneering group of early adopters set the template for much of our later work. And many of these nurse and health care leaders have moved into other corporations, consulting practices, and associations where they carry their circle experience forward.

The Wheaton Franciscans have elected a new provincial leadership team, and their story is continued in Chapter 5.

CHAPTER

Rotating Positions of Leadership in the Circle

A PeerSpirit circle is an all-leader group, in which positions of responsibility change and adapt as needed. The three most identifiable positions of *host, guardian,* and *scribe* hold the progress of a circle session while all participants hold the infrastructure.

A small Zimbabwean woman named Sikhethiwe (pronounced "Ski-tee-way") leaned forward in her handmade wooden chair and said to the guardian, "Stephen, ring the bell." Stephen rang a *tingsha,* held the pause a few seconds, and rang it again. All twenty-four of us, brown and white faces, young and old, paused in our talking under the thatched-roofed, open-walled meeting house in Kufunda village. After the second ring, our young host said to her guardian across the circle, "I don't know what to do next. What do you think we should do?"

With the rest of us quietly observing, Sikhethiwe (the host) and Stephen (the guardian) held a dialogue across the circle about where to take their leadership around a community issue we were discussing. After a few minutes, they decided to pose a question to the group: "Is everyone ready to vote on whether to offer leadership training to surrounding communities next month?" The group nodded. Sikhethiwe asked for a "thumbs vote," and soon the group had made a decision and was ready to move to a new topic, which was to be hosted by a new host and guardian. We took a break, and while most of the group scattered out into the sunshine, Sikhethiwe and Christina (scribe) spread flip chart paper on the floor

49

and recorded the important points of conversation and the decision the group had made. The sheets were posted next to the day's agenda for all to read.

This interaction is an excellent model for the three positions of host, guardian, and scribe within a circle:

○ The host and guardian work together in leading a meeting; the host's role is more verbal, though both are tending group process.

○ Transparency in circle leadership is helpful to the learning curve and therefore supported by the whole group since group members know that their turn to hold these roles is coming sooner or later.

○ The pause offered by two rings of the bell gives everyone, especially the host and guardian, a chance to reflect on the direction the conversation needs to go in order to reach a sense of completion.

○ The scribe volunteers to record highlights, insights, and decision points so that the essence of circle process is preserved and the group has a history of itself.

○ The thumbs vote asks those in favor to point their thumbs up, those with remaining questions to hold their thumbs sideways, and those who are opposed to signal with their thumbs down. Those with questions or those opposed are invited to explain their vote. It is a form of modified consensus building common in PeerSpirit Circle Process.

PeerSpirit invites an equality of presence, contribution, and responsibility that is shared out among all members of the circle. Rotating positions of leadership within this collegiality greatly enhances everyone's experience. The circle remains peer-led, and peers take on temporary positions of authority that support presence, participation, and accountability. Host, guardian, and scribe become the pattern holders. They lead from within the rim of the group and work together to assist in holding the social container, tending intention, and moving through the process.

The Role of Host

In the early years of PeerSpirit work, we experimented with flattening the triangle completely, with leadership roles disappearing into the rim. This didn't work very well because leadership would spontaneously emerge and people would take on functions that shaped group process whether or not these roles had been named. However, we didn't think that naming someone the "circle facilitator" accurately reflected what we were learning about the qualities of collaborative conversations in circle.

The word *facilitator* often connotes a position that is mostly outside the group. A facilitator comes in to help a group or organization but does not *join* the group or organization. In these early years, we were in the middle of developing a new model for circle process, and we didn't have a name for where we wanted to go. Then, in the international collegiality growing out of the From the Four Directions initiative, the phrase "circle host" began to come into play. We recognized it as exactly the term we needed. A circle host is like the host of a dinner party. The host cooks the meal, sets the space of welcome, and when people are gathered, both serves and sits down to partake of the feast. The host does not stand aside and observe while others partake. The host is not trying to facilitate other people's experience while remaining an outsider or expert. *The host joins the group process while maintaining and observing the pattern.*

The person serving as circle host provides continuity from one meeting or topic to the next and gently assists the microstructures of the conversation.

- The host sets up the room, placing chairs or seats in a circle, creating the center, posting agreements, intention, and so on so that participants enter a prepared space of welcome.

- The host helps the circle abide by its agreements and fulfill its intention.

- The host is granted temporary leadership authority by circle members to guide group process and work in conjunction with the guardian.

- Typically, the host and guardian sit opposite each other so that they can see each other and observe both sides of the circle.

This ability to serve the group and at the same time participate in the group is the essence of leadership from the rim. The redefinition of where leadership sits and how it offers guidance instead of asserting authority is the paradigm shift to which circle calls us. Leadership is understood to be a temporary authority, a stewardship of group process, a donation of one's skills, focus, and energy so that the collective well-being is tended and the inherent wisdom i[n] may emerge. Circle leadership assumes that everyone in the circle m[ay] position at some time in the process.

The role of host also acknowledges how hierarchy can helpfully and healthily appear in circle process: the triangle is always present—and always shifting. When people lean forward to help each other, to move the conversation forward, or to make a contribution—they assume increments of leadership. These are acknowledged, and then the process moves on. For an hour, Sikhethiwe is host; then Fide takes a turn, and then Silas, and so on. The circle is stabilized within this spirit of voluntary contribution.

In the council of community members at Kufunda village, the various topics in need of discussion were laid out for all to see—like pieces of a pie. Coming from another culture and country, we were serving as coaches to their adaptation of PeerSpirit circle. We had traveled to Zimbabwe to honor the challenges and strengths of circle self-governance and to help increase the villagers' confidence in their own circle skills. We would teach the Components of Circle and then lean back so that their leadership could lean forward; we would suggest and ask for their suggestions. This openness gave them opportunities to practice without a sense that they had to do things in a certain way: everything in circle became a lesson that served the ongoing cohesiveness of their community life.

After a break, Sikhethiwe led a short discussion on what had been decided during her hosting and then passed her role on to another person in the circle. Stephen handed the bells and the role of guardian to someone else. New leaders stepped in to guide and scribe the next topic.

Hosting in Conflict

There are many creative ways to host a circle. Our German colleague, Matthias zur Bonsen, was confronted with a challenging situation when asked to help a company in conflict host a circle of 140 distressed franchisees.[1] Matthias explains:

> "Private Tutoring is a billion-euro business in Germany. Students who do not make a passing score have to repeat the current year of schooling, so parents are motivated to help their children maintain satisfactory grades. There are two big companies that offer their services nationwide. These companies tutor students in groups of three to five.
>
> "One of these companies, which has around one thousand outlets throughout Germany, wanted to intensify the collaboration with

its franchisees. To achieve this, the company decided that the governing board that represented the franchisees needed to meet more often with management. And to make this economically feasible, it was proposed that the board size be decreased from twenty to six members and that those six be reimbursed for their increased investment of time. This required new bylaws.

"A small group of franchisees met with management and created a proposal for the new bylaws. And then the conflict began. Many franchisees didn't like the idea. They were afraid that their region wouldn't be represented in the smaller board. Put to a vote, the new bylaws received only 60 percent approval. An emotional, somewhat aggressive, and hurtful discussion between franchisees in their Web-based forum generated more confusion and resistance. For company management, letting the majority rule was simply not an option: the company did not want to lose the consent of 40 percent of its franchisees."

The company called in Matthias and his colleague, Jutta Herzog, who are well known in Germany as pioneers in the field of large group interventions. Since 1994, Matthias has written three books and brought Open Space Technology, Future Search, Real Time Strategic Change, Appreciative Inquiry and World Café to Germany; in 2007, he brought PeerSpirit Circle Process. After considering the situation, he and Jutta decided to host a circle.

Management invited all franchisees to a meeting from Friday noon to Sunday noon. This had never happened before. One hundred forty of them decided to attend. The most critical part of this conference was a whole-group dialogue about the conflict concerning the new bylaws to be held on Saturday afternoon. When using circle in a large group, hosting has to become very creative—it's like jumping from a dinner party to catering: there's more planning to make sure the quality of engagement will hold. Yet when every voice needs to be heard at first hand—and in this situation, that was essential if the conflict was to be resolved—the circle can expand to hold a large community conversation.

Matthias and Jutta designed a center with special significance to the group. They constructed a pyramid of sixteen red boxes, which was approximately 3 feet (90 cm) high. The box at the top symbolized the purpose of the company (including the franchising system). The four boxes in the middle level stood for its values. And the nine boxes at the bottom symbolized its goals. The whole group had worked on purpose, values, and goals in the preceding parts of the conference and understood the meaning of the boxes. Then Matthias and Jutta arranged 140 chairs in four concentric circles, like the rings of a tree.

Matthias reported, "On the box at the top of the pyramid we placed a microphone. This served as our talking piece. We explained the purpose of the talking piece and asked everybody to put the microphone back on the 'purpose box' after each person had spoken. (We thought that everybody who wanted to speak should be connected with this 'purpose box.') Then the dialogue began. Franchisee after franchisee came into the middle of the circle, took the microphone, and spoke."

He recalls, "In the beginning, the participants repeated their entrenched positions. Very slowly this changed. Some of the franchisees, who spoke in the middle time, were able to speak from their heart. This changed something in the group. The dialogue in the large circle lasted 105 minutes, and the energy level was high during this whole time. Then it became obvious that a solution had been found." Matthias and Jutta listened for the shift in group consciousness and consensus. They hosted the space for the circle process to do its work. They served as guardians. They served as scribes.

At the conclusion, for legal reasons, a vote was necessary: 137 out of 140 agreed to the bylaws change, with 3 abstentions and no votes against the solution. After this circle process, the mood in the group was euphoric. The franchisees had a pool party in the evening, and Matthias reported, "They danced, jumped in the water with their clothes on, danced again.... The circle had worked."

Guardian

The *guardian* is a unique contribution from PeerSpirit Circle Process that is now being adapted in other conversation modalities. As explained in Chapter 2, the purpose of guardianship is to hold a place for mindfulness and intervention in a circle meeting. The person serving as guardian is an energy watcher and observer of both spiritual and practical needs and often an intuitive guide for honoring conversational process.

- ○ The guardian serves as a conscious reminder of the energetic presence that joins people once they are seated in the container of circle process.

○ The guardian helps the circle fulfill its social contracts, timeliness, and focus.

○ The guardian is granted ceremonial authority by circle members to interject silence and recenter group process.

The holder of the bells rings the bell twice—first to call for a pause in the action and then, ten to twenty seconds later, a second time to end the pause. The guardian (or whoever has asked the guardian to ring the bell) enunciates the reason for calling the pause.

The guardian's role is to pay close enough attention to the nuances of interaction that he or she is prepared to intervene in helpful ways. The insertion of pauses ranges from calling for a stretch break to noting the passage of time to marking a space between speakers to making corrections of course—restating agreements, restating the topic or intention, and intervening in moments of destructive tension. Anyone can call for the bell and initiate the pause. The significance of this shared responsibility and how it democratizes circle process shows up throughout our work, over and over.

When someone is rambling on during a check-in that was framed as a chance to speak a few sentences of arrival, the talker has the talking piece and everyone is fidgeting. Here the guardian might wait for the speaker to take a breath, *ring* the bell, *pause, ring*, and say, "I call us back to understanding that this is a brief round in which to make sure every voice is heard as we begin." The person who is rambling may be momentarily embarrassed and is also usually grateful to have a graceful way to come to a conclusion and relinquish the talking piece.

Guardianship in Response to Conflict

At a university faculty training session, a classic need for intervention occurred late in the day. Everyone was tired and ready to be finished. Christina was teaching alone, and a volunteer guardian had just set the *tingsha* bells in the center, anticipating a break for dinner. A professor who had been hostile to the process off and on all day seized the moment and turned on Christina: "I don't get this circle stuff. In my way of thinking, you have abdicated your responsibility as leader. You've lost control of the group. We haven't made a single decision. What the hell are you doing here?"

The guardian looked panicky because she had no way to intervene. The room went into temporary shock. The youngest circle member, a department secretary who had been present as scribe, took on her personal power, grabbed the bells from the center, and rang them loudly. This gave Christina and everyone in the room time to sit up, pay attention, and collect their thoughts. When the secretary rang the bells again, she said, "We have an agreement about withholding judgment. And we are all too tired to talk about this now."

While the young woman spoke, Christina had a chance to think. She thanked the young woman and invited her to serve as guardian until the circle had truly disbanded. To the professor she said, "It is not my job to control this group. It is the job of the group to learn how to function as a collaborative circle. This is a training session. In any training, we wobble toward confidence and competence. Tomorrow we are scheduled to do more agenda-based work with shared leadership from your colleagues. It's my sense of the group that people have done all they can manage today." People nodded their heads. "So as host, I'm closing the circle. I invite you all to remember our agreement that what's said here remains here. Have a good supper, relax by the fireplace, and get a good night's sleep. Let's suspend judgment and show up here at nine tomorrow morning. Brenda, great guardianship. Please ring us out."

One of the skills of the guardian role is to practice naming the situation with neutral language. Neutral language requires the ability to talk about what's happening without instigating shame or blame. The guardian seeks to avoid personalizing or polarizing a moment in circle process by being able to call the group back to the infrastructure in place: the agreements, principles and practices, intention, and use of center for grounding. Brenda did this beautifully when she grabbed the bells from the center. She used neutral language and gave Christina time to compose a direct, yet uncharged, response. Christina's response is one of many that are possible. It was the host's wisdom that was being challenged in this instance, and the man was not likely to be easily placated. The faculty circle would need to learn how to manage his negativity without rising to the bait and to hold him accountable to their agreements.

In moments of tension, conflict, or surprise when the guardian needs to intercede, the pause is needed to help everyone get recentered on the rim and focus on the center to stabilize the circle container.

Several years ago, we were in a business setting participating in a circle check-in around the question "On the way to work this morning, what did you observe that made you thoughtful?" One of the participants spoke about the "crazy people" hanging out on the lawn of the city library where she had stopped to return some books. There was no intended malice in her statement; her remarks were focused on not feeling entirely safe around the library steps. An alert guardian saw a man on the other side of the circle wince and turn ashen. The guardian rang the bell for a pause and looked at her colleague. He gave her a barely perceptible shake of his head—apparently not wanting attention. Not sure what to do next, the guardian said, "I honor Debra's observation and invite all of us to be compassionate of the challenging lives of street people." The check-in continued with other anecdotal stories.

By the time the talking piece traveled around to the man, he spoke with emotion. "One of those crazy people on the library lawn is probably my twenty-eight-year-old son. He's schizophrenic. Sometimes he has a little room somewhere; sometimes he's on the street. He's not violent, but most people have no way of knowing that. Not a single day passes that my wife and I don't worry about whether or not he's taking his meds and staying safe. Sometimes on my way to work I drive around that part of town, by the library, under the freeway viaducts, just looking for him, to see if he's still alive." His voice shaking, the man continued, "Those 'crazy people' come from somewhere. They belong—or used to belong—to someone. When you can, look in their eyes and say hello. When you can, send them good wishes."

He passed the talking piece to his left. The woman whose turn it was to speak next didn't know what to say, and Debra looked stricken. The guardian rang the bell and let the pause linger in the room, rang again, and said, "Thank you, Frank, for the reminder that we all carry complex stories. And that we are all connected."

Debra leaned forward and said, "Oh, Frank, I had no idea you were carrying this burden. Thank you for telling us. And I promise you, I will see these people with more understanding than ever before."

The woman holding the talking piece took a deep breath. "Wow," she said. "That was big. . . . Are we really ready to move on?" Frank and Debra and several other people nodded, and the check-in round was completed.

Especially in moments like this, the bell serves as a voice in the circle. The guardian is watching for release of energy, for readiness to pause and readiness to resume. Though the guardian is holding the bell, anyone in the circle can call for a ring and pause. If Frank had been ready to speak right after Debra, he could have asked for the bell and shared his feelings immediately. Notice that even though a talking piece was in play, Debra leaned in with a direct response to Frank before the circle went on: the circle's conversational structures are intended to serve group process, not to dominate it. The art of circle practice is to hold the pattern loosely when that serves the moment and tightly when needed for support.

After all the members in Frank and Debra's circle checked in, the host, noting that the first agenda item was a conversation about budgets, asked the guardian to ring the bell and questioned the group: "This has been a poignant check-in. I'm not sure we're ready to jump into number crunching. Where would the group like to go next?"

Frank spoke up. " I am really fine— glad this secret is out in the open. I can move into agenda."

Debra spoke. " I'm having a thousand thoughts that are not about the budget. I'd like a little break." The group decided to take a stretch before proceeding.

This became a defining moment for the team, often referred to as "the moment we came together." Over the years, they continued to share authentically about their personal lives and to face challenging decisions with cohesiveness and depth.

In Kufunda, translating back and forth between Shona and English, we noticed that people were pronouncing the word *guardian* as "guide on." We were charmed and realized that they had captured the true essence of this role. The guardian is a guide.

Guides in the wilderness use skills that cover the full spectrum from first aid and camping survival to encouraging the awe that comes from immersion into nature. So in the circle, the guardian is a guide who watches for what is needed, from the practical to the spiritual.

Scribe

One of the challenges in circle process can be catching the *essence* of the conversation so that we can communicate this to others or notice when a decision has been made. In traditional meetings, someone is often assigned the note-taking function and decisions are moved, seconded, and voted on according to Robert's Rules of Order. In circle, too, there can be a need or desire for someone to take notes and record insights, decisions, votes, or consensus. How this happens in the flow of circle process and what is produced and shared (or not shared) vary greatly according to the nature and setting of each circle. When called for, the scribe becomes the third point on the inner triangle of leadership at the rim.

The person serving as scribe serves as record keeper or historian in circle process and may be the first one to articulate emergent wisdom, decisions, or completion.

- The scribe negotiates with the host and guardian regarding what is needed as a record of the process.

- The scribe is looking for essence, not trying to provide a transcription.

- The scribe uses writing tools as appropriate to the group: notepad, journal, laptop computer, or flip chart.

- A standing scribe and flip chart may be included in the rim of the circle, or a group may choose to hire a graphic recorder to create a chronology of words and images.

- The scribe keeps what is recorded confidential and ensures that this agreement is scrupulously observed.

The scribe function may also be ascribed collectively such that all participants have journals dedicated to noticing their own thought process during the circle's ongoing work. These journals may contain notes on the contributions of others that the writer wants to comment on or notes regarding decisions, options, directions, and personal reactions and reflections. Circle journals are usually eclectic private records that are shared voluntarily or not at all. And yet when someone has a question about what occurred a session or more ago, there's a record somewhere in the rim of the circle. Participants have stated the helpfulness of journal keeping as a way to jot down ideas and return to listening while waiting their turn to speak.

Some circle gatherings require no scribe, and to put someone in that role would feel awkward. However, even in the most casual ongoing groups, people may desire some kind of record of their journey together. In an annual women's retreat, Christina records the essence of people's check-ins and the final checkouts in her journal. The following year, she brings this volume back to help the group remember where it was a year ago. Our friend Cynthia is known throughout the community as a note-taker who enjoys scribing for the circles she's in. "It's just how I'm wired," she says. "For some people, writing can distract their attention, but for me, when I'm writing things down, it brings me fully present." Other groups have experimented with creating collages of their experiences, putting together scrapbooks, and using digital storytelling or Internet social networking.

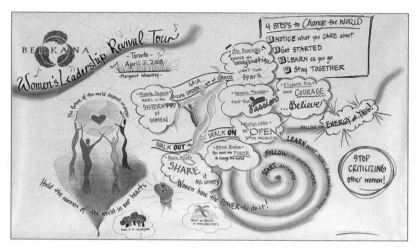

FIGURE 4.1

When Margaret Wheatley brought the Women's Leadership Revival Tour to Toronto, Ontario, a visual practitioner, Sara Heppner-Waldston, recorded the event in such a way that the memory of the evening would resonate whenever someone looked at her imagery (see Figure 4.1), and for those who were not present, the imagery could provide a sense of what had occurred. We need something to reattach us to the string of inspirational, thought-provoking, and heartfelt moments of circle. It's not a matter of being fancy; it's about anchoring the process of collaboration, which can become such a synergistic experience that we forget what actually happened because that wasn't the part of our brains that were most deeply activated.

When the host, guardian, and scribe meet before a circle meeting or when the group gathers around its intention, thinking about what is wanted from the harvest is an important frame for the conversation. In the drawing, the sponsor, event, date, participants, and major speech points are recorded. In a different circle, the history of a decision may be needed.

The leading-edge thinking about how to understand the "art of harvesting" these highly synergistic conversations has emerged from the Art of Hosting network. The Art of Hosting Web site (http://www.artofhosting.org/thepractice/artofharvesting) maintains an evolving downloadable guide to harvesting collaborative conversations that is an incredibly valuable tool. This work is being led by Monica Nissen of Denmark and Chris Corrigan of Canada.

Circle and Agenda

The host, guardian, and scribe roles are extremely helpful when circle process is combined with an agenda. There is usually a host of the meeting—one person who provides the kind of oversight mentioned throughout this chapter. The host sets up the space, offers a start-point, oversees check-in and check-out, and guides the overall process. Usually, the host also steps into a leadership role to steward each topic identified as an agenda item. The topical host brings needed information, communicates on paper or electronically, and designs a group process for his or her part of the circle meeting. None of this thinking is reflected in the usual flat sheets of agenda items, so the administrative circle at Fairview Health Services designed a chart that would serve the organization's needs (see Figure 4.2). We have carried this diagram to other organizations and invite readers to continue to use and adapt it to fit your needs.

As the agenda is constructed, time is allotted, and the need for scribing is determined, circle process blends the need for tangible outcomes with the softer elements of community building. For example, someone hosting an agenda item may negotiate by saying, "I need ten minutes to present the new space assignments for integrating two departments on one floor. I need everyone at our meeting to have a cubicle chart, to engage with comments and questions, and to take our chart back to your departments and get final feedback from those being shifted. Knowing we are going to get input from the staff being combined, I'd like to devote another ten minutes to generating ideas for creating an atmosphere of welcome so that this change is as pleasant as possible."

"Who's in charge?" is a question many people carry into a meeting; circle process leads us to ask, "How are we in charge?" This is the question that allows us to explore the relational core that binds us to one another in service to intention.

And then the deeper question "How are we *not* in charge?" invites us to honor the emergent wisdom collected at the center, experienced by the host, recognized by the guardian, preserved by the scribe, and held by all who are present.

Throughout this book we talk about circle as a container, holding space for each other in this form. We can provide this sense of holding space in person, over the phone, and even in written Internet conversations. However we do it, the roles of host, guardian, and scribe stabilize the environment so that our best offerings come forward.

Agenda Builder for the Circle/Session

Date: _____ Time opened: _____ Time closed: _____
● Circle Host: _____
   Guardian: _____

Sponsors by agenda items

● Item Host: _____ Item: _____
   Scribe: _____ Negotiated Time: _____
   Tasks, decisions, outcome: _____
   _____
   _____
   _____

● Item Host: _____ Item: _____
   Scribe: _____ Negotiated Time: _____
   Tasks, decisions, outcome: _____
   _____
   _____
   _____

● Item Host: _____ Item: _____
   Scribe: _____ Negotiated Time: _____
   Tasks, decisions, outcome: _____
   _____
   _____
   _____

● Item Host: _____ Item: _____
   Scribe: _____ Negotiated Time: _____
   Tasks, decisions, outcome: _____
   _____
   _____
   _____

● Item Host: _____ Item: _____
   Scribe: _____ Negotiated Time: _____
   Tasks, decisions, outcome: _____
   _____
   _____

© *PeerSpirit, Inc.*

FIGURE 4.2

Circle on the Telephone

Increasingly, as people use the telephone and computer-based communications for conference calls, "webinars," and online classes, they want to transfer the quality of face-to-face experience to these settings. We find that the infrastructure of circle thrives in an aural environment—the difference is that the cues are no longer visual: they are spoken. On many conference calls, the host is established by having sent the invitation or intention beforehand. If the roles are not yet established, the first questions become "Who is hosting today?" "Who is guardian?" and "Who is scribe?"

The host will describe a center that is meaningful to the group and present a virtual talking piece. For example, "I'm sitting at my desk, and I've cleared away all the paperwork and created a little center here that consists of our intention and agenda for this call and I just turned on the LED tea light from our last board meeting table setting. I'm putting a small glass globe in the middle for our talking piece. I invite the guardian to ring us in."

The guardian may say, "I've got the *tingsha* right here. I'm going to ring it about ten inches from my headset. Let me know if that's the right level of sound." Ring, pause, ring. "For our start-point, I'd like to offer a poem by Mary Oliver."

After the poem, the host picks up the conversation and invites check-in. "Thank you for the poem. And thanks to Bob for volunteering to scribe for us. If you hear computer keystrokes, I'm assuming it's you, Bob—let us know if you need help capturing something or want one of us to type when you're talking. OK. I've got our group photo displayed on my laptop. We're all smiling, and I hope that's true this morning as well. Let's check in from east to west around the question 'What energy from our last meeting comes with you into this call today?'"

One by one, people introduce themselves and simply say, "I pick up the piece," and when they've finished, "Piece back to the center." As conversation progresses, the talking piece may or may not be formally used, and if things speed up or if voices are having a hard time breaking in on the conversation, someone will say, "I'm picking up the piece! We need to slow down a bit here, so I'm putting it back in play."

At the end of the call, there is a brief check-out, and the scribe sends the harvested insights, decisions, and chronology of the conversation out by e-mail.

Holding the Space of Circle

As we practice, circle increasingly becomes an art of paying attention to ourselves, to one another, and to the conversation.

Our teaching colleague, Martin Siesta, was recently asked to describe the process of "holding space" that occurs in circle and other forms of collaborative conversation. He said:

"Holding space in circle means staying engaged and present with one another while we undergo a process of self-inquiry. We are listening and noticing each other's contributions deeply, with empathy, and managing our own judgmental stream, bringing ourselves back to presence. This is a form of love—and it doesn't have to be personal; it often occurs with strangers. When we love others in this way, we provide a space in which they can simply be able to feel what they need, to speak without worrying about how they will be perceived. It is a true gift. In some ways, it is seeing not only through someone else's eyes but also in a way that transcends this. Perhaps a great example of this is in the video of the Three Tenors—the original from 1990—when Placido Domingo is singing 'No Puede Ser' and Zubin Mehta is conducting the orchestra. When I watch and listen closely, I notice how by 'holding space' for Domingo, Mehta is able to call out of the performer more than he dreamed possible. It is amazing—and at the completion of the song, there is deep recognition between them of how they served the other."

That is the essence of host, guardian, and scribe in circle: they are holding space so that all present in the circle can reach inside ourselves and call out more than we dreamed was possible.

CHAPTER

Accountability Through Agreements, Practices, and Principles

In any group process, there are skills for participating and norms for functioning. In circle work, the skills are the practices and the agreements are the norms for operating. The principles provide the energetic movement in an all-leader system.

A California middle school (teaching grades 6 through 8) had been experiencing increasing problems with student attitude and vandalism. Near the end of one school year, the principal invited a group of parents, teachers, and students to meet over the summer months to address these issues. The group pared down hours of conversation into three stated agreements, intended to reinforce the kind of environment that would foster mutual trust and respect:

- Take care of yourself.

- Take care of each other.

- Take care of this place.

Before the start of the next school year, a group of parents and students created banners and signs with these three phrases and placed them prominently around the school: on the gymnasium wall, on the doors of classrooms, at the entrances to the bathrooms, and so on. The phrases were referred to in the

65

classroom, both by teachers calling students back to order and by students teasing each other into better behavior.

One rainy October day, the first fire drill of the year occurred. Several hundred middle school children and their teachers stood outside in the muddy soccer field waiting for the all-clear bell. Once the bell had rung and everyone filed back into the building, the principal walked the grounds making sure everyone was inside. He was the last to enter, and when he came in the main entrance, hundreds of pairs of muddy sneakers and flip-flops were lined up against the wall. The principal stopped, nodded to himself, and thought, "Hey, we're getting it...."

We heard this story sometime in 2003 and have told it dozens of times since because it so clearly illustrates the power of articulated agreements to significantly shift a group into cohesive self-actualizing behavior. The agreements, practices, and principles of circle components allow people to self-organize toward shared purpose and common good and free a group to become a better version of itself.

Agreements

Cooperation is far easier and more effective than enforcement. In any gathering of people, there are social agreements in play that allow participants to function together through understanding what constitutes respectful interaction. In many social and business settings, these norms are assumed and unarticulated. Assumption works just fine a lot of the time (like knowing which side of the road to drive on) and creates misunderstanding and social disaster when it doesn't work (like the terror of driving the wrong way down a one-way street, hoping you and everyone else can readjust without crashing). People are observant, and we've had a lot of practice being socialized. Assumption of agreements will usually carry people through a two-hour meeting, and social norms accumulate in any organizational or social setting until most folks sort of "get it" about how to behave and belong.

When people come into circle, where everything is designed to enhance clear communication, interaction is strengthened and stabilized by crafting articulated agreements for being together. Naming agreements, claiming what is in play in the social field, is a significant part of what shifts us into "held space" and a sense of interpersonal container.

The first evening of a women's leadership retreat on the Oregon coast, we were sitting around the dining table at the end of a delicious meal with eight high-powered women from Seattle and Portland. The faint sounds of surf in the background, candlelight, and the remains of a well-catered dinner provided the ambiance for a rich and enjoyable conversation of current projects and politics. When Ann left to build a fire in the fireplace in the adjoining living room and then rearranged the upholstered chairs into a circle around the hearth and Christina suggested that the group bring coffee and tea and come to the circle, the women were somewhat surprised. Once gathered, we rang the bell, recited the PeerSpirit agreements, and offered a question for check-in: "What is the most significant thing you could receive from the next two days together?" We introduced use of a talking piece so that the women could speak one at a time. We brought one of the dining candles to the coffee table positioned between us. The conversation deepened into council—a pattern of listening and speaking.

The next morning at breakfast, one woman said to the group, "When we moved from the table to the fire last night, I couldn't imagine why Ann and Christina were breaking up such a good time. I was thinking—wow, this conversation is so energizing, these women are so amazing, I could go home right now. Then, what happened in the living room with those agreements in place and that talking piece thing—I've never experienced myself and a new group going to the depths we touched last night. What are we going to do today?" Everyone laughed. We headed for the beach—to start by looking for the patterns in nature that sustain us.

Over the years, we have refined four generic PeerSpirit circle agreements to support the skeletal structure of overall circle process. In the first moments of a new circle, or in a brief or onetime meeting, we offer our PeerSpirit agreements so that the meeting can proceed quickly. If the group goes on from this introductory session, we encourage members to take the time to discuss these agreements and make the language their own. Agreements are created in response to the question "What do we need in order to be fully present to each other, to offer and receive contributions, and to fulfill our intention?"

PeerSpirit Circle Agreements

1. *Personal material shared in the circle is confidential.* Confidentiality invites authentic speaking and allows people to speak their stories with the assurance they will not be gossiped about beyond the circle group. It is worth spending time considering what parameters of confidentiality fit a group and ensuring that all participants share a definition of what is meant and expected of them regarding this issue. A person's story belongs to that person alone; it's not for anyone else to dispense, sell, or give away without permission, any more than we'd take a ring off the person's finger.

Conversation about confidentiality has the potential to create a profound sense of confidence within a group. It clarifies how we will be listened to and how we are being counted on to listen to others. This first agreement creates a boundary that builds a sense of community inside which personal sharing can occur and ensures that when someone takes a risk, the person understands how his or her story and other sensitive information will be held within the social container of this circle. Confidentiality is not one size fits all. We have helped a group of therapists design a circle where they could share the life stories they were hearing in their sessions for the purpose of peer supervision and where strict confidentiality had to be the highest-held norm. We have called the circle at public meetings where members of the press were present and we had to make sure everyone understood they were essentially speaking in public—that is, confidentiality could not apply.

2. *We listen to each other with curiosity and compassion, withholding judgment.* Curiosity allows people to listen and speak without having to be in total agreement with each other. This agreement invites circle members to use the center as a place to deposit stories, opinions, thoughts, and feelings. When people speak energetically to the neutral point of the circle's center, it reminds everyone of the power of this space, which belongs to everyone and to no one. Because the center creates a third point between people engaged in social interaction, we can lean in with curiosity about differences, ask questions, explore issues, discern what fits in the learning of the group—and suspend judgment, or at least notice our judgments and set that stream of thought aside so we can listen more fully.

Judgment is a form of mental defense, a way of guaranteeing that one's opinion or worldview is not about to be swayed. When curiosity replaces judgment as a thought process, it invites consideration of another's opinion and worldview. Curiosity and judgment cannot function simultaneously in the mind. When people choose curiosity, diverse opinion and life experience can be honored while people continue to listen to each other and seek their deeper wisdom. And through this practice, our compassion for ourselves and each other grows. Changing our hearts and minds in response to our deeper understanding of one another keeps the circle vibrant and creative. Our diverse voices become like spokes of a wheel attaching to the hub of our common purpose.

3. *We ask for what we need and offer what we can.* Generally, if a request fits the task and orientation of the group, someone in the circle will respond to help

carry it forward. If a request doesn't fit task and orientation, there will be a lack of interest. Circle members learn to negotiate what they can and cannot do and to hold intention for the direction of group energy.

This agreement also serves as a kind of balancing rod. If a few people end up carrying an inordinate level of responsibility for the circle's work or process and don't receive support from the whole, this agreement provides a way to address nonparticipation with neutral language. The group, or the guardian, can call for a conversation about shared responsibility and rotating leadership. Such conversations have the potential to clear up resentments before they erode the circle's cohesiveness.

4. *From time to time, we pause to regather our thoughts or focus.* This is the agreement that activates and acknowledges the role of guardian to create pauses on behalf of the group. When the guardian rings a bell, all action stops, at least for ten to fifteen seconds. During a pause, each person takes a breath, focuses on the center, and waits to find out what is going on. The guardian rings the bell a second time to release the silence and then briefly explains why he or she called the pause—perhaps for a challenge, perhaps for an insight, perhaps simply for a break.

Putting the pause into the agreements grants the role of the guardian an acknowledged authority to stop action. The pause becomes part of the circle's self-governance. The structural acceptance of intervention is a great teacher in circle process. Anyone in the circle can call for a pause, so guardianship is diffused and responsibility for the quality of group experience sits in the rim in profound ways.

The Wisdom Circle Agreements

Drafting circle agreements is a powerful task that can challenge a group to examine many underlying assumptions and social patterns. In 2006, when the Wheaton Franciscan sisters decided to embark on a yearlong experience of circle they named the Wisdom Circle, one of their first tasks was to designate a small group to draft their agreements. As is true in many orders of Catholic religious women in North America, they knew they needed a process to hold delicate conversations and hard decisions as their community faced declining enrollment and advancing age. They took seriously the writing of agreements, which the whole group eventually discussed and approved. The agreements they crafted are shown in Exhibit 5.1:

Exhibit 5.1

...le Agreements

- ...we ... to be respectful, honest, and creative in our circle conversations for the sake of our future together.
- Trusting that we have what we need to come together for our future, we ask for what we need and offer what we can.
- Each person speaks her own truth. We listen to each other with respect, freshness, curiosity, compassion, and sensitivity. Stories shared in circle conversations are confidential.
- Remembering that agreements are updatable, we will review the agreements each time the circle meets, and we will agree what may be shared outside the circle.
- From time to time, we pause in silence.

The Wisdom Circle agreements clearly contain some of the elements of the PeerSpirit generic circle agreements, yet the Wheaton Franciscans' wording reflects their own social culture and specific needs. These agreements were artfully typed on large paper, read aloud at the beginning of each Wisdom Circle gathering, and placed in the center to remind all participants of the self-governance they had chosen. Agreeing on their agreements was an elaborate process that took several hours and included considerable conversation council followed by a thumbs vote and a round of singing sixteen alleluias.

While this story focuses on religious women, we have noticed time and again that organizational issues are very similar and that in other settings, we wished we could suggest a round of "sixteen alleluias" when an administrative team or association board had reached clear guidance because the sense of satisfaction felt the same. The gift that the Wheaton Franciscans gave to us was the opportunity to return with such consistency over the period of our consultancy, to observe their process, to coach the circle form and watch its evolution and integration into their collective life.

One of the benefits of taking time upfront to craft agreements is that it allows some of the shadow issues of a group to come forward early on. By shadow (discussed in greater detail in Chapter 9), we mean those things that have not been previously discussed or ways that people have accommodated to one another that produce tension. Sometimes this is referred to as the "undiscussables": asking, "What topics are off limits in this organization? Fam-

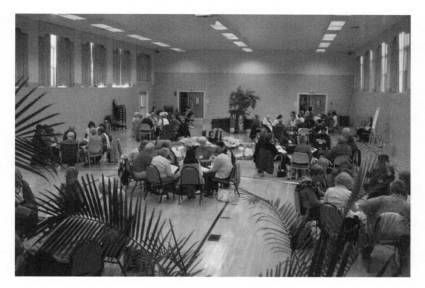

FIGURE 5.1

ily? Community setting?" opens up layers of dialogue. For example, the sisters questioned themselves deeply about the meaning of confidentiality and how to honor each other's stories without creating a sense of "secret meetings" that separated those present (generally every member who felt she had the physical and mental stamina to join the conversation) from more frail elder sisters who held an equal stake in the outcome. The conversation on confidentiality brought forward several issues and clarified intention for the Wisdom Circle. The sisters decided to maintain confidentiality for personal stories and to share the progress of their topical conversations with older vowed members and with covenant members (laypeople who are woven into the spiritual life of the community). They also promised that decisions would not be made in the Wisdom Circle without calling the whole community into session. This led to further clarifying of the intention of the Wisdom Circle as an experience of deepening community bonds and coming to know one another again after decades of service and living in small groups. Their experience was chronicled in their quarterly newsletter. Needed topics raised in the Wisdom Circle were then brought to the whole community at semiannual gatherings, such as the one pictured in Figure 5.1. And as confidence in their capacity for circle leadership grew, they hosted circle experiences for the elder sisters and covenant members. All this stemmed from the original conversations on agreements.

Agreements remain constant while leadership rotates. They become the core expression of a circle's self-governance, a sort of constitution designed to support the circle's intention and the ability of every member to contribute to that intention.

The Practices of Circle

Conversation of any kind, from casual socializing to structured dialogue, requires skill. In PeerSpirit Circle Process, we articulate three practices that strengthen verbal interaction. These practices are interwoven: it is much easier to do one of them when the other two are activated. At the beginning of a round of council, the host or guardian might recite the practices as a start-point and say, "We call our awareness to the gifts that come from attentive listening, intentional speaking, and contributing to the well-being of the group."

Attentive Listening

Attentive listening is the ability to focus clearly on what is being said by someone else. This means that we listen when someone else is speaking and avoid withdrawing into our own thought process to prepare agreement or rebuttal. We are not searching through our memory archives for a story of our own. In large or complex circles, such as the Wheaton Franciscan Wisdom Circle, it was very helpful for each sister to have a notebook on her lap so she could jot down thoughts for later reflection or reference without being distracted from listening. Their long talking piece councils could take several hours and include several breaks.

Attentive listening is a donation of energy to others that is sustained by a focus on the center. Attentive listening combines thought and empathy: the mind seeks comprehension while the heart seeks connection. The art of bearing witness to other people's stories and receiving others' thoughts and questions requires the kind of deep listening for which the circle is well suited. Listening in circle can transcend the cognitive and become a kind of mystical experience. We have sat in circles where people spoke in different languages, making cognitive comprehension impossible, and yet a profound essence of understanding emerged.

During a kayaking trip we guided among the Greek isles, we were befriended by an elder Greek fisherman who joined our evening campfires. Trip participants came from five countries and used English as our common language. And even though he couldn't speak English, Barba Mitsos sat thoughtfully through our evening circles. When the talking piece came to him, our Greek guide would translate his contribution. We were not sure what he understood of our stories, but we welcomed his help and his boat as we made our way through the week. On the last night of camping, Barba Mitsos said, through a translator, "You are good people. Thank you for coming to my olive grove. When you go home to your countries, tell your people of this place and its good people." Attentive listening invites a tenderness that can shift a circle's comprehension of its purpose and identity.

Intentional Speaking

Intentional speaking is the ability to contribute stories and information that have heart and meaning or relevance to the situation at hand. This ability arises out of the patience of waiting and watching for the moment when we know precisely what to say. We may feel a quickening of the pulse that insists we offer a certain thought, a sense of being moved to speak. When we are listening attentively, we base what we choose to say on a sense of receptivity alive in the group.

Timing is more transparent in circle process. In Chapter 4, when Frank begins to share the story of his schizophrenic son, he has established relationships in the group, and the moment offers him a context for fitting into the narrative that is occurring. If he chooses to step into his own readiness to share his story, he will find that he has support among his colleagues. There is alignment between his willingness to expose a vulnerable story and the group's capacity to respond in helpful ways.

As with listening, sometimes speaking can transcend the cognitive and take on a mystical quality. A number of years ago, we were privileged to offer a brief circle experience to a group of profoundly handicapped young adults and their caregivers. Two dozen of us were gathered in a classroom at a community college—one of several sessions that people could choose during a conference exploring issues of giving and receiving care. Shortly after we began our session, the school band began practicing in the courtyard, and we had to huddle close to hear one another. Our welcome and explanation were brief. We passed a talking piece, a small, easy-to-hold stuffed animal, inviting a response to the question "What is one thing you are learning at this conference?" The responses ranged from thoughtful—"I've never spent time with my client in a social setting before, and I'm enjoying this"—to humorous—"I'm distracted by the band—anybody want to dance?"

When we got three-quarters of the way around the circle, the talking piece was handed to a woman with severe cerebral palsy. She used a talking board to express herself and rarely attempted verbal speech. She held the talking piece a long time, rocking back and forth as if gathering the energy of all of our attentiveness. Finally, she stuttered, "I'mmmm hhhere," and beamed with pride that she had been able to contribute in her own voice. The band had stopped playing. The room was utterly silent. For a moment, our ordinary classroom had become a sacred space in which we had been able to receive what she so intentionally offered.

Attending to the Well-Being of the Group

Attending to the well-being of the group is the ability to consider the impact of our words and actions before, during, and after we speak. This ability arises from being present to the subtleties of circle practice. The first thing we notice in this environment is how sitting in circle listening to others activates a stream of thoughts, stories, and ways we want to respond to what is happening. The second thing we notice is that we can't respond to all these impulses—and that we need a kind of impulse control if we are to remain thoughtful participants. This sets off an internal process of conscious self-monitoring: we find ourselves running a mental checklist through our impulses before we contribute.

Agreements, principles, and practices corral some of our individual impulsiveness—like a tiny internalized time lag that allows for brief but necessary reflection: "Hey, do you really want to say that? Remember that stuff about tending to the well-being of the group? Remember that this is confidential? Maybe listening and not interrupting at this moment is the best way to show leadership right now." We practice self-monitoring by looking at the content of our contribution in relationship to the larger conversation, sensing the readiness in ourselves and in the group, and understanding our own motivations or hopes for sharing our comment. Self-monitoring questions might include the following:

- Is this an appropriate moment of receptivity?

- Am I speaking from competition or collaboration?

- What is my body telling me?

- How does what I want to do or say benefit where the group is?

- How do I phrase my contribution in neutral language and still speak my "truth"?

- Can I say this with integrity without disturbing the integrity of the group?

When attending to the well-being of the group, there is an important difference between self-monitoring and self-censoring. The infrastructure of the circle helps us in this discernment. If we're in a talking piece round, we know when our turn will come; we can hold the talking piece in a few seconds of silence and gather our thoughts; we can speak to the center and draw from the intention represented there. We can take the time necessary to say what we need in the manner most likely to be heard.

One weekend, Ann was part of a large training that was running late into the evening hours. The circle hosts had designed the closing round of the day as a talking piece council that invited each person to share an insight story from his or her experiences in the session so far. No suggestion had been made as to how long or short the stories should be. Ann was seated about halfway around the circle—tired and ready to go to bed. As the talking piece was making its way toward her, people's contributions were getting longer and longer. In her mind, Ann was having a little battle between her physical self, who was irritated and ready to sleep, and her circle host self, who knew the importance of allowing each person to speak. She vacillated between thoughts of sharing a short, thoughtful story of her own and simply speaking the truth of her exhaustion. When the piece finally came to her, she realized the importance of acknowledging the hour and her own stamina. "It has been a good day," she said, "and I am not a late-night person. I am doing my best to listen to each one of you and would greatly appreciate it if our comments tonight could be succinct. I'll share my story in the morning session when I can be more present." No one took offense, the second half of the circle went more quickly, and everyone had the opportunity to be heard.

One lesson from this moment is a reminder that in circle, impulses to speak something are often collective as well as personal. Ann named an experience shared by others, and by doing so in neutral language, people could ally themselves with her and admit their own tiredness while still choosing whether or not to tell their own stories. Listening, speaking, attending is the practice of wholeness. When we listen to the wholeness of the group, we know we must acknowledge, listen to, and speak from our inner truth even when it initially appears to contradict conformity in the group.

Three Principles

Amid the Components of Circle, three principles animate PeerSpirit Circle Process. Back in the early 1990s when we were articulating PeerSpirit Circle Process, we asked each other questions like "Who's the leader?" "How does power show up?" "How might it be shared?" "Who takes responsibility for what happens?" "How do we help each other see what needs to be done when we've been trained to segment responsibilities?" "Who decides when there is conflict or difference?" "What exists in circle that is greater than any one person?" "How do we name that presence?" From these questions, the clarity of the three principles emerged.

As is true for the three practices, the three principles are interwoven: when one is activated, the other two are also activated, and they work in coordination. Sometimes when introducing these principles, we almost want to use as preamble the phrase "We hold these truths to be self-evident." Every action in the circle supports these principles, and these principles support every action.

Rotating Leadership

Rotating leadership means that every person helps the circle function by assuming an increment of leadership. In PeerSpirit circling, leadership can shift moment by moment and task by task. Rotating leadership trusts that the resources to accomplish the circle's purpose exist within the group and that the energy of leadership is active in every member.

Shared Responsibility

Shared responsibility means that every person pays attention to what needs doing or saying next and steps in to do it. In PeerSpirit circling, responsibility also shifts moment by moment and task by task. Shared responsibility is based on the trust that someone will come forward to provide what the circle needs.

Reliance on Wholeness

Reliance on wholeness means that every person places ultimate reliance in the center and holds his or her place on the rim. Through simple ritual and consistent refocusing, the center houses collective intention and reminds people that the circle consists of all who are present as well as the circle itself.

The Principles in Action

Every four years, the Wheaton Franciscans elect a new leadership team, set forth a clarified and renewed mission statement, and attend to the business of their community. As the 2008 election approached, the vowed community voted to use circle process as its governance during Chapter. Chapter in religious communities is a formal process of discerning direction and leadership. The meeting needed to be conducted with an understanding of the community's religious life and the ecclesial dimensions of the Chapter, so Sister Brenda Peddigrew, a Sister of Mercy from Ontario, came to serve as facilitator, and we continued to coach the community's circle process. Sister Carola Thomann, the general directress of the congregation, arrived from Rome to oversee the proceedings. They were ready to trust the three principles with the most important of their meetings.

For the Wheaton Franciscans, as for most communities of religious women, Chapter meetings are a formal governance process to which delegates are elected. Meeting participants reflect in depth on the life of the community and try to discern the direction of the next four years of province life. After lengthy conversation in the Chapter of affairs, new leadership is formally elected in the Chapter of election to guide the community in fulfilling the Chapter's directives. Chapter is a time set apart from other work: meetings are a formal process with daily Mass, prescribed voting in the chapel, and lengthy discussions about current issues. In previous Chapter meetings, speakers had moved to the podium to address the group or a stood at a microphone stand waiting to be acknowledged by the facilitator or chairperson in order to engage in dialogue.

In the 2008 Chapter, half of the gymnasium was set in circles of six chairs around a common center, and the other half of the gym contained forty-five chairs in a gigantic circle around an exquisite center of candles and flowers and colored scarves. An outer rim of chairs invited nondelegates and lay covenant members to witness and sometimes participate. Sister Carola and two other members from Rome sat at a round table adjacent to the large circle. Though religious in tone and context, the form here is similar to stakeholder meetings or annual association meetings. There is a need for a full gathering, strategic discussion, decision, and commitment to a course of action.

The group ceremonially filed into the circle singing. There was no particular order as to who walked in first and who walked in last. Once everyone was seated, several sisters shared a prepared meditation. Leadership was rotating, responsibility was shared, and the reliance on wholeness was deeply set in place.

At lunch on the first day, Sister Carola approached us. "Are you the ones who teach this circle practice?" she asked. We nodded. "You invented this?" Christina responded, "Not exactly. People have been meeting in circles for thousands of years. We have studied the structure that resides within this very old form so it can be used in modern-day meetings."

"And the purpose is that each woman's voice can be heard?" she continued. We nodded again. "I think I like this. We will see if it can work all week." As the week progressed and complex issues of finances and programs came forth, the group alternated between large circle councils and small circle conversations. We acted as guardians of the process and actually said very little. In the evenings, we met with Sister Brenda, Sister Carola, and anyone in the community who volunteered to help design the next day's process. This was no longer a circle in training; it was a circle fully in its stride. After two years of working with the Wisdom Circle, the Wheaton Franciscans had clearly made circle process their own.

At the conclusion of the Chapter of affairs, the delegates adopted the following as their vision statement for the next four-year cycle:

> Grounded in the Light of the Gospel and our Franciscan way of life, we deepen our commitment through contemplation and action:
>
> ⊙ To leadership in issues of justice, peace, and integrity of creation
>
> ⊙ To conscious use and sharing of resources that are faithful to our values of sustainability, solidarity, and collaboration
>
> ⊙ To live compassionately and creatively in the chaos and brokenness of the Church and the world
>
> ⊙ To grapple courageously with the challenges of the changing face of the province
>
> ⊙ To integrate the Circle Process as a respectful holding of one another and as a form of shared leadership
>
> ⊙ We face what Life presents, returning only blessing that we might be instruments of peace, transformation, hope, and healing.

Then the delegates regathered for the Chapter of election. A subgroup of sisters who had designed the election process moved into their leadership roles. Election discernment began in the chapel with meditation and prayer. Names for leadership were placed in nomination through written ballots. The results were read aloud, and then the nominees had the opportunity to speak within the circle concerning their readiness to serve. Back and forth the process went as people carefully considered what it would mean to share responsibility at the leadership level.

There is a painful history in many religious communities concerning elections, and the Wheaton Franciscans used circle process and the three practices to keep the discernment grounded in faith and trust. Every effort was made to sustain an open and respectful conversation, especially among those who were willing to serve the community as possible leaders.

When the final ballots were cast in the chapel for the new leadership team, the individuals the community had selected were formally welcomed in front of the entire membership. PeerSpirit and Sister Brenda had given Sister Carola her own guardian bells. She rang them to begin the ceremony. Each member of the new leadership team proclaimed her willingness to use the principles and practices of circle as she moved into service on behalf of the Wheaton Franciscan province.

As is true in wider society, the new leadership team, of Sister Beatrice Hernandez, Sister Margaret Grempka, Sister Jane Madejczyk, and Sister Rose Mary Pint has had to make some very difficult financial decisions as the recession of late 2008 gripped the United States and the world. As a team and as a community, they have made these decisions by both grappling with numbers and statistics and leaning into the trust that circle leadership has bestowed on them.

As we completed our consultative cycle with these women, we remembered the first time we had walked into the provincial offices at the motherhouse. The central meeting room had a long oval table with a flip chart hovering at one end and a center filled with markers and sticky notes, fruit, and snacks. At the other end of the room was a circle of comfortable chairs—four for the council and one draped with a shawl and icon to represent the community, symbolically present in all the council's dialogue and deliberations. A candle burned there, calling these women to an experience of collaborative leadership in the heart of Roman Catholic hierarchy.

Although this story comes from a religious community, we were aware many times of how universal these challenges are for people working or living together. We have applied insights from our experience with the sisters to organizational settings and articulated insights from our organizational work back to the sisters. We have helped other organizations incorporate the symbolic empty chair to represent employees or staff nurses or clients, just as the Wheaton Franciscans held this space for community members during their circles. And sometimes in the heat of a business setting, we have looked at each other and wished that the wholeness provided by ceremony that is so deeply embedded in the Wheaton Franciscan culture could be available as a sectarian option. How differently our meetings would proceed if people could file in ceremoniously, if they felt they could bless each other at the beginning of difficult times, and if they would allow themselves songs of gratitude, praise, and recommitment as their time in circle progressed.

Ceremony doesn't have to look religious: it's what those middle school students did taking off their shoes—hundreds of them pausing in the foyer, bending down, and laughing and calling out to each other as they padded off to class in socks or bare feet.

CHAPTER

Circle, Step by Step

The overall flow of a circle meeting is directed by the components of start-point, check-in, and check-out. These three components set a social container for a clear beginning, a path of conversation, and a clear ending. They are easy to use and explain and can stand alone or serve as a transition to the full use of circle process.

Christina was shopping in our local town when a business card fell out of her wallet and onto the counter. The shop owner scooped it up, "PeerSpirit . . . interesting name. I'm Linda, president of the chamber of commerce. What exactly do you do?" After a brief conversation, the woman invited us to join the chamber and suggested that we attend a board meeting, to be held a few days later at a Chinese restaurant. That was a Thursday afternoon.

On Saturday afternoon, we showed up at a round table in a small meeting room at the back of the restaurant to join the shop owner and five board members. We were introduced as potential chamber members, attending as observers. The meeting began. It was August, and five tiny bouquets of flowers decorated the middle of the table—nice touch, we thought. "Thanks for coming out on a summer Saturday," Linda said, raising a tall glass of iced tea. "I propose a toast—for the good of the community and our commerce within it." Everyone clinked glasses. The agenda items were laid out for all to see.

"For the benefit of our guests," said Linda, "could we go around and each say something about how the chamber contributes to our business—one benefit of belonging? That would give PeerSpirit a sense of what we do." This check-in set a thoughtful tone that lasted through several agenda items. About twenty minutes into the meeting, a topic arose that veered into a rather delicate conversation about the financial tribulations of one particular business.

Linda leaned in and said, "If we're going to discuss this, can we agree to confidentiality?" She looked at everyone around the table—we all nodded.

The next agenda item led to a rather gossipy string of comments about one of the town characters. As the board members revved up, Linda leaned in again. "Could we speak about him with curiosity instead of judgment?" Again she looked at us individually until we all nodded.

We were amazed watching Linda skillfully introduce circle in bits and pieces. She never mentioned the word *circle*. She didn't use a bell or a talking piece. Yet she had chosen a round table and created a center in a completely unobtrusive way. She had introduced start-point by raising a toast to the intention of the chamber. She had used our presence as a rationale for check-in. And she had brought in agreements in the moment on an as-needed basis. None of the participants seemed to notice that the structure of the meeting was different—they were all engaged in content and let Linda tend to their process—yet it gave her a precedent. She could say at the end of the meeting, "Remember now, we agreed to confidentiality;" and at a future meeting she can say, "Remember that time we did a review of chamber benefits? Today, what if we do a review of…"

Of course, we signed on as members. We later had a background conversation with Linda, who explained that she had gone to the library Thursday evening and borrowed a copy of *Calling the Circle.* "I thought I should look at it before you showed up—and I decided to try out parts and see how it worked. Pretty well, don't you think?" She looked quite pleased with her experiment. Linda's hosting was one of the smoothest introductions of "a little bit of circle" we've ever seen—and we've told the story many times since.

When PeerSpirit trains people in the use of circle, we often say, "If you don't try anything else, try these three elements: start-point, check-in, and check-out. It's easy, it's helpful, and it works in virtually any setting." These are the components that open, initiate, and close the container of circle; they weave the group without having to teach the group.

Start-Point ~ silence

A start-point begins a circle in an intentional manner. In many meetings, the transition between walking into the room and beginning the meeting is practically indistinguishable. The leader just starts talking over the buzz of the group, announcing the first agenda item. One of the hallmarks of circle process is that it has boundaries—beginning, middle, and end. Start-point is an essential element that calls in the contained space for practicing attentive listening and intentional speaking that needs to occur, even if the full components are not named.

Start-points can be as simple as reading an inspirational quote, poem, or a meaningful paragraph from a book. Or they can be as elaborate as inviting people into a ceremony, such as filing into a hall. A start-point fits easily into the informality of the chamber board meeting. The culture of the Wheaton Franciscan sisters invited song and procession—not a common practice in organizational settings. Whatever is offered for a start-point, it serves to assist participants in shifting from social chatting into focused listening and speaking.

Start-points are part of common culture in public meetings and events. In the United States, we recite the Pledge of Allegiance, sing the national anthem at baseball games, and pray at presidential inaugurations and congressional sessions. Everyday rituals are widely accepted and expected and occur in every culture. We understand them as signals that shift our attention.

Offering the start-point is an incremental way to share leadership: Who will bring an opening thought for our next gathering? People often have favorite quotes, readings, or poems they are eager to share. The content of the start-point may lead directly into a check-in question.

In our neighborhood association, the year Ann was president, she called in the annual meeting by announcing, "What organizes us into a community is our shared water system and neighborhood maintenance, so I'd like to start by reading a poem about water—and I'm going to put this vase filled with our shared water and Louise's beautiful flowers in the center of our table." People stopped chatting and listened to the poem, and then she introduced check-in by saying, "I'm not sure everyone knows everyone else here, so let's go around the room, say your name, how long you've lived in the neighborhood, and one thing you like about living here."

People spoke briefly, "I'm Bill, I've lived here thirteen years, and I like that people are friendly." Nothing apparently profound came forward, yet the weaving was strong enough that the tenor and efficiency of the meeting was noticeably smoother than in previous years. People left the meeting saying, "My, that went well," without necessarily attributing the quality of their interactions to the weave at the beginning.

Check-In

The choice of question or story for a check-in sets the tone of the gathering. The host's contribution to the success of check-in is to offer a question that ties in to the purpose of the meeting. Questions about the benefits of the chamber of commerce or the length of time lived in a neighborhood set a tone that slows people down enough to realize that the meeting is beginning. The nature of the questions also set expectations that people will be moving fairly quickly into the major conversation or agenda items. A heartfelt question, such as "What do you love most about being part of this organization (family/community effort/ etc.)?" invites a deeper, slower weave and sets the expectation that the check-in is a significant contributor to what's to come. And whenever a question elicits a response revealing personal vulnerability, the check-in takes on a more profound quality—as is evidenced in many of the stories throughout this book.

It is helpful for the host and guardian to have a conversation about the length of time they expect check-in to take and the role they expect it to have in this particular meeting. They can hold this intention with each other and also hold the possibility that some surprising comment may enrich the group and shift expectations in ways they cannot anticipate as they go into the meeting.

Crafting questions is an art form. The choice of an opening question for check-in is a significant piece of preparation for whoever is calling the circle—the first time and every time. The question is like a flower that beckons to the bee, and the responses pollinate the ensuing conversation. The question can be designed to strengthen a sense of commonality or to shake loose attitudes and assumptions that may be preventing the group from considering options and seeing creative possibilities. Sometimes when we've been invited into a situation where tension and conflict are present, we'll surprise people by starting with a check-in question that invites them to perceive the difficulty in a new way, such as the following:

- What about this current situation can you imagine being grateful for in the future?

- How is this situation maturing your leadership capacities?

- What is one shift in attitude or action you could take that could potentially improve the situation?

Our Danish colleague Toke Paludan Møller says, "If I can only have two tools going into a room, I choose a good question and a talking piece." Intriguing questions serve to unlock a treasure chest of information, experience, and passion. Check-in questions can also invite stories that bring insight to the task at hand: "How did you come to be on this committee?" "Whom do you consider yourself

EXHIBIT 6.1

Attributes of a Powerful Question
○ Generates curiosity in the listener
○ Stimulates reflective conversation
○ Is thought-provoking
○ Surfaces underlying assumptions
○ Invites creativity and new possibilities
○ Generates energy and forward movement
○ Channels attention and focuses inquiry
○ Stays with participants
○ Touches a deep meaning
○ Evokes more questions
© 2003, "The Art of Powerful Questions," http://www.theworldcafe.com

representing?" "How do you see this piece of work contributing to your overall life path?" The possibilities for developing intriguing questions are endlessly varied and will shift groups in many directions. The delightful study of what constitutes a powerful question has been shared by many of us who are introducing collaborative conversation (see Exhibit 6.1).

Often when going to work with a new group, our longest search is for the right question—the one that will twirl the tumblers in the padlock where the group is stuck or will open perception to new and intriguing possibilities. Eric Vogt, Juanita Brown, and David Isaacs, founders of the World Café process, have posted a downloadable booklet, *The Art of Powerful Questions,* that is a classic reference guide and a gift to the rest of us. In it they write, "A powerful question also has the capacity to 'travel well'—to spread beyond the place where it began into larger networks of conversation throughout an organization or community. Questions that travel well are often the key to large-scale change."

In 2005, when working with Toke Møller and his dynamic community of hosts in Denmark, we asked him to send us home with a question that he would like to know we would be asking other Americans. He thought for a moment and suggested, "Ask, 'What else could America be?'" Versions of this question have traveled far and led us into stunning conversations across the fire of the center. "What else could this community be? This company? This school? This relationship?"

Check-in is a piece of circle practice that can work in almost every setting. Sometimes check-in is designed to lead to the main conversation; sometimes it is designed to serve as the main conversation. Working to help strengthen team spirit among nurse leaders at Craig Hospital in Denver, we brought one of our well-traveled questions to a breakfast cookout at Rocky Mountain National Park during a two-day training session and retreat. Craig Hospital is exclusively devoted to rehabilitation and research for patients with spinal cord injury and traumatic brain injury and has treated more spinal cord injury patients than any other facility in the world. So here in the great nest of mountains, with elk wandering by the edge of the campground and squirrels chattering in the pine trees, we formed a circle under blue skies and asked the question "What led you to become a trauma care nurse?" This time we expected the check-in to be the essence of circle experience and had allotted ample time for the group's responses and stories.

Terry Chase, once a patient at Craig and now its patient and family education coordinator, said of that event, "The authenticity of our stories and the quality of our listening that morning laid a foundation between us that I still remember when we're dealing with each other in the day-to-day of the hospital. That's when circle work was born in our organization."

Sometimes check-in can reinvigorate intention and commitment when a group has meandered away from its original purpose. A women's circle that had started out as a book discussion group focused on sharing thoughts, critiques, and insights gradually shifted to long check-in stories focused on the personal details of the women's lives. A few members began to drift off; several more became ambivalent about wanting to stay. When it was our friend's turn to host, she sent everyone a suggested check-in of three questions: "Why did I initially join this group?" "What has it given me?" "What do I want it to give me now?" The check-in rounds gave each member a voice and helped the women remember their intentions and explore their evolution. A few members felt complete with the experience and left with the good wishes of all present. The following month, a slightly smaller configuration returned to their focus on a common book with an opening round of check-in on their personal lives that was time-limited.

Sometimes a group can become so acclimated to check-in that the process turns into a perfunctory exercise. Check-in can lose its power to call people to presence. People may say something short and unrevealing, like "I'm here" or

"I'm fine." Meaning comes from the intention people bring to bear when they participate. If check-in questions are routine or irrelevant, perhaps it's time to shake things up. Elicit check-in questions via e-mail before a meeting to see what people would like to respond to. Invite each person to bring an object from home or the office that represents a special personal strength or skill and place it in the center with a story. Draw a card from a deck of words or images and respond. Be ready to be surprised.

Check-Out

Start-point and check-in create a clear beginning and set a meeting on a path of interaction. Just as it is important to open circle space with an invitation to participation, so it is important to consciously close the space. Check-out can be as variable as check-in: closing with quotes, readings, or poems; removing check-in items from the center of the circle with a brief thought, sharing a round of appreciation, or simply ringing a bell for a closing pause. A commonly used closure is to ask people to "share one thing you learned from our meeting today." If the meeting has been scribed, use the opportunity to harvest insights and to thank those who have stepped in to take on tasks or leadership roles. As soon as the check-out is complete, the group will erupt into social time, and everyone will notice the shift in energy.

Sometimes check-out can be the major conversation in a longer group process. Near the end of the school year, after a number of different collaborative meetings and conversations with elementary school teachers, we wanted to complete our engagement with them with an experience that might heal some of the tensions that had accumulated over the year and acknowledge that layoffs were occurring: this was the last time this particular group of teachers would all be together. We had introduced them to circle and to World Café. We had told the story of the California middle school—and they had adopted and posted those agreements around the school: "Take care of yourself, take care of each other, and take care of this place." They had developed their own staff agreements. We had hosted conversations on resilience in the midst of unrelenting change. The reduction in force announcements had gone out. Negotiations were still under way, and some people were uncertain of their employment status. We had three hours on the Friday before Memorial Day. We started with lunch.

Tables had been moved out of the community room, and we had set a center—a cardboard box covered with a tablecloth—in the middle with a big

bouquet of local flowers donated by a parent and dozens of photos of the teachers' students splayed out in a colorful spiral. We conducted a brief review of the
year, offered a few journal-writing exercises to ground them into their strengths
as teachers, and offered the invitation—this time for checking out: "Choose
one story of success you've had with a child this year." Every teacher spoke.
Every teacher had a story of great heart. They all slipped into their deepest
knowing of themselves as teachers. Things would be different, difficult; maybe
they wouldn't be back. But what they remembered and witnessed for one
another on that day was that they had made a difference in the lives of children.
The check-out took ninety minutes. There was no fidgeting—not one of them
wanted to miss a single story. For those ninety minutes, they celebrated themselves as the community of caring teachers they had been in a challenging year.

Pamela Austin Thompson, CEO of the American Organization of Nursing
Executives (AONE) and coauthor of PeerSpirit's booklet on circle and nursing
leadership, has one instruction for people interested in trying circle in organizational settings: "Practice—just start somewhere and practice," she says. "Shifting
a meeting into a more circular way of being still makes my knees shake, but you
just have to jump in and try it and know that sometimes it will work better than
others and that everything is a group learning experience."

In an organization devoted to fostering a culture of communication from the
administrative level to the direct care nurses, Pam uses some of the Components
of Circle in many of the meetings she facilitates for AONE. "One of the skill sets I
bring to the nursing community is how to convene people in a different way. Even
if we don't formally call it a circle, I always use check-in and check-out. I tell people,
'Check-in convenes us and check-out releases us.' Some people push back on the
formal methodology of circle because it feels foreign to them. So often I simply
introduce a component or two in the moment it's needed and then afterward tell
them, 'That's what circle is all about.'"

Adopting Circle as an Organizational Methodology

It's a business adage that "to get a better outcome, hold a better meeting." A
fine thought but not very instructional in the "how-to" department. Many
organizational leaders want *something* to be different: the effectiveness of
meetings, the strength of relationships in teams or units, the ability to envision together, the commitment to mentor leadership development. Various
components of PeerSpirit Circle Process have been successfully used as an

innovative group process shift to support these desires for different outcomes and greater success.

When Jerry Nagel, cofounder of the Meadowlark Institute, was invited to facilitate the board retreat for the North Dakota Humanities Council in June 2009, he walked into an association with a history of a revered founder who had carried a legendary vision of bringing humanities into the ranchlands. After a transition director, the council is now led by a dynamic young woman, Brenna Daugherty, who contacted Jerry with two desired outcomes for their annual board retreat: to reconnect the board with the mission of the Humanities Council and to reconnect the board and staff.

Jerry said, "The Humanities Council needed to decide what the organization is *now*. It also needed to define board responsibilities and commitments to the staff and the mission." The group met in a hotel room in the city of Minot in a hotel basement conference room. In one half of the room, Jerry set up a large circle (for three staff, twelve board members, and one facilitator), and in the other half of the room placed round tables for smaller discussions. "For opening check-in, everyone brought two objects to place in the center: one personally symbolic of the state of North Dakota and the other representing something about the humanities. The staff had created a truly beautiful center, and the storytelling that emerged allowed the group to know all its members on a more personal level. I closed by reading a poem."

It was a two-day retreat, organized as follows: day 1: circle, World Café, barbecue at the board chair's home; day 2: circle check-in with talking piece around a topical question, adjourning to small tables for strategic planning process, and closing with circle and poetry. "At the end of the business time, the board practically rushed back to circle, eager to get back into this kind of interaction. It was all new to the board members, but Brenna later reported that they all considered it the best board retreat ever and made a commitment to continue meeting in circle."

Even if only offered as a onetime experience, circle has the potential to change an organization by creating a sense of connectedness that had been lacking in the group. The host needs to be aware of this potential and have done the necessary prep work to provide support for the meaningful conversations that may be set in motion. That is why PJ, whose story was told in Chapter 3, took such a long time to go through her own preparation process before inviting other people into circle.

How Circle Integrates with Other Methodologies and Consulting Practices

We often combine our use of circle with World Café or Open Space technology when we see the need for the gifts these processes offer, and we work with and hear stories of other companies, networks, and seminars that are integrating circle into their specialties.

Creative Health Care Management

Creative Health Care Management (CHCM) is an international consulting organization that works exclusively in health care. Based in Minnesota, CHCM provides leadership, staff, and team development and work process improvements consistent with nursing care standards in settings both large and small. Over the years, it has integrated circle process into its seminars, invited us in for staff training, and successfully negotiated the transition from a strong founder to collective ownership of the company. One of the primary programs CHCM has developed is a three-day seminar called Reigniting the Spirit of Caring that focuses on caring for self and others and is designed to help care providers find renewed commitment to their work. Colleen Person, vice president and consultant, who was introduced to PeerSpirit through the Center for Nursing Leadership, brought her circle training into the heart of the Reigniting experience. She and cofacilitator Susan Edstrom understand the importance of circle in this program.

"Self-awareness is an essential component of a nurse's ability to reignite her caring—to revitalize herself and her commitment to nursing," Susan explains. "Circle fosters self-awareness as it enables people to see others as individuals and to be seen by others as individuals. This may not sound revolutionary to outsiders, but there is a subtle culture of anonymity in nursing." Susan notes that the generic roles in health care (patients often call out " Hey, nurse!" or "Hey, doctor!") can lead to a diminished sense of individuality. "This acceptance of anonymity can pervade units so that nurses know surprisingly little about each other and communicate only about clinical details. Their lack of story and broader communication contributes to a nurse-specific form of workplace exhaustion that this seminar addresses through the circle practices of listening with attention and speaking with intention."

CHCM contracts with a hospital or health care system for entire groups of colleagues to go through the workshop together. On the second day, Colleen and Susan ask participants to bring something personal to share—poems, photos, and mementos. "We watch the light bulbs go off as people realize they've worked with this other person—sometimes for twenty-five or more years—and had no idea that they had a creative side, a tender side, or even a family."

Once an organization sent all the nursing staff that had been identified as needing an attitude adjustment. "Circle was the essential intervention with this group," Colleen recalls. "The nurses' entire *modus operandi* was blaming their leaders, blaming the organization, and building a subculture based on self-righteous anger, judgmentalism, and victimization. On the second day, we called a circle. About two-thirds of the way around, as one after another they listened to their usual recitations of negativity, someone said, 'Maybe we need to think about how each of us is contributing to the situation at hand.' From that moment on, everything began to switch."

"Trust the process" has clearly become a mantra for Colleen and Susan. CHCM's use of circle process occurs within the context of its consulting spectrum and a number of specialized and profession-focused interventions and exercises. The women offer circle as one of the tools they know can succeed in the environments where they work, and they have developed a respectful relationship with PeerSpirit regarding the use of our materials. After over a decade of offering circle where no one had previous experience of the process, Colleen remains enthusiastic of its impact. "Nurses who have done circle do their jobs differently. They open up the social container for active conversation and develop the confidence to take increasing leadership roles."

It is not only nurses and not only health care that are changed by circle, though these are fields in which we are often called to work. Organizational use of circle provides a body-mind-heart experience that stays with participants and shifts the status quo. Circle can be comforting or unsettling; it can reinforce what's good about an organization, and it can raise previously undiscussed issues and lead into the deeper territory explored in Chapters 8, 9, and 10.

The Art of Hosting

The Art of Hosting and Harvesting Conversations That Matter is a loose international fellowship of people committed to offering "a powerful leadership practicum" for individuals, communities, families, businesses, and organizations. The organization's Web site calls it "a practice retreat for all who aspire to learn and find new ways for working with others to create innovative and comprehensive solutions. We are a growing community of practitioners, supporting each other to explore and accomplish what we most care about." The Art of Hosting grew out of Berkana Institute's From the Four Directions project in 2000–2001 and the Shambhala Summer Leadership Institute (now called Alia—Authentic Leadership in Action) when a critical mass of creative group process facilitators kept identifying their passion for using conversation as the foundation for social activism and systemic change.

The Art of Hosting invites participants to jump in and practice four basic conversational methodologies: circle, World Café, Open Space, and appreciative inquiry in an intense learning experience of two or three days together in retreat settings. Those of us on the hosting team are in-depth practitioners of one or more of these processes and take turns modeling the infrastructure of each form, teaching it during short instructional sessions, and coaching people to step into their hosting leadership.

We participate in Art of Hosting events sporadically as our schedules allow and appreciate how many who serve on the hosting teams carry the presence of circle. It is truly a cross-fertilization of models that reinforces the integration of circle elements in modern methodologies and theoretical teachings that increase our capacity to understand, withstand, and welcome change.

PART

III

The Art of Presence in the Circle

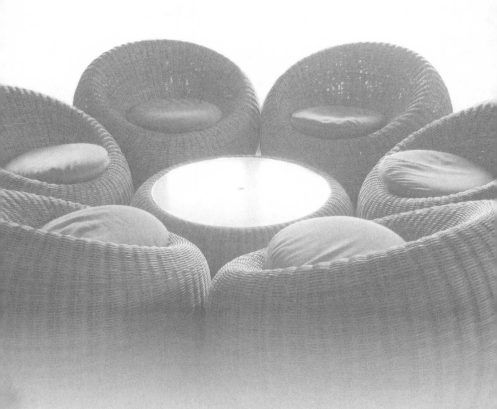

CHAPTER 7

Story as Core Communication

Story is a map of human experience. It has chronology, character, scene, and insight. A teller needs a listener; a story needs to be "caught" to be complete—and circle provides the perfect container for "catching stories."

Stories anchor learning. Human beings are storytelling creatures. The well-known twentieth-century anthropologist Laurens van der Post is said to have proclaimed, "Ninety percent of everything we know about being human we have learned through story." We are the only species that relies as deeply on communication of experience as on actual experience. You can teach a child to look before crossing the street by the power of a story—by explaining consequences and telling stories of what has happened before. Learning though association is part of van der Post's 90 percent: our chances for survival are greatly enhanced by this capacity to change our behavior through listening to the passed-along experiences embedded in the stories—of others.

The ability to learn vicariously, to communicate our accumulated knowledge and understanding, and to share both previous and anticipated outcomes is the essential definer of our humanity. Not only can we share what we know, but we can also share our dreams and aspirations and our grand imaginings of what the universe is and our place within it.

Understanding the power of story to create a self-educating and self-organizing community is as old as the circle. In *On Dialogue*, David Bohm notes the power of story in indigenous cultures:

From time to time, [the tribe members] met . . . in a circle. They just talked and talked and talked, apparently to no purpose. They made no decisions. There was no leader. And everybody could participate. There may have been wise men or wise women who were listened to a bit more—the older ones—but everybody could talk. The meeting went on, until it finally seemed to stop for no reason at all and the group dispersed. Yet after that, everybody seemed to know what to do, because they understood each other so well. Then they could get together in smaller groups and do something or decide things.[1]

Bohm is describing an experience people have in circle all the time. The willingness to see story as a partner in circle process depends on our understanding of its power as a teacher and our trust that people will grasp the metaphor. Assuming that van der Post is correct, people learn more efficiently, more holistically, and more indelibly through story than through any other form of communication—whether the story is spoken or written. We are practicing our belief in the power of story throughout this book—illustrating the infrastructure of circle and bringing concepts to life through story.

Story Shared

In the fall of 2008, the Tacoma, Washington, Fund for Women & Girls, under the auspices of the Tacoma Community Foundation, provided a grant to support facilitated circles for women living in extreme stress and poverty. These women were selected by social service providers as having enough stability to show up for seven consecutive weeks. The intention question of the fund in its fiduciary role as grantor was quantitative: "How many women would enroll in schooling as a result of the investment of the grant?" The intention question of Catherine Place, a small Catholic women's center that coordinated the participating agencies and helped solicit facilitators and participants, was qualitative: "How might the circle experience lead to greater personal stability and encourage education?"

PeerSpirit offered two days of circle host training for sixteen women leaders from agencies ranging from Goodwill and the YWCA to the Tacoma Urban League and several drug abuse treatment houses. Our question was both qualitative and quantitative: "Could we effectively prepare these hosts to embrace the circle concept and trust the circle to hold the women?" The newly trained hosts left the practicum with a sense of excitement and anticipation, carrying the Women's Leadership Circle Kit developed by the Berkana Institute and PeerSpirit. Though each participant was eager to experience the circle as a social container, they also had many unanswered questions about how they were going to work with their respective populations. Courageously, they stepped into hosting and guardianship and followed the format and conversational topics laid out in the kits. We reunited with the circle hosts after the completion of their seven-week programs to review how the experiment had gone.

While honoring the confidentiality of their participants, the hosts shared experiences from their circle groups. The enthusiasm in the room was palpable. Here are some of the hosts' reports:

> "The Hispanic women in our circle came together from half a dozen different countries. Women from different Latin countries don't usually mix socially, so we weren't sure how the diversity would meld. But the stories did it. The women told the circle about experiences they had never whispered aloud because the circle offered support and not judgment. After the third session, something shifted because we noticed that they were doing things together outside the circle meetings, such as going shopping at Goodwill as a group."

> "In our agency, getting the women not to physically fight or emotionally abuse one another has been a huge challenge. So, of course, setting agreements was a big deal. However, once they began to share their stories, we saw violence disappear. Women bully each other when they perceive scarcity—which has been everywhere in their lives. The circle structure bypasses that dynamic, and if bullying came up, they called each other to the agreements to intervene."

> "Even with women who were slightly more stable financially, the biggest barrier to education is low self-esteem, a woman's sense that she's not capable of learning or that she doesn't have the right to better herself. The circle began to serve as an esteem builder, with a dozen outside voices pouring confidence into one another."

A universal statement from all the circle hosts was that the success of their circles was at least partly dependent on the fact that quality child care had been available during circle meetings. "No woman can relax into any kind of story sharing or listening if she is concerned about her child's well-being. This was crucial to the program's success," said Judy Mladineo, program director for Catherine Place.

In addition to their enthusiasm about the depth and quality of stories shared, the circle hosts reported that from one-fourth to one-third of the participants enrolled in a next level of education for themselves—ranging from food handler's license to driver's education to English as a second language to the GED and even community college. Perhaps one of the strongest statements about the program's success is that many of the circles elected to continue meeting after their seven-week cycle ended.

Story Defined

Just as circle is a slightly more structured form of communication that employs understood rules of engagement—such as speaking one at a time, using the center, and listening without judging—story is a slightly more structured use of language that employs narrative structures of chronology, character, scene, and insight. Not every word out of our mouths is story: story is the narrative heart of language. The stories from the Tacoma experience enable us to look at the four characteristics of all stories. Story has a *character*—one or more persons who are the focus of the narrative. It has *chronology*—a beginning and an end. It happens in a particular place: the *scene*. And it offers an *insight* or lesson.

Some of the stories from the Tacoma experience involved the *scene* of arriving in this country penniless, unable to speak English, and getting raped or beaten. The individual *characters* experienced similar *chronologies* based on their lack of economic and educational resources. The *insight* that most of them experienced in their circles is that other women were experiencing similar challenges. Together they could offer one another verbal encouragement and even support in things like child care, bargain shopping, and meal sharing.

Story is a powerful medium. It *creates relationships* in that other people become real to us through story. It leads to insights we cannot access through thought and opinion because our emotions, as well as our intellect, are activated. We read statistics such as "less than 25 percent of women entering drug rehabilitation houses recover from their addictions." That is a fact. Our minds take it in, and we categorize it as "not a good thing." However, when we hear Elissa tell the story of being in treatment for the fifth time, wanting to stay drug-free yet having to return to live with her drug-using partner because she has nowhere else to go,

generous, strong

green silk scarf - field/ground, strength, not the figure of a neckline but the warmth or comfort.

we want to help. Facts do not lead to action as often as a poignant story that bonds us to another human being. Through story, a statistic becomes a face, a personality, a woman with a heartrending life who hasn't given up on herself.

Story leads to *insights* that we cannot access through thought or opinion, facts and data. It was a risk for the Tacoma Fund for Women & Girls to trust a process as "soft" as circle. They hired a professional evaluator who surveyed and interviewed the women before and after. They were relieved at the statistical percentage (80 percent) that enrolled in next-step schooling during this time. This data support the heart of the experience—that the women gained confidence by sharing and hearing each other's stories.

In the WE-CAN Women's Circles Project Report, the evaluator noted:

> Despite the challenges, the co-conveners reported that the circles had clear benefits to both the organizations that convened the circles and the participants. A primary benefit to the convening organizations was forming new partnerships with other organizations. These partnerships increased the capacity to fill a gap in the availability of supportive services for women. The key benefits to participants were that the circles offered a safe place for women to come together, tell their stories, and experience a supportive community of other women to help them on their life-changing journey.

Making Time and Space for Story

Understanding how rare it is to have our stories witnessed with support and without interference, on the third day of our training seminars, the Circle Practicum, we invite participants to take the afternoon off for reflection, rejuvenation, and preparation for an evening of Story Council. By this time in our process, the group has studied circle components, the art of working with energy in circle, and creative responses to tension and conflict. We have combined cognitive theory, stories, and experiential learning. The closing day will focus on setting a clear intention for integrating circle into their professional and personal lives, so before that shift into application, we gather for an evening to honor story.

Maybe it's spring at Stanford Valley Farm in the rolling hill country just up the coast and inland from Cape Town, South Africa, with duiker grazing in the pastures. Maybe it's summer at the Aldermarsh on Whidbey Island, Washington, with miles of sand flats and tide pools on the nearby beaches.

Maybe it's autumn in the color-blazed forests of Canterbury Hills at the edge of Toronto, Ontario. Or maybe it's winter on the snow-sculpted beach at Oceanstone Inn south of Halifax, Nova Scotia. Over and over, the Story Council is the apex of our time together. Everyone is fully present, the synergy is at work, and there is enough familiarity with one another to want to share authentically. We are here. We are together. We are held in the flow of the seminar, in our sense of community as peer-spirited learners, and everyone in the group is ready to lead from the rim.

In the Story Council, we send a talking piece around the circle three times. Something different happens in carefully held circles when the talking piece is passed around more than once. There is a stretch break in silence between each round, and a different guardian serves each round. The group hosts itself through the question, usually an open-ended invitation, such as "What story is on your heart right now that you would like witnessed in the safety of this particular group?" or "Now that you're here, what is the story you'd like to speak to this fire?" Sometimes a common theme emerges; sometimes we notice our eclecticism. Always the sharing has been profound.

When people are speaking with a powerful level of intention and others are listening with a corresponding level of attention, the quality of story creates a possibility for healing that engages us at the heart level. It is exactly this heart-felt quality of engagement that will be so hard to explain once people leave the retreatlike environment of the training session and head into the mainstream settings where they will offer circle process.

A Story Council takes time. It is a donation of presence to one another. The experience of being heard does not come from direct response or advice; it arises from the pure act of having one's story received and held in the center. Someone speaks of a hidden joy or a terrible burden he or she has been carrying, and as the person lays it down, it is as though the heart of the group—residing in candle-light, residing in a vase of flowers, residing on the placards of their intention state-ment—receives it respectfully and does not interfere with the speaker's journey toward insight. The circle provides a kind of alchemy—to transmute sorrow, to highlight joy, to open empathy where there had been enmity.

In the practicum in Cape Town, we sat with two members of the Xhosa tribe, an older Afrikaner man, several English–South African women, and an Indian–South African woman—a microcosm of the country's diversity. Their stories of the apartheid era spilled forth into the center, and we were aware that this may have been the first time they had sat in such intimate diversity and heard, one after another, the burdens of their shared history—including the pain of privilege as well as oppression. In that moment, the stories of wounding started to become the stories of healing.

This ability to transmute experiences into healing is hard to explain in the boardroom, the office, or the community education room—and yet healing through heartfelt listening is needed everywhere. If the conditions are created to sustain it, listening and healing will emerge. Chapter 10 is devoted to three such stories.

The Four Gifts of Story

In meetings that rely on agenda, Robert's Rules of Order, and fact sharing to move things forward, story may be received with a "get to the point" attitude. At a seminar for elected officials sponsored by the Luke Center for Leadership in Salem, Oregon, Christina found herself in a group of people for whom data and information were more comfortable than narrative. "Data is code," said one city engineer. "Data is story in another form. When I look at the numbers, what I see is what you call story. The progression of events—how we got here—is clear to me, and I get excited to present the data to others thinking they'll understand. Some do, some don't."

"Yes," said a city planner, "for me story means a member of the public standing at an open microphone and droning on about some particular concern while I'm looking down at the figures and thinking—I don't care how heartrending you're being, we're not gonna put a stoplight at that corner, 'cause the money's not there!'"

Christina's question to these managers was "How could we make space for both the language of data and the language of story?" If the intention is to communicate, then our role as communicators is to become as skilled as we can in each language. Just as circle and hierarchy can work together, so story and data can work together. Here are the facts; here is the story; here is a group process that allows us to offer and hear every contribution that leads toward creative problem solving. She taught them the four gifts of story, and they practiced on real situations in their communities. And Christina learned a new way to view facts and figures.

Let us explore the four gifts of story.

1. Story Creates Context

Context is the setting in which experience happens, so that listeners can come into the world of the story and identify with it. It provides enough framing information so the listener can track appropriately and begin to understand the impact or importance of the story more fully.

A large city school system had to make budget cuts when the funding to keep the current system operating was no longer available from state and federal revenues. Everyone was stressed as the impact of the shifting numbers became obvious. After-school programs would be cut, and six grade schools and two high schools would need to close in the next few years. (This is the context.)

The school superintendent, Dr. Jamie Braslow, was hired in part because she seemed able to enter systems in this kind of transition and work with the volatile reactions of concerned parents and community partners. (This is context that has expanded into story: the superintendent is a character, a real person with skill and background, and the other players in the decision—parents, students, community partners—are being called into the scene.)

2. Context Creates Relationship

When context is set, story starts happening to real people, and those people are in relationship with each other—and also with the listener. We start to care about the situation and what's happening to the folks in the story.

The facts remain the same: the budget cuts are unavoidable, the charts and graphs and spreadsheets are all in the room—and now, so is story. An impassioned mother speaks into the microphone at a community meeting, "Zora School is named after Zora Neale Hurston. It started out as a colored school during segregation. As our city, schools, and neighborhoods became integrated, Zora was the only elementary school inside a black neighborhood that welcomed other students to come to us instead of our children being bused elsewhere. This is history. You cannot close this school!" (Now character, scene, and event combine to create tension in story: we want to know how it's going to turn out.)

3. Context and Relationship Create Vicarious Learning

We put ourselves into the story. We evaluate characters' actions and reactions and anticipate how we would want to behave if we found ourselves in a similar situation. We prepare ourselves for wiser action through imagination, empathy, and discernment: whom do we want to be like if anything like this ever happens to us?

As we observe or engage in this unfolding event around the school closures, we have the opportunity to reflect on community values we may not have thought about recently. We have the opportunity to imagine ourselves in the decision maker position and what input we hope Dr. Braslow is bringing into consideration. We identify with various characters who seem to be speaking and acting as we would want to act, or we practice not acting the way some characters are acting. (As listeners—or readers—we used vicarious learning to transfer insight from this story to another situation that bears a resemblance to this one.)

4. Vicarious Learning Creates Cohesive Action and Expands Consciousness

Though specific in detail, story serves as a universal teacher. The actions of characters expand our sense of choice and our ability to identify with people with whom we may not have previously had affinity.

In this story, the superintendent opened the decision-making process to a World Café and asked 150 community members to think with the board. In the café, community members were encouraged to explore "out of the box" ideas while continuing to honor the necessary budget constraints. When options are explored in an open conversational process, they carry the four gifts of story along with them. Even those who are disappointed with the outcome have a greater understanding of how it was reached.

This is the key: people want to be included in the story. We are much more likely to find ways to support disappointing outcomes—of which there are many in the world right now—when we have been included as much as possible in the story of how information was gathered, what conditions leaders have faced, and who and what were taken into consideration. When people understand how choices were made, they can become carriers of story able to explain the character of the characters, the scene behind the scene, the chronology of events, and the insights of the process.

Circle and Story on the Mountain

Often the most profound impact of story in circle occurs when taking people—managers, lawyers, ministers, consultants, business owners, human resource directors, nurse leaders, and a range of creatively self-employed women and men—out of their usual environments to live in circle on a wilderness quest. With Ann's dedication to nature adventure and environmental education, Christina's dedication to journal and memoir writing, and our mutual dedication to helping people make great leaps in the direction of their dreams, goals, and contributions, we have taken the circle back to where it came from—a fire for the night and the power of story to help us make our way.

It is dusk; it is dawn. Sun rises; moon sets. Silence is the conversation. In the shallow valley, the guides come to the Threshold Circle for their evening drumming and praying ritual. Somewhere nearby, each quester is alone—fasting from food, drinking only water, and focusing on the intention and question he or she has brought to the mountain.

There have been several days of eating, hiking, and sitting together in circle to prepare for this solo time. There have been months of communication and preparation and intention setting. There have been phone calls "in circle" between the guides and each quester. There are agreements, there is center, and there are guides and guardian. Each person has the essentials for living outside—sleeping pad and bag, tarp, water, and clothing. Cell phones and car keys are handed in for safekeeping. People have eaten a healthy diet leading up to the fast. There are many moments of ceremony.

Alone, the questers begin to understand that everything stands with them: the rocks, the trees, the wind, the sun and stars, the weather, the mountains, the big and little birds, the big and little creatures. There is time to breathe, time to remember. Through traditional and self-generated ceremony, they explore the larger questions of their lives.

All of us can hurry along from day to day and make a good enough story to steer our way through ordinary events, and sometimes life offers us extraordinary events and we watch our story fall apart. It is necessary for one narrative to shatter into nonsense so that another narrative can emerge to make new sense. At these times, we step aside from busyness to remember that surrender is part of strength, that stopping is part of going forward, that disintegration is part of reintegration, that giving up an old story can be the source of the next story. And we remember that for thousands of years, the circle has held our kind as we turn to the solace of nature with our questions.

The check-ins on wilderness quests before and after solo time are deep and unhurried. There is no place else to go; there is nothing else to do. The talking piece moves round and round: we each speak to the center; we each listen at the rim. We find the universal questions that fuel our individual stories. It is said that if we really understand what is given us on our solo time, we will understand our whole lives.

We two women who vowed to mainstream circle process are also dedicated to taking people into nature, reawakening the fundamental understanding that everything is interconnected—nature and technology; spirit and practicality; past, present, and future. The purpose of the ceremonies embedded in the quest is to experience a willing death within life: to let go of mental constructs and the humancentric and technocentric environments we have made and allow nature to offer us rebirth. This is done by emptying ourselves—of food, distraction, relationship, comfort—and noticing what is present and presenting itself to our wonderment. At puberty, the child dies into the young adult; at marriage, the single self dies into the partner self; at parenthood, the partner joins with the child to raise the next generation; at points of professional shift, the old path dies into the new path; and the adult dies into the elder. Combining an immersion into the natural world with the support of community and time for solitude, a wilderness quest is a powerful way to take the next step in one's life.

Story and circle are essential elements of questing. Telling one's story to a community and listening to others' stories inform the new life being shaped. The power of story in the quest circle is to have a community witness the emerging self and bring it into existence. This happens in the quest, and it happens as the quest shows up in initiatory moments in our working lives. The mountain can metaphorically come to us—in the boardroom, the office cubicle, the community hall, the living room.

If we step into circle as presence beyond methodology, new stories can be born. Members of an embittered team can let go of their grudges and reclaim respect for one another. A dogmatic leader can release himself or herself into shared leadership. A floundering company can find the courage to restore its identity and establish a new direction.

We are all in a period now where our survival depends on our ability to rectify the issues that divide the human family. Whatever else we are doing in the decades of our lives, in the busyness of our work and daily routines, the need to keep mending the world is the story within the story. The storycatching level of circle experience is not about answers and fixes and policy shifts—though that may come out of story time. Storycatching is about opening our hearts to strangers, colleagues, neighbors, friends, and family and being moved by the human spirit in all its confusion and courage.

CHAPTER

Activating and Responding in a Social Container

In Western culture, we are trained to focus on communication through words. We study the nuances of language and analyze other people's communication, from e-mails to major speeches. Yet everyday experiences remind us how much is being communicated beyond words: we sense other people's moods, we feel welcomed or not walking into a room, we know when to leave a threatening situation. Nonverbal cues of communication are intensified in a circle where we pause and face each other. Understanding and harnessing the circle's energetic patterns is an essential leadership skill.

Amid the snap of table legs folding and the chaos of moving chairs, the radio on the young man's belt suddenly crackled into noise and a somewhat garbled bosslike voice boomed into the empty, large, lower-level conference room. "Casey, what the hell is going in 1108B? You there?"

The young man grabbed for the volume control and turned his back as though we couldn't hear him if he weren't looking directly at us. "There's two ladies down here moving all the tables," he said. "They ordered a chairs-only setup."

"Do you have the paperwork?"

"No, sir. Can't find it. Can't find Lindsay either. She's got the clipboard, and it's fifteen minutes to showtime."

"Are they the facilitators?"

"Yes, sir." He looked tentatively over at us, as if to make sure.

"How are they going to run their slides in that arrangement?"

"No slides, sir—they moved the projector out of the middle of the room. They want a coffee table. There's a candle, sir. They say its battery-operated—just an LED light."

There was a pause that felt like a four-letter word uttered silently to himself, then a final order, "OK, do what they want. I'll send Tyrone to help you put it back together during lunch." The radio went dead. We continued moving the tables.

"You just out of the military, Casey?" Christina asked.

"Yes, sir—ma'am." He blushed.

"You know, a lot of professions are run on a kind of military model. In hospitals, they talk about officers—the chief nursing officer is the big 'kahuna,' and the floor nurses are called the 'front line.' When you have to trust your buddies—whether it's in combat or in an emergency on a nursing unit—a lot depends on how you talk to each other during the calm times. All the stories you share about where you come from, who you love back home, what you're gonna do when you get out or stateside—they help you know each other so that when you just gotta bark orders, somehow everyone knows what to do."

"Yeah," he said, eyes lighting up. "It's like we're all one body. Like we got eyes in the back of our heads and twenty legs. Like we're Transformers or something"—he looks to see if we know what he's talking about—"those toys that turn into robots?" We nod, grateful that our office manager's son has brought some models to entertain himself on days when he's out of school and playing in the back room. For a few seconds, we're hip. "Is that what you're doing here?" he asked.

"We're reminding people what that feels like," Ann replied, "how important it is to tell stories and share information when there's a little respite—so that we *can* move as one body when we know what's needed next. This circle is like when you all squatted in the sand and huddled to talk—only more comfortable."

"And less dangerous," Christina laughed, "at least most of the time. It's what we call 'making the social container.'" Casey's radio sputtered again, and he was gone.

Using the word *container* or *containment* to talk about social space is a shift in vocabulary occurring as a result of group processes, such as circle, World Café, and Open Space, that work with intention, attention, and practices of listening and speaking. A container is something designed so that something else can be placed within it. A box contains its contents; a circle contains its conversations and relationships.

There is a physical and energetic vulnerability to sitting in circle. We are facing each other, usually without even a table between us. Our soft bellies are exposed, our expressions convey emotional nuance, and our body language is in full view. Our personal energies begin to link up and overlap and influence each other so that even before the first word is spoken, before the bell rings, and before the host starts check-in, we have taken in a lot of information about how we are. We absolutely count on this ability to "read" a group, and most of the time we don't talk about the intuition or information coming in at this level or even acknowledge that it's occurring among us.

We're mammals. We have a finely developed amygdala (sometimes called the primitive brain) that works like a Geiger counter, always testing the levels of danger and safety in our physical surroundings and in our social field. Casey knows what that Geiger counter is like: he's alive because of it. We sigh, watching him go: we won't hear his story today—this is not his circle, but we hope he has one. We hope there is a place where his story can be heard and where he feels contained and supported in exploring his truth.

Containment as an Aspect of Group Process

Because the container of circle is both carefully designed by modern-day hosts and attached to the archetypal lineage of circle, the quality of conversation and our expectations of what we can bring forward are intensified. Becoming aware of the social container is a new experience for many people arriving in circle. In the ring of seating and the tangible presence of the center, the imperative to participate hangs expectantly in the air. For some people, circle space is immediately comfortable: when they see the container, they are eager to enter the conversation. We have watched people come into a room where we've prepared for circle and sit down, emotional with relief, later reporting that they experienced an immediate sense of "I've been looking for this space." For others, the obvious intentionality and requirements of participation are initially uncomfortable. We have watched people hesitate at the doorway of rooms such as 1108B, looking ready to bolt and mumbling, "I must be in the wrong place."

People are responding to two things: the container, which is physical, and the containment, which is energetic. These two aspects create the field for interaction and the invitation for synergy. The container holds it all—the seen and the unseen, the tangible and the felt experience, the agenda and the mystery. As hosts, guardians, and participants, understanding social containment increases our comprehension of what's going on and our confidence that we can sustain group process in the midst of circle's ordinary and profound energies.

Energy, like weather, is constantly shifting and largely visible through action and reaction. Weather can be calm or stormy. Weather contains and releases power. When the wind shifts, when lightning is about to strike—we know it and take cover. When the storm is over, we emerge gratefully into the sunlight. People tend to feel more confident on "good weather" days than on "bad weather" days. Attentiveness to weather is wired into us—and so is attentiveness to energy. When we step into circle, we are bringing our personal energy into collective energy and creating the weather of the circle. The interaction of energy between people is as natural and normal as weather. There's one difference: not only are we watching the weather—we *are* the weather.

Becoming Aware of Our Personal Hoop

All living things emit a subtle electrical field that emanates into the space around them. Every person is dressed in an electromagnetic "space suit" produced by our bodies. This suit of space extends to an average distance of one to two feet beyond our skin in all directions and has a permeable and expanding and contracting boundary. You don't have to go very far down the rabbit hole to consider this; just walk one city block at noon and notice how people dip and swerve around each other; notice the difference between standing in a park and standing in a crowded elevator. Expansion and contraction are influenced by what is around us in our environment—the electrical charges we receive from others—and by the thoughts, moods, and feelings going on inside us—the electrical charges we are sending into the interpersonal space around us. Weather around us, weather within us. Add to that the careful attention to sitting down, facing each other, and turning up the receptivity, and you get the weather of circle.

The first energetic practice of circle is to step into the social container aware of what is going on inside our individual container so that we can be more conscious of what we are contributing to the space around us. We encourage people to see the ring of chairs as a doorway and to step through that threshold intentionally; to put down papers and bags and to pause to take a few breaths.

This is the first check-in—with yourself. How are you right now? What do you notice? Are there aspects of your thinking and feeling that you want to alter before engaging with others? Are there thoughts you need to tuck away so that you can focus? Are there feelings you need to share with others so that you can be present?

In certain North American Native traditions, the electromagnetic field is described as a "personal hoop." People are taught to be accountable for what enters and leaves their hoop. A few seconds' pause at the rim of the circle allows us to center ourselves in the middle of our own space suit and to be aware of the persons to our left and right who will be our closest energetic partners as our hoops touch or overlap. Energetically, a circle is comprised of a number of overlapping and expanding and contracting hoops. Whether or not we talk about these things, our brains are hard-wired to send and receive energetic signals and to have a very clear spatial understanding of where we are in relationship to each other—energetically and physically. Ten seconds in a nanosecond world is time enough to make a big difference in how we enter the social container, look around, and greet each other. We are the weather in circle—so let's offer each other the weather we want to enjoy.

Weather rises in us and moves through us. Sometimes we use this metaphor as a check-in question when we want to get a quick understanding of the energy in the rim. "What's your personal weather?" and around goes the talking piece. People respond in a word or phrase: "I feel partly cloudy." "Sunny and breezy." "Overcast and hoping to clear." "High-pressure zone, looks good on the outside, churning at high altitude." A lot of information and diversity emerges through this one question.

And circle teaches us that the sun, the fire at the center around which we are orbiting, is always shining beyond the weather. We notice this when taking off in a jet: when we get above the clouds, we enter an eternal sense of expansiveness, a presence of sunlight or starlight that makes weather irrelevant and dwarfs human concerns. While most of our attention is focused on the weather playing out between us, it is helpful to remember that we are never without light; we, and circle process, are always upheld. Our experience is a question of perspective, and when we know this, it's as Casey said, "we become one body with eyes in the backs of our heads and twenty legs. Like we're Transformers or something." If a young veteran is thinking about such things, so can the rest of us.

Preparing the Physical and Energetic Container for Circle

Once we are committed to personally showing up energetically, we need to arrange the literal space for ourselves to show up within. Many public rooms contain an aura of spent energy that's been unconsciously left there by thousands of previous meetings. The air seems stale, as though everybody exhaled his or her exhaustion on the way out the door. Rows of recessed fluorescent lighting emit a barely audible shrill whine. Windows are barred with slatted blinds. There may be no view, no windows at all, no natural lighting.

OK, it's not ideal, and we *can* do circle here. We can do it because the strengths of the energetic social container will mitigate the drawbacks of the physical container. We can do it because the beauty in the process, the ways people become real to each other in even a few moments of authentic speaking and listening, can compensate for the industrial carpeting and the bare beige walls of foamcore and plasterboard sound barriers. After a while, we won't notice so much *where* we are sitting so much as *with whom* we are sitting and the quality of what's actually happening.

When convening a circle in a new place, especially when we've flown in to offer preconference training or a seminar in a corporate setting, we try to enter the room while it's still empty. We want to notice what the space feels like without people in it and have a chance to adjust the seating and lighting to be as conducive to circle practices as possible. We clear away clutter around the edges—piles of papers, dirty dishes, or distracting boxes. We have been known to throw tablecloths over the whole mess when necessary and to commandeer plants and floor lamps from the halls or lobby. We raise the shades and let in natural light if we can. We open windows or doors and create a flow of air before people arrive. If we are alone, we stand in the center of the room and clap our hands a few minutes to release stagnant energy and make space for the energy we want to call in.

We ask ourselves, *What would make us feel welcomed and relaxed in here?* Then we prepare that kind of space for others. Surprise is fun: bringing flowers into a sterile environment, offering bowls of fruit and nuts for refreshment, putting on music—upbeat to generate energy, melodic to calm energy down. We work with the chairs or seating arrangement—making the shape as circular as possible and finding something the right size to serve as the center of the energetic wheel.

The first impression of circle is important. We create a kind of interior design of chairs, flip charts, coffee table and talking piece, and possibly a beverage cart at the edge. Once we have the rim in place and the backdrop beautified, we focus on establishing a meaningful center. We carry with us a number of objects that can be placed in the center and ask our hosts to bring things that are meaningful to this particular group. We are thinking about focus—something beautiful and authentic to look at—and we are thinking about the amount of energy that will soon be channeled toward and through the center space. These elements create the physical level of rim and center. What makes a circle a circle is the energetic level of what's about to happen. The circle is created by everyone's relationship to self, to the center, and to the rim.

Understanding the Energetics of Center

The essential role of center becomes even more obvious when considering the energy generated within the social container. Energy is an intermediary relating between one thing and another, always in a state of transition and never the same: energy seeks attachment to something and freedom to move on. In circle process, we want energy attached to center to stabilize the wheel, and we want energy to stay in flow at the interpersonal edge, to not accumulate on any one person.

A young PeerSpirit colleague, Roq Gareau, speaks of envisioning the circle as a bicycle wheel where every person is sitting on the rim with an energetic spoke attached to the hub at the center (see Figure 8.1). Roq says:

> "In circle, you activate your spoke. There's no hiding. The wheel depends on each spoke, each person, being energetically present. If I am saying one thing and being another, others can tell. When there is an energetic wobble in me, there is an energetic wobble in the circle—a wheel with a loose spoke cannot turn true. When there is strength in me, there is strength in the circle. I hold my place on the wheel, with the center as the source of strength, and offer myself as the source of balance."
>
> This is a useful working definition of containment and attachment in circle and defines the energetic work of everyone on the rim.

The center is serving as *transpersonal space*—a place that belongs to everyone and to no one. It is the space of the collective where the third principle—"Ultimate reliance on wholeness"—is made tangible. Imagine the circle as a tiny village with a center plot of grass. This common ground was used as the safe place where everyone could put their cows for safekeeping so that they were protected from predators by the outer rim of family huts. The ground belonged to the village as a shared community asset. In circle, commentary, instead of cows, goes into the middle. Here we protect each other's contributions from predation and understand that we form an outer rim of personal hoops contributing to shared intention. We protect this space, we honor it, and we speak to the center.

Sometimes people stare at the center while talking and listening; sometimes people look at one another. Where people look is less significant than where they send their energy. The practice of energizing the center focuses on sending and receiving each other's words through the space of our common ground. This can be a difficult practice to understand, as it shifts us of out of strictly *interpersonal space*, a familiar social context that occurs in many settings. In the exchanges of interpersonal space, two or more speakers are perceived as playing verbal tennis: one speaks and serves the ball to the other; the other speaks and serves it back. The goal is to keep the exchange in play until someone wins the point or the volley is complete. We know how to engage in rewarding dialogues. We may need to reimagine how the center and circle allow conversation to go even deeper: we lay the tennis ball down gently in the center.

The Role of Center in Conflict Resolution

The practice of talking to and listening from the center allows people to express divergent thoughts, feelings, and opinions and keep on listening. When we are energetically engaged with a strong center in place, the scope of conversation can expand into new territory. We can shift from the comfort of like-mindedness, in which we seek agreement and commonality as guarantees of social safety, to curious like-heartedness, where new perspectives emerge from thoroughly exploring differences. To hear one another through our differences, we need a transpersonal holding spot, a way to spread out the conversation as though it were a treasure map and curiously examine the thoughts, feelings, and stories that carry us forward to the fulfillment of intent.

Understanding how to use the center's transpersonal capacities has allowed us to help a father and son overcome a major disagreement about the young man's college behavior, to help church congregations talk about homophobia, and to help staff teams admit to bullying in the workplace and invite new behavior and accountability. Other friends and PeerSpirit colleagues

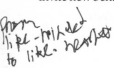

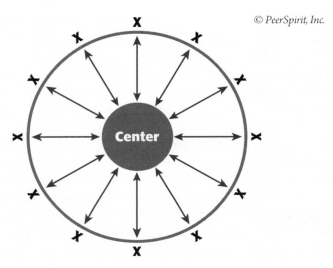

© *PeerSpirit, Inc.*

FIGURE 8.1

have hosted conversations between Palestinians and Israelis; between Protestants and Catholics in Northern Ireland; and between townspeople, tribal members, and farmers over land use rights. The more highly charged a conversation becomes, the more important the use of the center becomes.

Most human conflicts arise from a passion that has not had space to be fully expressed or witnessed by the other side. The father and son cannot change their relationship until they have heard each other out; conservatives and gay people cannot let go of their differences until they have each been listened to; the Catholics have to be heard by the Protestants and the Protestants have to be heard by the Catholics; and so on. The literal and energetic presence of the center in circle allows us enough room so that those holding conflicting views can begin to loosen their attachments to their position. Only then can the agreement "We listen to each other with curiosity and compassion, withholding judgment" truly take hold.

Imagine that everyone on the rim has an arrow—not a weapon, but a pointed view—as in Figure 8.1. As people speak, they throw the arrow far as their intention extends. So if they are energetically speaking to the center, their arrow lands there; if they are speaking to someone on the opposite rim, the arrow flies across the room. The goal is to fill the center with arrows—not to fill people's laps. In the center, arrows feed the fire and build like-heartedness—the sense that we can disagree yet still be respectful of one another.

Because the archetype of circle is present, language that comes from this lineage can communicate the essence of the center's power. "Speak to the fire," "Don't cross the fire with your anger," and "Feed your story to the center" are all phrases that will work when the circle is energetically hot. These reminders help people direct emotions, opinions, and declarations toward the center and each other.

The core practice of conflict resolution in circle is our ability to anchor our individual reactions in our personal hoops and anchor our intentions to the center. "I don't understand my son, *and* I will listen." "I don't understand how the Israelis can build a wall through my village, *and* I can look for something that allows us to reach across that wall." Anchoring our energy to the center creates a container capable of holding great sweetness and absorbing great tension. This anchoring has a profound impact on people's experience of subtle and subjective elements, such as a sense of safety, inclusion, spaciousness for story, and the ability to respond appropriately to conflict.

When the circle's energy is anchored to the center, we can trust each other to be passionate and respectful. And the energy of the arrows goes both ways: we need to honor the center, and we need to stay in our hoops. As we practice this, we can release lots of energy and not threaten the stability of the container.

During a check-in at a gathering of twenty-five leaders in financial planning, we were about two-thirds of the way around the circle, with each person putting an object in the middle that represented his or her relationship to the profession. There were photos and feathers and small stones and meaningful objects from desks back home. Then one man pulled a large, jagged rock nearly the size of a soccer ball out of a cloth bag. He held it over his head as if he were going to throw it from his seat about fifteen feet into the center. "It's time for us to make a big splash!" he declared boldly. "It's urgent out there in the world. What are we waiting for?" He waved the rock in the air, and people winced a bit to see what he would do. He paused for a few seconds and then lowered the rock over his heart. "Let me speak for myself," he said more calmly. "I am ready to make the big splash with my life. I feel urgent. I am here because I want to make the big kerplunk." Now he lowered the rock to his lap. "I am seeking community. I am seeking courage—and support of my courage." His voice cracked with emotion. He got up and walked to the center and carefully set the rock down.

He had noticed that his energy was overshooting the center and pulled it back, stabilizing himself in his own hoop, and switching into "I" statements. After this restabilization, he could make a heartfelt contribution to the quality of check-in. Though his words were challenging, we heard him because he shifted his energy.

The Energetic Roles of Host and Guardian

In the social containment of circle, the role of the host and guardian is a seamless collaboration—like a Möbius strip—in which each person assists the other in tracking the energy within the group process. A Möbius strip is a one-sided three-dimensional object (see Figure 8.2). The simplest way to make one is to cut a strip of paper, twist it once, and paste the two ends together. *Voilà!*—a circle, and an environment, where there are no leader or follower positions: all is in motion—host, guardian, and all participants.

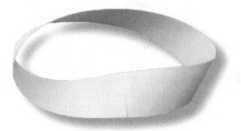

FIGURE 8.2

By sitting across from each other, the host and guardian carefully watch the other side of the circle. They provide a compass of leadership that tends to activate others around the rim to step into their own leadership. Just as the guardian's bell is a voice in the circle, energy has a seat in the circle, and the host is hosting it.

Hosting Energy

This doesn't mean that the host is in charge of energy, only that the host is attending to energetic attachment and flow within the circle as well as the attachment and flow of conversation. The host is volunteering to tune in to the larger, invisible hoop, using the personal filter of his or her own experience as a test for the collective experience, and to test these perceptions verbally: "I'm thinking we're done with this topic. Do you agree?" "I need a break. How about you?" Or, as is modeled in Chapter 4, the host may openly ask the guardian or the group for assistance when stymied by group process: "I'm not sure what to do next. What do you think?" In the Möbius strip of interaction, the three principles of rotating leadership, shared responsibility, and reliance on wholeness are always in play.

Our colleague Roq expresses his understanding of hosting energy in the following way:

> "When I am hosting, I practice using my self-experience as a barometer for group experience. I give special attention to my own hoop, tucking away as best I can whatever doesn't serve the circle. I register what's going on with others through body language, voice tone, and sense of engagement. By asking questions, I learn how clear I am—or not—and so my practice improves.
>
> "As host, my response to what is happening is different than other participants' as I am asking the center, 'What is most needed?' And sometimes what's needed is not my usual way of participating. For example, if people are staying in their heads around an issue that requires that we move to our hearts, I will take the risk to shift into vulnerability to break open the pattern for the rest of the group. Or sometimes I have needed to go sharp, to show up with my clear anger. This is not my personal style at all, but I've chosen fierceness when it seemed we needed to relight the fire. This anger has been an arrow to the center—naming something that we were avoiding or trying to help the circle get in touch with productive outrage."

Roq's clarity is important here: the host's focus is to preserve the intention, and sometimes for that to happen, the weather has to shift. If a group has been stormy, it needs some calm; if a group has been languishing in the sunshine, it needs a lightning bolt to wake it up to purpose again. Hosting at the energetic level requires a willingness to shift moods, to detach from comfort and help the energy attach at the center and flow at the rim. The guardian is a partner in this practice, and so are all the participants. Everyone is moving around the Möbius strip.

Guardian of Energy

The role of a guardian and the use of the bell as an interceding voice modulate the energy in the circle's social container. As the guardian watches over the energetic level of group process, he or she holds the bell, (chime, singing bowl, or other neutral sound maker) and rings it to pause interaction. When the bell rings, everything stops. The purpose of the pause is to give all participants a little time and space to inquire what is happening inside themselves at this very moment. It is an invitation to regulate one's own nervous system: Am I agitated or calm? Withdrawn? Paying attention? Taking responsibility for myself? When the bell stops action, we have time to check in with our personal hoops, to recenter the self and then recenter with the center. The group becomes a living embodiment of the rim-and-center diagram. When the guardian rings the bell a second time to release the pause and speaks to why the pause was called, the guardian becomes the spokesperson for the circle's energetic needs. Remember that anyone can ask the guardian to ring the bell and announce the reason for the pause.

The time to normalize and support the practice of pausing is when the circle is moving along smoothly. To establish this, we often ring the bell during a check-in or other round of talking piece at the quarter turns and say something like "We're a quarter (half, three-quarters) of the way around. Let's take a breath, hold the center, and prepare to hear the remaining voices." In this little ritual, people learn not to react personally to the bell. We notice what it takes to self-regulate: to be a little surprised, perhaps to feel a little interrupted, and then to choose to come back to self-center. We can choose to be curious about what's happening instead of immediately jumping into judgment of self or other.

When the bell rings in a moment of calm or ceremonial marking of transition points, we have an opportunity for tapping into spaciousness. The group comes to expect and often enjoy both the sound of the bell and the experience of the pause. In addition, ringing the bell at transition points, such as completing a round or shifting from one topic to the next, honors the energy that has been generated, anchors it, and marks the shift into the next thing.

The bell also reminds us of the intermediary nature of energy as we move through the pattern of a circle meeting and helps keep the social container clear. When the host or any participant asks, "Could we have the bell?" it gives everyone a chance to take a breath, to stretch, perhaps to have a break before moving on. When we are so focused on speaking intentionally, listening attentively, and tending to the well-being of the group, we need a little release of attention—the way coughing moves through an audience between movements of a symphony or songs in a set. It's mostly nervous energy. The release is not dismissive; it creates a boundary, a way to set one thing aside and welcome another.

If you're on the water in a kayak, there are times to paddle and times to rest. The voice of the bell calls us into a little eddy, to rest in the swirl that's not rushing downriver or caught in the current. Participants know that the guardian is watching the waters; that the rest of us can stretch, relax, take our paddles out of the water, look around, and then start paddling again, refreshed.

Holding the Container in a Storm

As a highly skilled kayaker, Ann is a great student of weather. She knows the first faint changes in wind, current, and clouds can mean the difference between getting safely back to shore or being caught in high seas. When paddling, she is our weather guardian, attuned to nuances that the rest of us don't yet notice. We may have started out on a calm, sunny morning, and then conditions start to change. There's no stopping the weather. It is by its very nature changeable: the winds will come up and the tides will ebb and flow and the calm will return.

When looking back at on the weather of circle, there is often a similar sense of inevitability: energy will intensify and subside, we will feel incredibly connected in heart and mind, and we will feel nearly torn asunder. As long as we keep leaning into the conversational structure and tending the social container, we will find our way back to calm seas. What makes these experiences of weather and wobbliness worthwhile is that successful self-governance is ours to celebrate. Circle is an experience of being truly grown up, capable of managing the impulses of our own internal reactions and handling the impulses and reactions of others—not perfectly but satisfactorily.

Throughout this book, the illustrative stories focus on conversational infrastructure so that we learn to trust our capacities when the weather changes, when the Geiger counter suddenly starts clicking, when our hearts race with the bigness of what's occurring—and we're right in the middle of it. Energy shows up in the circle because it is a container. Energy shows up in us because *we* are containers.

Though it had been accumulating and dissipating in a project team for several months, there was a moment when tension between Diana, the human resource representative, and Doug, the technology expert, came to a head. Diana had the talking piece at the end of a round of idea generation, and Doug interjected a comment just as she was making her point. "I get it, Dee. Can we just move on?"

Diana stopped, disconcerted and surprised. "Dammit, Doug. You've interrupted me every time I've talked for the past week!"

"No, I haven't," Doug countered.

"Well, you just did it again. The purpose of this thing is to give me a chance to finish my thoughts without interruption." She shook the talking piece, a chunk of polished agate the host had brought for use that day, at Doug. She took several deep breaths and went red in the face. The host and guardian looked at each other across the circle. Several people stiffened a little. Group energy shifted into "level orange."

Doug, not noticing, plowed on with his next comment. "I don't get why you're so touchy. I'm trying to get something done in this circle process, not just process!" He pushed back his chair as though wishing to eject himself from the rim. The invisible arrows had just been thrown with force across the space—and the guardian and host had been caught off guard in the few seconds of heated exchange.

Mike, the host, recovered and asked for the bell. "Hey, Susan, ring that thing!" he called out. She did. Everyone paused and looked to him for guidance. "OK," he said, "I think there's an issue here we'd better talk about—and I'm not sure what it is. Are you two willing to go there?"

Though it may seem counterintuitive, it is most helpful to slow down when tension rises instead of speeding up. Tension is a yellow light—if everyone speeds into the intersection, there's going to be a crash. Pausing the action allows everyone a chance to put on the brakes and let the momentum roll to a safe stop. Energy is rolling around like a loose hubcap. People need to take a breath and make sure they are grounded in their own hoops so they can hold the rim, hold the center, and see how to contribute to whatever is going to happen next. Mike may not know exactly what's going on, but he is wise enough to call the conflict forward, to see the tension as something that requires group attention.

"I'm willing," said Diana. Her voice shook with emotion, and she started to tap her foot nervously on the carpeting, looking increasingly agitated.

Agitation is a signal that a lot of energy is running through someone. Diana may have been agitated before Doug interrupted her; maybe no one noticed, not even herself. This is not group therapy: this is business. We have an expectation—or at least a tendency to hope—that whatever is going on in the background for Diana, for Doug, and for any member of the group will be pulled into their hoops and tucked away so that we can proceed with the anticipated topics. Sometimes this is possible; sometimes it's not. We all have in our personal hoops a little trash bin where we can deposit the imperfections of interaction and our reactions to them and keep them out of the way so we can move forward. Even if it is business, or the Parent-Teacher Association or Monday night at the League of Women Voters, our histories and vulnerabilities are with us—we need to get the banana peels out of the way. And then something happens, a slipping point, and the trash bin turns into a careening Dumpster that breaks out of our personal hoop and into the space of the group.

Mary, the woman seated next to Diana, reached over and squeezed her forearm gently. "It's OK," she said. "It's OK."

The woman doesn't actually know whether it's OK or not. She's made a calculated choice to try to help Diana ground her energy by offering a comforting gesture and phrase. She's hoping to interrupt the circuitry of agitation and invite Diana to compose herself.

Doug turned to Mike. "Can we do this in five minutes?"

"We can try." Mike paused to gather his thoughts. "We've got a basically good circle process going here. I don't know what's really irritating the two of you; maybe it's a bigger issue—maybe it's the tension between thinking and doing. So, first Diana and then Doug, let's see what—"

Mike's sentence was cut off by a throaty cry from Diana, who exploded into an angry diatribe about how circles are manipulative, cults of personality, how she feels like a pawn, how the men take all the space. People sat shocked, surprised, and unsure what to do next. Adrenaline was pumping through everyone's veins. Alert level went to red. Susan's hands twitched holding the bells: when to ring? Should she interrupt? This felt horrible, but maybe Diana was "asking for what she needed" by dumping her load. Mike gave her a nod. She rang the bell loudly—jarring their ears, but the sound penetrated Diana's harangue. She stopped talking and burst into tears. "Whoa," exclaimed Mike. "I've got no clue here, guys." The group sat frozen in place listening to Diana cry, totally uncomfortable.

Nevertheless, the circle is holding. Everything is happening in the only way it can happen—even though all kinds of impulses are firing off in people's minds and bodies, even though "fight or flight" is pumping through the amygdala, people are hanging on to the infrastructure while they figure out how to restore the social container.

The flash flood of Diana's trauma is contained, has moved through. What feels threatening is the unknown. The wisdom of recovery from this event has not yet emerged. The only thing that can get this group in trouble right now is if people jump out of the energetic presence into judgment: being critical of Diana's falling apart, of Doug's insensitivity, of Mike's clumsiness, of their own ineptness and the stupidity of trying this circle stuff anyway. . . .

The guardian rang the bell again, more gently in the stillness, leaned in and spoke clearly and firmly, looking around the group and making eye contact with anyone who would look back at her. ["Everyone in this circle has a job: hold the center, stay on the rim. We'll figure this out together." There was a palpable energetic shift as people calmed themselves through Susan's instruction.

Meanwhile, Diana hunched over her lap trying to pull herself together. "I'm so sorry . . . I'm so embarrassed . . . I'm so sorry . . . Don't look at me . . . ," she recited.

"Gosh, Dee," Doug exclaimed, "I didn't mean to bring on anything like this."

"Can I touch your back?" Mary inquired. Dee nodded, and Mary placed a hand between Diana's shoulder blades. "It's OK," she whispered again. "Truly, it's going to be OK. Is there a story behind these feelings?" Diana nodded but did not look up. Mary continued, "We need your help, Diana, to put the circle back together. Can you tell us what's going on inside you?"

Leadership has rotated, responsibility is being shared, and the group is relying on its wholeness being restored. There is a host, a guardian, and a friend. Diana's agitation is lessening, and now a sense of electrical discharge is floating around looking for where it needs to land next. Grounding out. Energy wants to attach: so the guardian's instructions are helpful reminders to put the lightning in the center—don't take the hit.

First Diana and Doug took their arrows from the center and threw them at each other. When Diana exploded, all the others took their arrows and threw them up in the air. Mike and Susan have caught their arrows and reattached them to the center. Susan's instructions invite each participant to catch his or her own arrow and reestablish the stability of the wheel. Diana's arrow is broken in her lap; Doug's is behind his back—he's not sure he's coming in until he knows he's not the scapegoat.

Mike was breathing again, drawing from the center to steady himself. He looked around the group. "OK, people, let's take a minute and do an energy check. I think Mary's right: hearing the story will put the circle back on track. I am willing to listen to whatever Diana has to say as long as she doesn't shout at us. Everyone can make a choice: stay if you can, leave if you need to; the rim will hold, and we'll call you back later." Everyone stayed.

As host, Mike's decision to let people choose to stay or leave was a risk. What if everyone had left? How then would they have put the circle back together? But the choice itself was significant, and now that things had calmed a bit, they were curious, and supportive. They did have a pretty good circle process going—and they wanted it to keep going.

You may be thinking right now, if this is what's going to happen in circle, I don't want to be there. Well, this is what happens anyway, with or without circle. People get their feelings hurt, old patterns break through, resentments mount and never get resolved; five years from now, Doug and Diana could have no idea where the enmity between them started. Without a container for a conversation that never happened, maybe they've built up factions and polarized the office environment. Maybe they've become less than their best selves and don't even know it, though their coworkers gossip about their dysfunction, how they don't seem suited for the positions they hold, and why administration doesn't replace them is anybody's guess. Circle didn't cause this eruption: it is simply dealing with it openly, and something important is being cleared in the moment.

People are learning to be present during another's volatility and not get into the drama, not take it on. As they integrate their experience in the circle this morning, they will be able to apply it in other areas of their work and lives. Diana blew up: nobody fought back. Diana crumpled: nobody tried to fix her. Even in her emotional state, Mary and Mark are working with Diana as a colleague, asking her to tend to the well-being of the social container, to help mend what got torn, to bring her story forward so that people might understand and move on.

"Let's have another breather," said the guardian. She rang the bell softly. A kind of relief and readiness settled over the group." Energy alert deescalating. The bell rang again.

Diana sat up and stared at the center. She spoke of her high school girls' volleyball coach who used the circle to create a cult of personality around himself. "We were like followers. We would have done anything he asked," she said. "It was so scary. He took all that adolescent intensity and fed off it. He never touched me, but I wanted him to, and that scared me even more. I thought I was going to hell. He said we were going to state." Mary kept her hand on Diana's back.

This is not business as usual. No one came into the meeting that morning anticipating tension, disruption, time-out from the agenda, or being asked to witness human suffering; it just happened. It happened because the circle was strong enough for it to happen. The web between these people will be even stronger as each person has a sense of increasing interpersonal courage. Circle calls us to show up and be ready to witness the troubles that collect in each other's hearts. And so the clouds break open, it thunders, it rains. The storm goes into the center—and the rainbow eventually comes.

The host and guardian did not immediately know what to do—and that's all right. There is no formula. Slow down. Pause. Focus on the center. Make a helpful gesture. Discover the way forward by trusting the wisdom in the room.

Ten minutes passed from the first exchange over Doug's interruption to the end of her story, and then Diana was able to look up from the center into Doug's face. "First of all," she said to Doug, "you are not him. It's not anything you did wrong, I just got triggered. I'm sorry."

Doug exhaled. "Well, I'm glad you don't think I'm like him. But I am kind of a control freak, and I coach my youngest daughter's T-ball team. I'm impatient. I'm the guy who likes to get things done. It makes my day to have a long to-do list in my Blackberry and just tick those items off like a speed demon. This circle process is way out of the box for me. I wasn't expecting this."

"Me neither," said Diana. "It's taking everything I've got not to run out of here and resign from the team because I'll feel foolish for the rest of my life."

Mary spoke. "No way, girl. We need your perspective. And every single person in this circle has something inside them we never told. I can think of two of them myself right now." Heads nodded. "You just went through the wash cycle for all of us."

"You OK then, Diana?" Mike asked. "Let's take a ten-minute break, stretch, open the windows in here, get a cold drink. Then we'll come back and see what we need to do next."

"Can I say one more thing?" Diana unfurled her fingers from the smooth, round stone. "I still have the talking piece," she said, and this time she smiled. "First of all, thank you. Thanks for just listening. For not making me feel weirder than I'm making myself feel. And Doug, I don't think we're going to have ongoing tension, but if I do frustrate you, just have the guardian ring the bell, and I promise to get to the point."

Doug laughed with relief. "I can do that," he said. And everyone rose up, eager for a break. Now they are all in current time. Now they are reattached to spaciousness.

This is a vulnerable moment in circle process. The breakthrough is so fresh that it needs everyone's consciousness to hold it honorably. During the break, tension will turn into relief to have found a way back to camaraderie. However, too much joking or raucous energy can restimulate or minimize the situation. Diana will most likely need reassurance for a while that people still see her as a fully contributing member of the circle. She will need support not to turn her emotions into shame, and right now, she may just need a little space. The group members will need to reference this moment and to speak their individual lessons from it, but that will be done better after the energized weather settles a bit.

As host, Mike will resume hosting the conversation planned for the morning. Everyone will be present, and the work will go more smoothly. He will take a bit of extra time for check-out, knowing that the usual question, "What is the primary lesson you will take away from this session?" may elicit more profound reflections than usual.

CHAPTER

Why Circle Takes Us to the Shadow

The strength of the circle environment allows a broad range of human interaction and provides enough structure so that people have insights that increase their capacities. This includes unconscious material that comes forward for healing. As we gain experience, circle helps hold and integrate the natural complexity and diversity of human beings.

We get very busy in the spheres of our lives, focused on a hundred things we consider essential and important. Yet when we slow down, as circle slows us down, the issues submerged under our busyness rise to the surface. Sometimes this is a gentle process—like looking around a circle of friends and thinking, *Wow, I really belong. These people—we care about each other,* and feeling our hearts open and threads of storyline weave into our check-in. Sometimes what's going on in us is a shock—like listening to a circle of colleagues checking in with one negative comment after another and thinking, *Boy, are we exhausted or what? We can't even tap into something hopeful to say to each other,* and feeling overwhelmed. We slow down. We start to listen to our inner story and the stories around us. We look around, and sometimes we see clearly who is in the circle with us and sometimes we recall a figure from the past or sense an aspect of ourselves we have not claimed or a reflection that seems cloudy and disturbing. This eruption of personal history and the psychological veil that fell over the present was modeled in the story of Diana and Doug in the preceding pages. These are all aspects of the *human shadow.*

This use of the term *shadow* originated with the visionary work of Swiss psychiatrists Carl Gustav Jung and Marie-Louise von Franz, who used the word to refer to "the parts of ourselves that we have been unable to know."[1] Jung and von Franz theorized that every person develops both a known and an unknown self and that the known self casts a shadow self, just as we cast a shadow when walking in sunlight. This concept has been broadly integrated into psychological thinking and has recently spread into more common usage as a way to talk about the confusing issues that arise whenever people get together.

That's the key idea: *issues arise when people get together.* We've been noticing this since the first stranger wandered into the firelight, sat on the wrong rock, and committed a social faux pas. How do we create and sustain community when we are all imperfect? How do we handle our volatility and vulnerability and keep focused on the purpose of the group? To address these questions, we start with an assumption: *most of the time, most people are trying to offer the best of themselves to a group's experience, and we stumble and fumble and thwart that process unintentionally.* Part of the resilience of leadership at the rim is becoming aware of how these dynamics show up and helping ourselves and others get through the rough spots and get on with our vision, intention, and appreciation of each other's presence. Circle brings us experiences of great depth and fulfillment— the ways our stories move our hearts, the courage and authenticity called forth in each other, the deep satisfaction of a process gone well and celebrations of accomplishment. All these experiences help us trust the circle to hold us as shadow comes forward.

How Shadow Shows Up

The minister of a mainstream city church was dying of cancer. He kept bravely showing up at work, racing against time to leave his legacy. However, Reverend Larry was an extremely private person, and he had not explicitly told the congregation what was going on. Some people noticed his loss of weight, his dwindling energy, and his shift in leadership style as he became more directive about those things he felt compelled to complete. Some people continued to see him as he was and were oblivious to these subtle changes. Those in the governing council, who knew of his condition, were sworn to secrecy.

Lorraine, Larry's wife, was also under tremendous pressure. She coped with constant shifts in their daily lives, driving to all his radiation treatments and doctors' appointments, cycling through stages of grief without a place of comfort and collapse for herself. Sometimes she even believed that Larry could overcome this disease through faith and willpower. And sometimes she pleaded with him to deal more openly with people, to ask for help, to talk with their young adult children, to let her tell a few friends. His response had been, "I've prayed about this, and this is how I want to handle it. I will tell the congregation when God tells me to. Meanwhile, I'm asking you to trust my process and stand by me."

This is a situation rife with *shadow*—everyone is doing his or her best to honor the reverend's wishes, consciously or unconsciously, and to hold the community together and prepare for what they know and don't know the future will hold. This is a true story whose context has been disguised to protect privacy and honor confidentiality: it is an amalgam of several consulting situations.

In PeerSpirit, we define shadow as any covert energy residing in the group—in other words, the undiscussables. *Covert* means "covered": things that are in hiding. So when looking for shadow in circle process, helpful questions include these:

- Are topics being avoided?

- What assumptions or behaviors are not addressed?

- What power issues are not explored?

- Who does not own their power, avoiding invitations to shine in the shared leadership of the group?

- How am I involved in these behaviors or reactions?

The purpose of addressing shadow is to make it overt. *Overt* means "open": things that are fully revealed. So as we acknowledge shadow, helpful questions include these:

- How are we expanding our courage to speak authentically with each other?

- What do we already know about trust, and what do we want to preserve about trust?

- How am I willing to show up and be fully myself?

- What infrastructure of circle process needs to be called forward so that we can address this together?

As soon as we name something and lean in to look at it together, we shift it from covert to overt energy.

This shift is the essence of shadow work, individually, as a group, and as nations, religions, and cultures: we have the capacity, by dealing with shadow, to expand the territory of our consciousness and shrink the territory of our unconsciousness. If we are to progress toward a just world for ourselves and all beings, we must recognize the imperative for increasing human consciousness. Circle plays a profound role in our abilities to expand consciousness: it brings us to each other and holds us together while we grow.

Reverend Larry does not know that he has shadow issues about his own dying. He assumes that he is handling his cancer in the clearest way possible and that he is helping his congregation by holding back the news week by week until "the people have to know." In this congregation, which is practicing circle as part of its committee structure, governance council, and interest and study groups, the circle can help—as soon as the veil of silence is lifted.

Though he doesn't ever truly drop out of facilitation mode to share his most authentic thoughts and feelings in circle conversations, Larry considers himself a thoughtful host and guardian. He believes, as a minister, that his role is different from anyone else's and that is it not appropriate for him to ask for or reveal anything that might stress his flock. (This is his *interior shadow*.) Larry's value on self-moderating leads him to be quite judgmental of people who "take up too much space" or "suck energy out of the group." (This is his *projected shadow*.) Larry has a hard time explaining himself to the bishop, and people who know him at church would be surprised to learn of his submissive streak. (This is his *transference shadow*.)

Interior shadow is doing something that we don't see ourselves doing. The church sexton speaks in a tone of voice that others consistently perceive as aggressive, yet he doesn't hear it himself and gets defensive when it's mentioned. "What? This is just how we talk in my family. We're Italian!" The organist has a tendency to nod compulsively in apparent agreement whenever Larry or another male authority speaks in circle and rolls her eyes whenever a woman speaks. If someone asked about her body language, she would be astonished. "I am absolutely sure I'm not doing that. It's totally not like me. Why would I do such a thing?"

Going back to the definition of *shadow* from its Jungian source—that we have both an accepted and a forbidden self—these covert behaviors most often stem from adaptations we made in childhood while doing our best to figure out who we really are. In the sexton's big Italian family, having a loud voice was accepted as how a person established a place at the table; for the organist, as a vulnerable child of a violent father, agreeing with Papa and discounting Mama was required to navigate safely through childhood. For Larry, the youngest of three sons, not asking and not telling was a family norm. The father sat at the head of the table and expected good daily reports from each child. "Tell me how well you're doing," he'd say. That's all he wanted to hear; that's all Larry and his brothers told him. Any areas where he did not excel went into his forbidden self.

Of course the sexton shouts. Of course the organist complies with men and distances herself from women. Of course Larry is telling the congregation how well he's doing. It's so obvious—to us. We can see another person's shadow, and if we are calm and clear and hold to the principles and practices of circle, we can help others see their own. And they can help us see our own.

Projected shadow is putting onto other people those qualities that we don't know how to deal with inside ourselves. These projections may be positive or negative. A positive projected shadow assumes that Reverend Larry is so capable that he cannot make a mistake and his decisions should not be challenged; a negative projected shadow sees any perceived flaw in judgment or action as proof that Larry is not worth following.

Positive projection stems from a desire to feel safe, to hand off leadership and responsibility to someone else and assume that the other person knows what is best, always does what is right, and so on. This is sometimes referred to as "putting our gold onto another." Negative projection arises out of fear of disappointment that someone is letting the group malfunction, is not taking proper care of people, has become competitive instead of cooperative, is too egotistical, and the like. This is sometimes referred to as "putting our garbage onto another." Positive does not necessarily mean good, and negative doesn't necessarily mean bad.

The issue of discernment arises here because *in projection, there is a grain of truth*. Someone *is* being a healthy leader—and we are challenged to consciously support the person by taking our own part in leadership. Someone *is* being competitive—so how do we restore his or her cooperative spirit and take our share of leadership without slipping into competitive behavior ourselves?

The release from projection may consist not of changing our behavior or others' behavior but of changing the energetic charge that accompanies it. We can appreciate each other's qualities and not attach a sense of "Help me, Obi Wan Kenobi" to our admiration. We can see someone's competitive edge as a point on the wheel, a necessary diversity, and not attach a sense of "Darth Vader is in the room" every time the person speaks.

Transference shadow is projecting onto a person in the present unfinished business from a person in the past. A man walks into a room, and something about the turn of his head suddenly reminds you of the relationship you had with your grandfather. A woman steps through a door into sunlight, and you know she's the love of your life, veiled in the relationship of the high school sweetheart who got away. Transference usually carries a lot of energy and a strong drive to be able to complete something. As long as transference remains unconscious, completion is impossible, so the energy builds. In Larry's family, his father decided his sons should be a doctor, a lawyer, and a minister. Larry can't remember exactly how his vocational selection occurred; it was just always there: a choice made for him that he assumes was made by him. And when father figures, such as the bishop, come into his life, he looks to them to make his choices and rebels against their authority at the same time.

Like Grandma's attic, shadow contains all kinds of unclaimed material, jumbled together and gathering dust. And like little kids let loose to play-act, we hang old stuff on each other as a way to get to know it. Projection and transference are unconsciously dressing up someone else in our unworn clothes to see if we'd look good in them or coping with the fact that the reflection we see in the cracked and peeling mirror is not another person but us. Over time, doing the work of shifting shadow creates people who are more whole, more compassionate toward the human condition, and more able to lead. Our presence in circle is driven by a call to wholeness. We cannot clear shadow on our own. We need each other to surprise us into retrieving bits of our forbidden selves.

Transference and projection rule much of our world—both at the interpersonal level of shadow storied throughout this chapter and in the larger collective issues that come into circle for healing in the stories of the next chapter. And this is not a new situation. It was William Shakespeare who spoke through his plays of the need to become aware and accountable for the wholeness of ourselves. So in the play *Hamlet*, King Polonius advises his son Laertes, "This above all: to thine own self be true, / And it must follow, as the night the day, / Thou canst not be false to any man." Exactly—and what a journey that is!

Bits of Shadow in Everyday Life

Shadow is what complicates our abilities to respond clearly to interpersonal issues in the circle (and any other group we are in). A conflict without shadow is significantly easier to resolve—and more rare. One church secretary buys supplies at a big-box store; the other buys supplies at the local stationer's: one

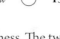

is trying to save money; the other is trying to save a small business. The two can more easily work out a compromise if they remain aware of their motivation, agree on both sets of values, and have a fairly easy working camaraderie. If they get into a conversation that draws on deeper issues (how one secretary's grandfather ran a small store that went under in the Great Depression, how the carbon footprint should guide the church's purchasing decisions), they will need to watch for shadow.

Most of us bring unconscious material to the places where we or others get stuck in a group. For example, when Reverend Larry's church was renovating its building, a major benefactor was an older woman in the congregation. Born and raised in this church community and married here sixty years ago, Mildred then raised her children in the church and buried her husband here. Still vibrant and thoughtful in her mid-eighties, she sat on the renovation committee, enjoyed using circle process to offer creative solutions to various challenges, and contributed her much appreciated sense of design. Yet shortly after the renovations began, she suddenly closed down, withdrew a significant financial pledge, and stopped coming to the meetings. Everyone on the committee was greatly distressed and tried to talk with her about what happened, but Mildred seemed both adamant in her emotional reactions and unable to state what could restore her sense of belonging.

Finally, one day, a younger member of the committee noticed Mildred struggling with her arthritic hands to open the newly installed doors to the community hall. After several tries, she gave up and walked away. The committee member went immediately to her side. "Millie, were you having trouble with those doorknobs?"

The older woman looked puzzled and then burst into tears. "I just had this thought: why help pay for a church that doesn't want me in it anymore? I couldn't shake the feeling."

The younger woman put her arms around her friend. "We love you here, Millie. We can change the doorknobs!" Because Mildred couldn't discover a practical source for her discomfort, it went into shadow, becoming both unconscious behavior and projection that led to a complete breakdown in the relationship. As soon as the shadow part of the issue was brought to light, the solution became obvious. "Oh, I feel like such a silly Millie," Mildred later confessed in circle. "I didn't even register the connection to those dang-blasted doorknobs." Everyone cheered and put her in charge of testing every bit of the renovation for ease of use by the young, the old, and the frail.

How to Tend Shadow in Circle Process

Tending to shadow is an aspect of the third practice of council, "tending to the well-being of the group," and the third principle, "ultimately rely on wholeness." Shadow tending is not so scary if we do it regularly and use the infrastructure of circle to hold the conversation—speaking to the center, using neutral language, making "I" statements, sharing responsibility, and trusting the spirit of the group that is already established. You'll notice that in the following exchange no one gets blamed or shamed, and people speak from their own experience.

The church's financial committee (which was not aware of Larry's illness) uses an agenda-based circle process to manage the budget and human resources of the congregation. The guardian occasionally rings in a pause and asks people to reflect on how they are beneath the layer of business. "Is there anything in how we're working together or handling the responsibilities of stewardship that needs clearing?" A talking piece is passed, and each person holds it thoughtfully, whether speaking or not.

This time Larry spoke up. "I haven't been saying much lately, and I don't want my silence misconstrued. A lot is happening away from the church that I'm not ready to talk about, and I know that I can look tired or distracted. Thanks for giving me the space to just be here."

A few minutes later, a woman said, "I'm so glad you spoke, Larry. I have been worrying about you. I thought it had to do with me. Let me know how to support you."

Although the issue isn't finished—it's shifted from covert (closed topic) to overt (open topic)—Larry's statement gives him and others in the group a way to bring up the topic again. Perhaps a few meetings later, someone will say, "Remember when you said you're looking tired and distracted, Larry? I'm wondering if we could talk about that some more because my concern is growing." Or Larry might say, "Well, it's time to talk about what's been going on with me." And if Larry had not spoken, any member of the circle could have referred to the matter using neutral language and exploratory "I" statements.

According to Jungian theory, shadow accumulates as children put away aspects of themselves that they cannot make fit in their families or cultures. Whatever is not approved of or unacknowledged can slide into the forbidden self. For example, anger may be put away when a 40-pound child cannot figure out how to express that emotion safely in the presence of angry 200-pound adults. The resulting personality is a compliant child whose anger will erupt elsewhere—perhaps bullying younger siblings or becoming an overly permissive parent to his or her own children. What is classified as "not fitting" may also be talents that cannot be used in original situations—a musical or artistic child in a family that doesn't value the arts, for example—or assertiveness in a girl or tenderness in a boy in settings where only traditional attributes of femininity and masculinity are supported. We all have shadow; and a significant part of life's inner journey is to help ourselves and others reclaim our lost parts. This search for reclamation is happening in every interaction of meaning: it doesn't matter whether or not you think you want to deal with your own or other people's lost parts—they just show up. If we can't see them in ourselves, we project them onto others.

Doing shadow work begins with converting our own covert thoughts and behaviors into overt thoughts and behaviors. The first aspect of shadow work in circle is to ask ourselves, *What's showing up in me that might be shadow?* Christina says, "I often felt like a stranger in my family when I was a child, so I have to watch out for thought patterns of not belonging in groups and not project old insecurities onto current situations. Of course, the positive that grew out of that experience was creating PeerSpirit Circle Process, which helps people claim their belonging and grow together!" Our wounds often become our gifts.

Ann says, "I can be extremely sensitive to criticism and hear it as a much bigger, louder remark than intended. So I need to take a walk in nature and then come back and explore the scope of the remark from the point of being recentered in myself. The positive side is that this gets me out in nature, where everything is accepted, used up, and transformed into something else." The first step in leadership is to know our own vulnerabilities and strengths—what causes us to slide into our own emotional potholes—and what we have learned works to help us get out of them.

Many ongoing groups invite journal writing into their collective process: each person keeping some form of narrative of his or her experience. When these journals—contained in notebooks, laptops, or handheld devices—are respected as private records, they provide a way for each person in the circle to do some shadow clearing before (or while) working with dynamics in the group. This does not mean that every circle stops to process individual shadow or becomes a therapeutic environment; rather, it means that every member owns his or her vulnerabilities and strives to stay conscious of them so as not to undermine group process, intention, and activity.

So after Larry's comment to the finance committee, another member may write in his or her journal, "What isn't Larry telling us? I assume it's significant, or he'd just go ahead and say it. It triggers my old fears about family secrets. Part of me wants to grab Larry by the lapels and make him tell me—right now! My foreboding gets bigger and bigger.... And knowing that, I can manage my own tension. What if he's transferring out? What if one of the kids is having trouble with drugs? What if he or Lorraine is sick? Divorcing? OK—that's the disaster list. Now the question becomes "How will I take leadership in helping them? In helping the community respond?"

Shadow is not a failure of group process; on the contrary, it is integral to group process. No matter how focused a group may be on a task or how foreign a concept shadow may be in a particular setting, when people come together, the drive for wholeness and healing is always a subcontext in relationships, circles, organizations, and communities. We cannot avoid it. Part of leadership in circle is to know that shadow sits with us and to develop healthy ways to name, respond to, and work with shadow elements that will inevitably show up.

A men's group associated with the church has a dark rock that is part of its center. Every now and then, the men pass it around "to turn over the stone" and look for anything that has been hiding that they want to speak to the center. A women's group that has accumulated a basketful of circle accessories has a small, stuffed toy elephant that the members pass around to ask the question "Are there any elephants in the room that we want to talk about before they get any bigger?"

Of course, someone needs to be willing to crack open the egg of silence and start the conversation. There is always tension when addressing shadow. Once issues are raised, the group cannot go back. All participants are about to learn something potent and empowering about themselves, individually and collectively. Different levels of capacity for acknowledgment, of readiness and willingness, are likely to exist in the group. For most people, reactions to embarking on an exploration of shadow work range from uncomfortable to terrified. And yet it is exhilarating to come through it. Shadow work gives people the chance to experience a kind of psychological alchemy: we have spun straw into gold, transformed not knowing into knowledge. This is tremendously empowering. A group that has addressed shadow and come through it, as Doug and Diana's story in Chapter 8 illustrates, is a powerful group.

Hosting the Shift from Covert to Overt

Addressing shadow issues is generative in the life of a circle. It articulates points of divergence and still aims for the greatest common good, even from different points of view and even with great passion. As long as intention is clear and visibly represented in an energized center; as long as a respectful environment is maintained, conflicting points of view can be ultimately empowering and confidence-building for everyone in the group. No one can sleep through the eruption of shadow in the circle: the host and guardian are working in tandem, and everyone needs to be present—not necessarily participating verbally but holding the container of the circle with a firm belief in the ability of circle infrastructure to provide support though this moment of difficulty.

Back at the church, the governing council had been having side conversations about people's discomfort at being asked to keep Reverend Larry's illness a secret. Finally, Hank, the council president, called a meeting at his house on a night when his wife was attending her book club. All six colleagues gathered. Hank put a copy of the church directory, a photo of himself playing golf with Larry, and a candle in the middle of the coffee table. Valerie volunteered to be guardian and pulled a bar chime out of her purse. As a start-point, Hank spoke an opening prayer for guidance and dedicated the meeting to Larry, his family, and the church community. He opened the circle with a statement of intent: "I know that several of us feel uncomfortable even having this meeting without Larry present, and I know that we feel uncomfortable being asked by Larry to keep his illness a secret from the congregation. I believe we are at the end of our abilities to maintain the status quo, both because Larry's illness is progressing and because we are starting to see our community struggle under his silence. I called this meeting so that we could have a place and time to respectfully share our own feelings before we try to be clear with Larry or others—at least, I need that clarity. Our usual agreements are in play—especially confidentiality. Let's check in, listen to each other, and discover where to go from there."

Val said, "I'll check in first so I can focus on serving as guardian. I am so relieved to be in this conversation even though I don't know what we will decide. I've lied to my husband twice, saying nothing is wrong, and I hate that! I love Larry, and I'm getting mad at the position he's put us in."

member said, "Larry is the pastor. He has his reasons and his faith.
sting any time asking myself whether or not I agree; I'm just doing
ked. That's what I'm going to continue doing—and I'm here tonight
to basically say I don't think we should be having this conversation. God will
watch out for us. There's still a possibility Larry will get better and the whole
thing will blow over."

The next member practically grabbed the talking piece. "He's not getting
better; he's getting worse. Larry's not going to have the stamina to stand in front
of the congregation for much longer. We need a plan when this whole thing
blows up. We are not prepared to hold this church together during Larry's
passing."

Before she could speak, Maureen began to cry. "He's dying? Who says
he's dying? Why would God take him from us? We need him. We have to get
everyone praying for him—we have to believe in miracles; that's what faith is
all about." Val rang the guardian bell. Everyone paused. She rang it again.

Hank said, "Thank you, Val. I remind people to keep focusing on the center, to lay down our different reactions in ways that we can all keep listening.
Let's finish the round of check-in and then decide how we might take our own
leadership in this situation."

Obviously, this group now has to work through its own shadow and differences. There is no going back beyond the breaking of silences. One of the
ways Hank is using circle process is calling people to place their emotions in
the center and reminding people of their ability to keep listening while holding
diverse reactions and points of view. The presence of shadow and leadership
challenges for the governing council are becoming clear. The council's reactions
are a sampling of the range of reactions that will surface in the larger community. Hank was wise to create a space and time when people could stay with the
process until they came to their own clarity or at least a resting point.

We later asked Hank how he experienced his circle-hosting capacity that
evening. He replied:

"What you said—that the only way 'out' is 'through'—sure became
obvious. At the end of check-in, I was sitting in the pause of the bell
wondering, *Now what? We are at such different places.* I remembered
you two saying to trust the process, so I just thanked everyone for
being so honest, noted that we were not yet clear, and asked that we

commit to another round of talking piece council. I kept remind
us that the wisdom we need is in the group. We will know it whel
arrives. Our job is to be patient, to listen, to have compassion for Larry
and one another, and to trust the process."

At this delicate moment, the governing council could have fractured into
decoy conflict—fighting internally instead of keeping the focus on Larry's illness. The elements that helped were Hank and Val's careful hosting and guardianship, the group's track record of good internal relationships, and the call back
to intention. It was an emotional evening, and it looked like the council might
not reach a decision when Val took a breath and said, "I think every emotion
and reaction going on in us is also going on in Reverend Larry and will also
go on in the congregation. I now feel strong enough to sit with Larry while he
has feelings and strong enough to sit with friends in the community while they
have their feelings. What I have learned about myself tonight is that I'm willing
to be there in the hurt that is coming. I mean, we can't avoid grief, and after this
conversation with you, I'm not afraid to face this. I cannot imagine how hard
it is to be in the dying stage of life. I want to be accepting with Larry; I want to
encourage him to trust us with his story. I want to be there for Lorraine and their
kids. And most of all, I want us to look back on this time in our church life as a
growth process that matured our faith."

Maureen leaned over, rang the chime resting in Val's lap, and said, "I think
wisdom just arrived. Thank God."

The group sat in silence awhile; then Val rang the chime again, and Hank
said, "While Val was talking, I thought, let's start at the end, let's go to that point
where we look back on this time. Then let's look at what conversations and
experiences need to go into creating the community we have the potential to
become."

One of the other men said, "Great idea, but I cannot go there tonight; I'm
wiped out. But maybe this is how we can talk to Larry: ask him to be in that
vision with us as part of his legacy. We can reassure him that he can share his
situation and we'll deal with whatever happens."

Visioning is actually a powerful tool for gaining perspective on shadow.
How would I be if I weren't stuck in this place? How would we be together if
we weren't afraid to talk about Larry's dying, our own dying, the planet's dying?
Carl Jung posed a paradoxical question about shadow: "How do you find the

lion that has swallowed you?"[2] Going into a visioning process allows the circle to acknowledge the lion, acknowledge being swallowed, and acknowledge our capacity to sit in a tree and look down into the situation and out to the far horizon for help.

Three days later, the council met with Larry and Lorraine. First the council members listened to the couple; then they expressed their heartfelt concerns and readiness. A week later, Larry spoke of his illness from the pulpit, and the council stepped forward and made a statement of love, sympathy, and purpose—creating a social container for this new part of their community story. The council hosted an all-church meeting on the following Tuesday night that consisted of three parts. People first gathered around tables to share thoughts and feelings; they had a social break for dessert and coffee; and then they shifted into a World Café session with three rounds designed to help people use their long-held circle practice to address the questions "How do we want our church community to look back on this time?" "What can we contribute to this experience?" and "What help do we need?"

It was not easy, and it was a powerful, maturing time. The congregation shook with emotions. The church lost some members who chose not to stay in the process and gained some members who wanted to be part of a community capable of doing this kind of collective shadow tending. All participants were given opportunities to be in house circles and occasional all-congregational circles to keep talking through their learning about grief and aiming toward the vision of themselves being created through this loss.

Why People Avoid Shadow Tending

Much of our shadow material is held in its corner of unconsciousness by an embedded threat that makes us afraid to reveal ourselves to ourselves. This threat is an unconscious "or else." You shout your way into the conversation *or else* you don't have a voice in the family; you support Papa *or else* you'll get a beating; you tell the people how well you're doing *or else* you don't deserve their faith in you. The "or else" is an internalized warning: "Don't you dare change this behavior!" The threat is what drives these behaviors into the unconscious and is also why pointing them out can trigger surprising reactions of defense, shame, rage, or fear. It is a huge leap of faith to believe that you'll be heard if you whisper, that you won't be punished for aligning yourself with the women in the group—or for Larry, that he could ask for help and still be regarded as fully capable. When somebody pokes your "or else" or you poke theirs, you know it. What actually happened may be small: "Hey, Giorgio, could you lower your voice?"—but the internal reaction of humiliation is so emotionally volatile that we struggle for control over our impulses, seeking to understand why the interaction felt so huge. When the request is reasonable and the reaction is unreasonable, we've got shadow.

Our personal experiences of shadow are often explosive. The "or else" that triggers us has been pushed down for a long time and emerges with great force, spewing anger, gushing tears, howling terror, judging withdrawal. These energetics are hard to manage, and whether the container of the circle will hold strong or shatter depends on our abilities to hold ourselves steadily to circle's infrastructure of safety in the midst of energetic storm.

In Diana's story in Chapter 8, when transference shadow overwhelmed her, she spewed as best she could into the center and was able to become conscious about her old story. The circle host helped hold the rim; so did the woman sitting next to Diana, and so did Doug—he didn't escalate to match her, even though he was confused and defensive. Everybody contributed in some way to Diana's ability to let go of history and come more fully into the present. In the years of PeerSpirit work, this is our most common scenario: circle can hold outbursts of shadow if the person can erupt without doing violence, and the person can ride through the shifting process if the circle will just hold the container.

However, our media images of shadow behavior heighten our fear because it most often portrays shadow as uncontrollable. We see the Incredible Hulk, a mild man who turns into a raging, green monster whenever he gets angry; or a drama queen, who disrupts social and circle settings with unpredictable narcissism and the venom to command her way; or a sociopath who tracks and torments innocent people, outwitting their attempts to save themselves at every turn. This is extreme shadow without social container or self-control. Throughout the years of our work, most of our experience with shadow in circle confirms people's abilities to make courageous and healing breakthroughs. It is true that a circle's container can shatter when the structure is abandoned or when individuals are unable to remain attached to practices of council and their agreements.

The circle can hold shadow work on the condition that even in chaos, everyone maintains the infrastructure. Anger, yes, and this does not include uncontrollable rage projected at another member of the group. Intense emotion, yes, and this does not mean hijacking the group away from its collective purpose in order to fulfill one person's purpose. Over the years, we have seen shadow erupt and people respond with creativity and strength that allowed the circle to hold, to reform, to enter ceremonies of healing, or to help a person realize the need to leave.

Reverend Larry's funeral was full of grace. The conversations that had started during his illness continued and deepened. People had profound experiences in their house circles. Val later said of these, "We spoke at a level of authenticity that went almost beyond words. Spirit was palpable in these moments. We were energetically changed, and I cannot tell you how. Even if I told you the story—which I can't—you wouldn't have the transformation we had; it's like something whole and holy came out of us, through us, for each other."

Then, with a knowing smile, she added, "Of course, now we are facing the shadow of how to welcome new members who haven't been through what we've been through and not make them feel less for it. And finding a new pastor—wow, that was a shadowy trip! The search committee took forever, trying to find someone who could match our sense of ourselves. We wanted someone who could build on Larry's legacy and not try to be him. We called a woman—so that's a fresh voice in the pulpit."

Resilience in the presence of shadow cannot be formulaic because human beings are not formulaic. The nature of shadow is that it shows up differently every time and differently in every person and so requires that we handle it differently as well. The more disturbance comes into the container, the more strongly we need to hold ourselves and each other accountable to the agreements, to direct charged emotions energetically toward the center and not toward each other, to call on the guardian to call for pauses and slow us down as we move through the eye of the storm, and for willing leaders to be sitting in every chair.

10

Circle as Support for Collective Healing

Circle can transform familial, community, and societal issues by receiving stories in a community of listeners. Three stories in this section illustrate the intergenerational healing of a family, the healing provided by addressing issues of race and gender in a southern city, and the ability of traumatized citizens to shift their reactions to violence in the midst of social turmoil.

When the ancestors came over the hill and into the circle of firelight, the circle socialized them into communal groups and became the container for the deepest conversations of awakening human consciousness. Staring into the flames of the cooking fire, relieved to have made it through the rigors of another hunting-and-gathering day, questions rose up in them, and they told stories that made their world. *Who are we? How did we get here? Who or what made this world for us? How are we related? How do we educate our children and initiate them into the tribe?*

And as they developed a sense of *insider identity,* they also developed a sense of *outsider identity:* some people belonged, and some people didn't. *Who are these others? How did they get here? What do we do about them hunting our antelope? Shall we push them out? What if they win and push us out? Do they know things we need to know? Would it be better to ally our tribes and intermarry?*

Cooperation or domination, war or peace, trading or taking, kindness or cruelty have always been part of the conversation and part of human reality. What fuels our capacity for violence of any degree, from vicious language to making war, is our ability to mentally construct insider and outsider identities.

143

The consequences of seeing the world divided into "us" and "them" has shaped human history: it is our *collective shadow*. If "they" are not "us," we don't need to have the same regard for them that we have for our own kind. If "they" are not "us," we can shun, rob, rape, kill, destroy them, the "other"—and it is not the same thing as doing it to ourselves. "We" are civilized people; "they" are savages; "we" are God's chosen; "they" are heathens. On and on this thinking goes, accumulating collective shadow. Unconscious behavior, projection, and transference occur on the macro level as well as the micro level. And in circle, we can heal some of these macro issues by the kinds of conversations we are willing to have and the settings in which we are willing to call the circle. In this chapter, we will look at how circle has worked to heal family and intergenerational shadow, community and social history shadow, and shadow in war.

Talking the World We Need into Being

We have made stories and taken actions based on stories that create and sustain the world as it is, including sustaining the shadow of injustice, suffering, and violence that hangs over humanity. As Christina says in *Storycatcher*, "When the power of story comes into the room, an alchemical reaction occurs that is unique to our kind: love or hate, identification or isolation, war or peace can be stirred in us by words alone. The power of story is understood by the powerful, yet the power of story belongs to all of us, especially the least powerful. History is what scholars and conquerors say happened; story is what it was like to live on the ground."

We have the opportunity in circle process to heal our old stories and to make new stories that lead to different actions and create a different world. This is the essential task of our times! Understanding the power of story and the container of the circle give us life skills that have profoundly transformational potential. We can talk the world we need into being and then align our actions with our vision. This is what our ancestors did at the fire, and if we are to become ancestors to future generations, this is what we will do today.

Doing personal shadow work raises confidence in our abilities to shift social unconsciousness toward more holistic, accountable, and enlightened behavior. We begin to trust: if we can work through this shift at the personal and interpersonal levels, we can work through it at the collective level. To become peer leaders who can help transform our families, organizations, communities, and wider world, we need to practice our capacities as shadow shifters.

As circle practice takes hold in organizations, community groups, and families, it creates a social container strong enough to bring conversations out of hiding. The questions under the statements, the longing under the doing, the story under the check-in, the confusion under the confidence comes into the metaphoric firelight offering us the possibility that we may heal our collective wounds.

Healing the Family Lineage

In October 2008, Rubén Castilla Herrera, a community development consultant in Columbus, Ohio, put out a call on the Art of Hosting electronic mailing list asking if anyone was practicing this collaborative model in Portland, Oregon, and available to help host a circle of extended family members in need of significant conversation. Steve Ryman, a hospital administrator from eastern Oregon and dialogue consultant in the Art of Hosting network, responded. The two men designed the gathering by phone and e-mail.

Rubén's younger sister, Ruth Marie, was dying of breast cancer at age forty-eight. They were the two youngest in a large Hispanic family of eight siblings, nineteen grandchildren, and a dozen great-grandchildren. Dispersed over several states, they had not gathered as a group in decades and had never had a conversation about their histories, their identity as a family, or the impact of life events on who they had become.

Rubén later explained:

> "Our mother developed breast cancer when she was pregnant with Ruth Marie and was advised not to carry the baby to term. She had a mastectomy and gave birth to Ruth Marie but died two years later, in 1962. So we don't remember her, though the older kids do. My father remarried quickly—he had eight kids to take care of from a toddler and four year old—me—to teenagers. I don't know all the details, but he was shunned by our community in Texas and so moved to Oregon following the migrant stream. Everyone adjusted differently in this new town and our new mom, and soon the older children broke away and scattered, and all kinds of secrets went underground.
>
> "We became a family without a core identity or home, especially after our father died. We had not been together as a whole since 1982. Ruth Marie and I, perhaps because we didn't remember Texas or our

mother, set out on a search to discover our roots. I went back to Seguin, Texas, and interviewed people and always talked through everything with Ruth Marie. When Ruth Marie got sick, we both felt as though we were reliving the experience of our mother, that Ruth's illness was part of the search and path, and she wanted very much to use it to reunite the family."

The cultural anthropologist Angeles Arrien relates a belief that when a baby is born, the ancestor spirits hover over the crib and ask, "Will this be the one to heal the lineage?" In their family, Ruth Marie and Rubén set out to be the ones.

Rubén became the caller of his family circle, and Ruth Marie became the holder of intention. They agreed on a date for a weekend family reunion, with a three-hour circle in the heart of their time, and sent out the invitation. Rubén wisely decided to turn over the hosting and guardian function to Steve and to sit as a participant at the rim with the rest of his family. "I am the youngest man," he said, "and it is a Latino family. Only after my oldest brother said yes did I know it would happen."

Incrementally, the family shadow began to shift: the acquiescence to cultural norms, the prescribed roles of the brothers and sisters, and the sense of who has authority were all shaken loose by "the babies'" calling the family together. "They let us get away with it, of course," said Rubén, "because Ruth Marie had cancer. How could they deny her last big wish?"

Steve spoke to us of his role:

"With the exception of Rubén, no one had any previous circle experience. There were around thirty-five people coming and the potential for a lot of intensity. Rubén and Ruth Marie were being criticized because 'it wasn't their place' to call for a conversation. Nevertheless, all the family members came. Some of the older brothers who were pretty resistant to the idea arrived late; one came when we were already halfway through. It was awkward to weave them in, but we handled it by staying at the deeper level of conversation we'd already reached and pulling the patriarchs along into honesty. I rang the bell several times, and we really used the center—it was a great place to focus when the conversation got awkward or emotional.

"One thing that touched my heart was watching the men struggle with their emotions. Several profound apologies were made. Another late-arriving brother no one had seen for years. I don't know if they even knew he was coming. He talked about how far away he'd grown from the family and how much he wanted something different."

We asked Steve to comment on his experience as an Anglo outsider sitting as the holder of the container:

> "I was on the edge of my seat the whole time, leaning forward, listening carefully—my whole body was involved in the process of listening. There was so much emotion in the room, and it felt like part of my role was to let their feelings wash through me, to keep my heart open, to make eye contact with the one who was speaking. At times it felt like I was even modulating my breath to theirs to help them move more deeply into open-hearted space."

This is shadow cleansing without drama. Steve's ability to simply hold the space allowed family members to reach the deepest potential of their interaction: compassion and grief. Volatility was present, yet through a kind of spiritual willpower, Steve helped them ground into their baseline longings for healing. It was a moment of alchemy, a collective experience of shifting unconscious material into the light of story.

Steve concluded:

"After the circle, Rubén thanked me, but we didn't do a lot of debriefing. The focus was on the family's experience. My service was to be invisible. The family went back to socializing, getting photos taken. I slipped away—and I didn't need anything more than that. What an honor to have been their witness, and to experience my ability to host at the level of presence.

> "The lesson for me is that the family slowed down together to the point where what needed healing could now heal. In circle, when the portal opens to where healing is possible, a different kind of time takes over. It was a big group; we started late; we were sitting in a hotel conference room; Ruth Marie took a long time to tell her life story and medical history; several people came in late. When the talking piece started around, I was afraid there wasn't enough time or enough set-up. I soon realized that none of that mattered. A spiritual readiness took over: the family saw the moment and seized the opportunity."

Spiritual timeliness occurs when all parties to an event are ready to allow the event to happen. When readiness resides in the circle, the drive for connection overcomes the unconscious behaviors, projection, and transference that have created disconnection. This is not always true, but when it happens, everyone is aware of being in the presence of grace.

Rubén recalls:

"After our circle, driving home that night with Ruth Marie, there was such a sense of oneness and relief. Despite all the hidden stories and stuff that has happened in our family, we could come together and do this. Why didn't we invite this sooner? It takes someone to have the courage and someone to help hold the invitation. Whoever comes are the right people. We are all living now with a sense that something profound has happened in our family, even though we don't quite know what it is."

Calling the circle was a culminating moment that Rubén and Ruth Marie undertook for their own healing and on behalf of their family.

"We knew we had had a mother who loved us in those early years and we couldn't remember her. And those who could remember her never talked about her. So we did what we could to recapture that period in our family life. When I went to Texas, I asked people, 'Tell me stories of my mother, tell me stories of my father, tell me about your relationship with them and with us.' I took the common things from all these interviews, to Ruth Marie, and we pieced our lives together."

Ruth Marie Castilla Herrera died on April 19, 2009, with Rubén and other family members holding her hands. During Ruth Marie's last two weeks, family gathered in circle around her at the care center. There were always at least two and as many as twenty-five people around her. Rubén remembers:

"I was called on Wednesday, April 15, 2009, in Ohio, and family members said I needed to come as soon as possible. They were certain that she was waiting for me. I arrived on Friday, April 17, to a circle around Ruth Marie's bed of family holding gentle vigil. This time Ruth Marie was in the center.

"In the next two days before she passed, there were many stories told about our family. My oldest brother was telling me stories about our mother that I had never heard him speak. On the morning of her passing, I saw him crying and talking softly to Ruth Marie, and it was as though he was talking to our mother. I kept hearing him say 'Mom.' Forty-seven years later, he was mourning the loss of our mother through our sister. Ruth Marie and I had spoken about this happening. This was the gift that she told me she would leave us. It was a true gift. It was as though my questions were answered and I had found what I had been searching for. It was at that moment that I knew the power of the circle, of conversation, of coming together with intention and purpose."

The story continues. Rubén recalls:

"Ruth Marie had asked at our October family circle if I would eulogize her. When I had visited her again in March before she entered the care center, I asked her what she wanted me to say. She said, 'Why don't you just come together in circle?'

"So that is what we did at the celebration of her life. This time I hosted the circle. It was a large circle and included many new people and children. This time we knew how to hold the space. I listened to new stories about Ruth Marie that I had not heard before. Again, another brother asked to be forgiven for some words he had said earlier. There was a profound statement from an eleven-year-old nephew who spoke from the next generation about what Ruth Marie's life meant to him. There were many moments of silence.

"No one commented about the circle that day; we just did it. For months after, I received notes and comments about how powerful it was. Connections and conversations are self-organizing among us. We are talking to each other and listening more. It's as though something has been lifted from our hands, our minds, and our hearts. Sometimes it just takes a while. Ruth Marie and I know this."

Her last words to Ruben, spoken over the phone before he got on the plane to stand beside her as she died, had been, "Remember the circle." They remain dedicated to sharing the healing of their family with as large a group as possible.

Here we, the writers of this book, ring the bell, pause, breathe, and observe a moment of silence to honor this story.

Healing Community History

In 1999, we were invited by Dr. Mary K. Sandford, at the time associate dean of the College of Arts and Sciences at the University of North Carolina, Greensboro (UNCG), to bring PeerSpirit Circle Process to a yearlong conversation and experience she was organizing called the Race and Gender Institute. Mary K. called us to say, "This institute has been functioning as a kind of remedial summer school for faculty who have failed to change old southern mores in their language and behavior around race and gender. If you've been 'bad,' your dean refers you to detention. When it came my turn to host the institute, I refused to apply a punishment model; it just doesn't work."

Mary K. picked a small group of forward-thinking faculty from several departments and started reconceptualizing what the Race and Gender Institute could be and how it could serve the university and community. "Two things were coming into alignment," she remembers. "Redesigning the institute and the college program committee were both my responsibilities that year. So we offered race and gender as the programming theme throughout the academic cycle."

Mary K. and her committee invited a diverse group of twenty faculty whom they expected would be willing to explore these issues. They hired PeerSpirit to start and finish the year, facilitating two, two-day retreats. We were privileged to see them take their first risks as a group and then to witness the creative and bold ways they had extended shadow healing to the university and community at large.

People who had been accepted for inclusion in the institute were supported by their departments, assuring additional responsibility beyond their teaching load and were generally excited to be in the conversation. They were also highly guarded as they entered the conference room and took a seat in a circle of chairs. In those first forty-eight hours, they had to forge a new way of being together in an environment famous for ruthless judgmentalism. They had to break free of personal preconceptions of one another and face their internalized notions of race and gender. This circle would set out intentionally to heal the participants' individual and collective shadows through the experiences of honesty and to explore ways to extend their learning forward.

After introductions and the mention that they would be developing their own version of PeerSpirit Circle Process, they were given a small note card and asked to write down something from their own life experience that at this moment they could not imagine sharing with the other people in the room. They sealed these statements in envelopes and held them close. The first shadow shift: people

EXHIBIT 10.1

Working Agreements for the Race and Gender Institute
○ We share a commitment to the process and to being "here."
○ We agree to maintain a relaxed, nonjudgmental atmosphere.
○ We agree to identify the specific foci of our group and planned activities.
○ We agree to share with one another our experiences and the impact of our sessions together in our classes and in our daily lives.
○ We agree to show respect for people's personal stories and keep them within the circle.
○ We agree to have the freedom to not know and to be absolutely wrong.
○ We agree to rotate leadership by asking members to volunteer to plan, organize, and facilitate monthly meetings of the group.
○ We agree that all members will share responsibility in the setting of the agenda.

carry stories into circle that they do not intend to share. What we share and how we share, what we withhold and how we withhold, are choices that build or diminish shadow in a group. People continually assess their levels of comfort and risk and whether they are willing to commit themselves to authentic interaction.

The group then listed attributes of social container they felt would foster enough trust that they could imagine making freer choices than simply withholding stories from one another. With a host, guardian, and scribe in place, we crafted a set of working agreements and intention that would allow people to grow in truth-telling and imagine themselves in leadership roles around these issues (see Exhibit 10.1).

After dinner we reconvened for the opening check-in. The intention and agreements were posted on the wall. The conference room had been transformed into a quieter space: a candle on a low table, a circle of floor chairs and pillows. The halls of academia were far away. And though it was an unusual arrangement for many present, they sat down willingly in the experiment. Each person had been asked to bring an object to place in the center that represented <u>a moment in time when the consequences of the person's race</u> or gender became clear. Someone read the agreements, pausing and letting the importance of the commitment sink in. Someone else rang the guardian bell. The group took a spontaneous long breath and dived into honesty with tears and laughter.

The next afternoon, one of the African American participants said to Christina, "Just so you know, I didn't come here with a nine-month commitment in mind—it was more like ninety minutes. I told myself I would not participate in another session of 'educating white folks' to the realities of color. When the agreements got in place, I was willing to extend another ninety minutes to see how the check-in went. I was the last to speak—and by then, I knew I could be here for the year. It wouldn't have happened for me without this circle stuff."

A few months later, the circle supported one of its members, theater professor Marsha Paludan, and her students in mounting a production of Emily Mann's play *Greensboro: A Requiem.* Mary K. said, "The play is about the Ku Klux Klan opening fire into a group of marching demonstrators on the streets of the city of Greensboro on November 3, 1979. Just as Marsha sat in the honesty of the Race and Gender Institute circle, the student actors prepared for their roles by sitting in circle with Marsha. They did powerful work around racism in order to be able to portray both people of color and white supremacists on the stage. There was a lot of edginess in the town because it was the twentieth anniversary of the actual shootings. There was some question about whether or not the Klan might show up on opening night and repeat the violence."

When using circle to shift consciousness at a community level, many elements are activated. Those who call the circle cannot predict or control these reactions. They can, however, hold their own intention clearly and their energetics strongly. They must also practice asking for the help they need and inviting others into intentional speaking, attentive listening, and supporting the well-being of the whole. A well-timed conversation can diffuse a lot of tension.

In October, a few weeks before the premier, the Beloved Community Center sponsored a coordinated event called the Night of a Thousand Conversations. It had prepared a video that combined fifteen minutes of television coverage from 1979 with survivor and witness statements, gospel music, and social commentary. It made one hundred copies and asked for one hundred volunteers to invite at least ten people into their homes to watch the video and have a conversation on its impact then and now. They were also asked how their lives as citizens had been affected.

Mary K. explained:

> "In 1979, there had been much criticism of the police for not being present at the march and slow to respond after the shootings. So of course, they made quite a show of presence at opening night of the play—squad cars out front, officers standing in the aisles—a bit of a siege mentality. Putting on my anthropologist hat, I stood on the stage before the perfor-

mance and spoke about our hopes to contribute to cultural healing. And because all the institute people were there and Marsha had worked in circle with the cast, we were able to create a kind of circle atmosphere during the 'talk back' at the end of the play between the actors, playwright, drama professor, and audience—including a number of survivors.

"The daughter of Reverend Nelson Johnson, a leader who had been stabbed during the demonstration, stood up and said, 'I've never had the opportunity to publicly tell my parents how proud I am of them for standing up for what they believed in.' A student from California said, 'I didn't understand before what people here in the South really went through, what it took for you to "overcome someday." Now I know.' And for months after that, people would stop me in the grocery store and tell me stories about their memories of the shooting, the impact on their lives, the things they were thinking about now. I felt like a walking circle space."

There are long-term outcomes to the work the Race and Gender Institute did that year. The members of the institute began using circle in their classrooms and in their faculty and staff meetings. In traditional meetings, they adopted the host-guardian configuration, sitting across from each other holding the energetics. The programs they sponsored were instrumental in establishing an African American studies major at the university. At the end of that year, the provost spoke in awe of what had been accomplished and acknowledged the central role of circle in all that had occurred. And in 2005, an independent "truth and reconciliation project" and "truth and reconciliation commission" were established to further the community healing. Rev. Nelson Johnson told Mary K., "None of this would have happened if it weren't for what you did through the Race and Gender Institute." So it was a seed.

The institute provided experiential evidence that deep issues of shadow could be intentionally brought to PeerSpirit circles for discussion, action, and ultimate healing. The topics had the potential to be explosive, and yet the institute members' experience was that everything could be said within the rules of engagement the group had outlined for itself. Nothing was stifled, and within the structure of circle, there was no need for violence or drama.

Some of the members of the institute still teach at UNCG, while others have moved to different universities and organizations, changed careers, or retired. And yet that circle isn't over. Everyone who experienced something during that year is still influenced by it—the circle members themselves and also the students, the folks in each other's living rooms, the police who stood guard that night at the play, the survivors from both sides of the conflict, the attendees at lectures, the college administrators who weren't sure what they'd unleashed, and the strangers in the grocery store who just had to share their stories. This is the great leap of faith in the world of circle: our speaking and listening contributes to one another, and beyond the small rim of personal feedback, as among those twenty faculty, we can never gauge the full impact we have put into the world.

Mary K. stared out the window, seeing something in her mind, and said, "I remember watching the news coverage of those shootings while I was in graduate school in Boulder, Colorado. And I thought to myself, *How could anyone live there?* with no idea that I was on my way to exactly that place to do exactly this piece of social justice work. Having grown up in segregated Arkansas, it horrified me to see this nasty piece of the Old South still happening in 1979. I have learned in my adult decades that after any milestone—voting rights, desegregation, the election of President Obama—we need to stay awake and active. We need to have continuing conversations about race and gender that keep society moving toward healing our ancient wounds. It's not over—and that's the human journey."

Whenever we need encouragement, we remember the observation that Mary K.'s predecessor in the field of anthropology, Margaret Mead, spoke from her experience: "Never doubt that a small group of thoughtful, committed citizens can change the world; indeed, it's the only thing that ever does."

Here we, the writers of this book, ring the bell, pause, breathe, and observe a moment of silence to honor this story.

Healing Lives amid War and Violence

Bev Reeler is a white citizen of Zimbabwe, a country where unemployment has run as high as 90 percent (the government being the only entity left in the country with money to pay employees), where systems of production have broken down, and the social infrastructure of the country is in shambles. In 2002, the governmental policy of internal land invasion, evicted all white farmers, causing the collapse of commercial farming and the displacement of tens of thousands of people from rural communities. Burdened by an untreated HIV/AIDS epidemic, near-universal poverty, and inconsistent food-growing capacity, the life expectancy of the country's eleven million people has plunged to thirty-three years. Once known as the "breadbasket of Africa," the nation has been devastated by years of intense political strife (amounting to an internalized state of warfare), with arrests, torture, and assassinations used to control access to power and even voting. The lion of shadow has swallowed Zimbabwe, and yet the spirits of individual people seek to endure.

Under these conditions, Bev has dedicated her life to calling circles of healing. Since 2004, these Tree of Life Circles have been taking place in the hidden corners of the countryside, in the face of continued violence and fear. Bev calls them "small sparks of hope and love shining in the darkness."

We met Bev and heard about her circle work when we visited Kufunda village in Zimbabwe in May 2007 and have included her in the list of Zimbabwean friends and colleagues we watch and pray for from afar. Most of this story is told in her words as she writes to let the outside world know what is happening in her beloved and tormented country.

Rays of late afternoon sunlight filter through the open sides of the thatched rondeval,[2] painting gold across the shining earth-brown faces in the circle. These are the Shona people, the primary tribal group of Zimbabwe. They have spent the last three days together sheltered in a Miombo woodland,[3] leaning against house-sized granite boulders, sharing their stories. This group has traveled from Epworth, a high-density suburb of makeshift huts and tiny plots of dirt yards and home gardens at the edge of the capital city of Harare. Political violence has left their lives shattered, their homes burned, and their community in tatters. Over three days, they have shared stories they have never told before.

All their stories are told in a circle with a talking piece. In the first circle, when the participants introduce themselves, they make agreements about how they choose to live and work together (Exhibit 10.2). "The agreements they choose are always the same," says Bev:

Exhibit 10.2

Working Agreements for the Tree of Life Circle
○ To treat one another with love and respect.
○ To treat all in the circle as equal.
○ To listen without judgment or comment.
○ To be trusting and truthful.
○ To keep the stories that are told in the circle confidential.

Here in the sunlight, the quality of their time together depends on maintaining these agreements. After they return to the shadow of sociopolitical violence they come from, their lives depend on maintaining these agreements.

"Sitting in circle is a simple behavior," Bev notes, "but it is in total contradiction to our present world experience. To spend time with one another in this way is a revolution in itself. Circle is a way of breaking the stranglehold of fear, distrust, and isolation so that a more wonderful part of ourselves can come into being.

"We start by speaking of our grandparents and great-grandparents, tracing the paths they traveled to Zimbabwe. Among the Shona, many find that others in the circle share the same totem (traditionally an animal or bird) or that their ancestors followed a similar path to Zimbabwe (from Mozambique, Malawi, or Tanzania) or that they come from the same rural areas or that their traditional belief systems are still held in the family or that their families have become divided over new belief systems."

About her own family's journey, Bev says, "My great-grandfather arrived as the first city architect, and my family has now lived for five generations in this country as architects and engineers. But most important of all, we have deep roots in this African soil and have become part of these amazing people."

In these Tree of Life Circles, Bev and others have carefully crafted a healing process, *where* the presence and metaphor of nature is part of what allows participants to handle the pain in their own and others' stories. Bev sees the connection with nature as a way for people to reconnect with their history:

"Our shared humanity becomes clearer and clearer to each of us as we observe how nature is interconnected.

"People spend time outside the rondeval looking at the trunks of the forest trees. They notice the bends and twists, signs of fire and drought, and compare the scars that mark the trees' growth into maturity with stories of their own childhoods. People speak of trials and difficulties, of sorrows and joys and of those who have loved them. They hear how their stories carry the same themes and realize they are all connected. The Tree of Life becomes a powerful symbol in these circles. The trees are living participants who hold our backs, provide shade and fruit, offer twigs to start the cooking fires, and connect us to our lineage stories.

"All Zimbabweans know that trees carry ancient healing medicine. The wisdom of old spirits is whispered when the wind stirs the leaves, singing long-forgotten stories. In the peace of sitting under the Msasa trees, breathing the natural pulse of the earth, the terrors of war begin to drain from our bodies, and we can feel our hearts beating with a rhythm we have always known.

"We speak of the forest that is Zimbabwe and of how it has been damaged, chopped, burned in these last years of violence. I hold the rim of witness while the others share stories of how this has been for them. An elderly carpenter speaks with great dignity of being beaten and burned; grandmothers and granddaughters speak of rape and humiliation; young men who are laborers, counselors, teachers, and preachers speak of being tortured and of the pain and abandonment, fear and guilt they have felt and of the deaths they have seen. The talking piece goes round and round, and the listening circle bears witness to horrific experiences they have never spoken before."

In the quiet sunlight of the forest in this place of temporary respite, the people around the circle shed their tears of mourning. These circles are addressing the deepest layers of collective shadow: humanity's capacity for systemic violence, for warring against itself. For all humanity's brilliance and creativity, for all the graces of art and craft and ingenuity, for our ability to make consciousness and religion and science and technology, we are the only species on the planet capable of premeditated and carefully designed cruelty. In this disastrous breakdown of life in Zimbabwe, Bev offers in response: the circle.

Tree of Life Circles began in August 2004 when eight activists selected by their communities were bused to Lake Chivero, near Harare, to spend five days together with Bev and her colleague Sonia and a wonderful team in the National Park cottages. The eight had all been recent victims of organized violence and torture and were understandably anxious to find themselves in the bush with people they hardly knew. In the following days, these traumatized people lived and ate together and shared the stories of their experiences, taking their first steps of transformation from victim to survivor. This was the first Tree of Life workshop in Zimbabwe, and the members of this chosen group have become the core facilitators of the process as it has begun to spread throughout the country.

Bev explains:

"Of that original circle of eight, Abby, Namu, and Rodgers are still active members and facilitators of the Tree of Life family. The others have had to leave to earn their living or move to South Africa to survive but are still in contact. In the intervening years, these three have led lives of inspiring dedication to healing. It has been a difficult process. All of the participants have been targeted by the government, so moving them around the country and finding places to meet has provided its own dangers. There have been times we have had some funding and longer periods without. There have been periods of ducking and diving and living on the edge. But throughout all this, these facilitators have stayed connected to the newly created Tree of Life circles. Each circle they have sat with has had eight participants—by now over three hundred people have sat in these circles. They have kept in cell phone contact, mourned the deaths of circle members, tracked them through arrests and torture, and celebrated their survival and success. A small and growing network of survivors has been formed across parts of the country. From this network of circles, two other survivors, Jane and Gift, joined the team in 2008 and have lent themselves unstintingly to the work of healing.

"In June 2008, we hit an all-time low when Tonderai Ndira[4] was murdered with seven of his activist friends. We had to find a safe house for Nhamo, who had been Ndira's friend. Then Gift, a Movement for Democratic Change government official, lost his seat in the elections, had his house burned, and was jailed. The other facilitators had to stay in hiding. When Gift was released, we moved him to a safe house and began to meet in circles again to keep up our morale, moving around police blocks and taking our chances to ensure we were connected. Our resolve began to grow again.

"We needed to get our own funding and ensure we could carry on with this process, as it was something we all believed in, so we dreamed our dream and it began to unfold. AusAID gave us funding to keep going for six months, and the Research and Advisory Unit,[5] our partner and support, began to deal with the money.

By the end of 2008, Tree of Life Circles had become a cohesive organization that offered twenty-five workshops for communities and grassroots and human rights organizations in the first four months of 2009.

Bev continued:

"In a time when the political status of our country is so ambiguous, the monolithic darkness begins to show its cracks. Shafts of light move through the shadows. And suddenly we can move in different ways. The Catholic Commission for Justice and Peace, the International Organization for Migration, the Uhuru boys (student activists), the City of Harare Resident Association, the Alternative Businesses Association, the UMA (a group of pastors), to name a few, are all now ready to begin the process of healing, and we are ready to guide new facilitators to take the process to their communities and organizations—and so the circles will multiply." The Tree of Life Circles have demonstrated that there is a process and a set of tools that can be used and built upon. Thanks to the generic nature of the organization, it multiplies and requires only the temporary support of trained facilitators to foster the leadership that emerges from the group experience.

Out in the woodlands, after a day of mourning, something different often happens. People bring out drums and mbiras and sing and dance and laugh, as if a huge weight has been lifted. It is as if the isolation they have felt has dissipated. Life is connected again, to this circle of people, to these trees and rocks, and to the spirit inside them that had been lost in their terrible journeys.

By their last day in circle together, people have changed. They look at themselves as a forest, as trees that stand together, and they see how they have taken their scars, survived, and grown again. They have discovered what incredible resources they have had at moments when all seemed the darkest. They have spoken the names of those who have been there for them in times of need and acknowledged their strength at times they traveled alone. This forest is full of fruit, of strength and courage and endurance. They begin to understand their survival and the great learning it has brought them and the incredible people they have become.

Says Bev in her witness role:

"A strong young man spoke in the circle: 'I heard my four-year-old daughter tell her friends as she sat in my yard, "Matemba from next door burned down our house"—and I wanted the sentence to end "and my father sorted him out [taught him a lesson].' For I spoke of revenge to my friends, and we were collecting knives. But today I know that I want my daughter's sentence to end another way. I want to hear her say, "and my father was part of the healing." My heart has changed.'

"This afternoon, they have been speaking of power: of the effect of abuse of power in their lives, in their homes and their schools and churches, in their country and their history. And now they begin to speak of another sort of power, that of a circle, carrying a common intention. A new way of working together begins to emerge. They look at how they can bring this into their lives and their communities, and they feel the strength of these connections. They walked in a silent procession up to the rocks, where, in a small fire, they burned what they wished to leave behind and shared their dreams for the future. And the granite boulders echoed with their songs and prayers, their dreams and their laughter."

Something Mahatma Gandhi said speaks to this work: "We must let the Law of Love either rule us through and through or not at all."[6] This is what the Tree of Life Circles are doing in Zimbabwe: choosing to let the Law of Love rule by bringing people's broken hearts to one another and claiming peace over retaliation.

The seeds of Tree of Life are being taken into the hands of other Zimbabweans, and a quiet forest is being planted across the country. These extraordinary people, who have experienced the most challenging onslaught to their lives, have agreed to carry forward a process of healing and empowerment rather than one of vengeance. Through the dedicated work of all those who have carried the vision of reconciliation in the face of all sorts of hardships and difficulties, who have prepared themselves to learn and take risks, the web of circles begins to hold them.

Here we, the writers of this book, ring the bell, pause, breathe, and observe a moment of silence to honor this story.

IV

Circle as Paradigm Shift

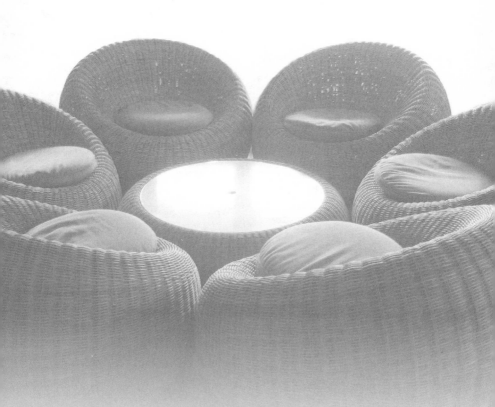

11

Organizational Experiments in Circle Governance

Organizations with a commitment to systemic change and alternative structure may use circle as their self-governance.

Circle's use as a dynamic, positive force for changing the world is rapidly evolving. In May 2009, Christina attended a two-day conference on Peace and Social Justice Issues sponsored by Catholic Women Religious. In a workshop on emergent social issues offered by Fran Korten, editor of *Yes!* magazine, she asked those of us in the audience to reflect on three questions:

- What did you notice on the fringe of society fifteen years ago that is now in the center?

- What do you notice on the fringe now that you hope will move to the center in the next fifteen years?

- What are you willing to do to contribute to that happening?

Christina walked to the microphone and began talking about the shift in circle work in the fifteen years between founding PeerSpirit, Inc., in 1994, and the conference of eighteen hundred women and men in May 2009. She spoke about circle being a fringe movement reentering society through consciousness-raising groups, through experiences like the California-based Women's Summer Solstice Camps (1985–1996), through organizations like Women Within International and the Mankind Project, through the Council of Wilderness Guides and the School of Lost Borders, through Ojai Foundation and its teachings in *The Way of Council*, through John Seed, Joanna Macy, and Pat Fleming's work with *The Council of All Beings*. She then spoke about how circle has now taken hold in indicator professions such as education, religion, health care, and the nonprofit sector. "That was our goal," she said excitedly. "We knew circle would work at the edge—and we believed it was equally needed in the middle." At the end of the session, people clustered around and talked excitedly of their own experiences with circle, moving from the edge of their lives toward a more central and accepted practice

Circle as Agent of Cultural Shift

What was on the edge fifteen years ago that is now in the middle?

The story goes that the origins of the Polish Solidarity movement started in 1970 when Lech Walesa and a few colleagues began meeting secretly around the docks of Gdansk, preparing to take on their government and through these protests deal with the interference of the Soviet Union in Polish national affairs. A handful of rebels versus the Soviet Union! In September 1980, Solidarity called a national strike based on nonviolent principles. One year later, Solidarity called its own national congress and elected Lech Walesa president of an alternative government, "a self-governing republic." In 1989, a Solidarity-led coalition government elected Walesa the prime minister of Poland. And from 1990 to 1995, he was president of the country he helped liberate: from the edge to the center.

Wangari Maathai, the "Tree Lady of Kenya," was a college professor of biology when she started responding to the hardships of rural women's lives by suggesting that women plant trees for food, firewood, and shelter. In 1977, she started the Green Belt Movement, consciously seeking cultural shift. "The planting of trees is the planting of ideas," she said. "By starting with the simple step of digging a hole and planting a tree, we plant hope for ourselves and for future generations." Of the first one hundred trees, twenty-eight survived. She persisted, and so did the trees. In 2004, she was the first black African woman and first environmentalist to win the Nobel Peace Prize. By 2008, the Green Belt Movement had planted 38 million trees and began aiming toward one billion new trees. From two dozen seedlings to a greening world; from the edge to the center.

Margaret Wheatley often tells such stories to remind audiences of the power of small, self-organizing groups. She says, "Every story like this I hear begins with the same phrase: 'Some friends and I started talking. . . .'" Each of the three organizations whose stories complete this chapter started down the path to cultural shift by a few key leaders entering just such conversations that led to their perceiving their own potential. As a result of these sparking conversations, each organization has embraced a profound underlying question that grounds its exploration:

- ⊙ What if we used circle process in determining how a national board guides the merger of two well-established entities with the intent to think differently about the management of finances and develop a holistic concept of what comprises wealth? (Financial Planning Association)

- ⊙ What if we used circle to restructure the nature of schools and education, starting with our own school? (Ridge and Valley Charter School, New Jersey)

- ⊙ What if we brought circle and dialogue into the management of a health care center and into the relationship between health care provider and health care receiver? (True North Health Care Center, Maine)

Each of these organizations lives the circle as an administrative form of governance in its day-to-day operation with awareness that incremental progress is a path toward exponential leaps. Every time that the Financial Planning Association national board meets in circle, the Ridge and Valley Charter School refers to its teachers as guides to the children's learning, and when True North Health Care Center administers itself in circle, a new way is forged: from the edge to the center.

How PeerSpirit Came to the Financial Planning Association

In 2000, the International Association for Financial Planners and the Institute of Certified Financial Planners decided to merge into one association, the Financial Planning Association (FPA), whose primary aim is to promote financial planning and advances in the financial planning profession. Initially, the executive directors of each association became codirectors, and the two boards merged without relinquishing numbers.

Former board president Elizabeth Jetton recalls of that merger:

"The two organizations just glued themselves together with the shared belief that it was time for one association to emerge from the process, but there was no process for that emergence to occur. Our first meeting was at a big conference center with Robert's Rules of

Order, a gavel, and chairs facing a panel of staff and directors. We raised the question 'Who are we going to be now?'—but there was no way to talk about it in the format of the meeting. It was a very painful year, with lots of facilitators coming and going and a sense that to discover some kind of cohesiveness we needed to get away and talk with and listen to each other. So for the summer board retreat of 2001, we went to Grand Targhee Resort in the Tetons."

At that time, Guy Cumbie was president of the board, and Janet McCallen was executive director. Guy, Janet, and a subgroup on the board were starting to look at how to develop FPA as a community. However, the internal sense of community in the board had not yet jelled. Jetton continued:

"I don't even know how it happened, but when we walked into the room at Targhee, the chairs were in a circle, and Meg Wheatley was there to facilitate the board retreat. We didn't have any circle skills, no principles or guidelines had been laid out, and no one was prepared for the shift. Some of us sensed that the new arrangement of chairs would open up the dialogue, but we didn't know if the circle was the leadership *technique du jour* or if it was going to stay. Some people wouldn't even enter the circle. They just stood behind their chairs with their arms folded in defiance. Meg was a strong facilitator and a needed bridge for us. I remember we talked about how we were all leaders, how we could better engage in dialogue this way, and we did a lot with flip charts and voting by placing paper dots on various resolutions."

Though FPA had a strong thought leader and an innovative staff leader, it had underestimated the amount of preparation and pre-work required to shift the paradigm of self-governance and create an amalgamated culture out of two highly defined preexisting associations. The board had been to its first mountaintop. The board members left Targhee still in conflict about the efficacy of circle and unsure how to integrate their experiments in collaborative conversation into the national structure. They planned to host a large World Café at their annual meeting scheduled for San Diego, September 12, 2001—a meeting that never occurred.

The board, staff, and meeting planners who had already arrived in San Diego woke on September 11 to watch the terrorist attacks on New York and the Pentagon on TV. "We were grounded together—trying to serve our clients and members in the face of chaos and tragedy," said Elizabeth. "The timing of the board meeting in the midst of such a shock, the recent experiences of Grand Targhee, and the work of the newly assigned Community Strategic Team may have allowed the board to accept the idea of more collaborative structure for a new way forward. The trust and bonding that occurred during those days when we were stranded far from our homes were profound." The board leaders then boldly called a series of World Café gatherings to host large group conversations with state chapters[1] and had successful experiences with the membership while continuing to struggle with circle process among themselves.

During this time, before we at PeerSpirit even knew they had adopted circle process and were struggling with it, the board members were doing the hard work of pioneering without understanding where to reach for the infrastructure that could stabilize the process. They were trying to invent the infrastructure as they went along. They desired collaboration and the ability to work in circle, if they could only figure out how to make the circle work for them.

In the summer of 2002, Meg Wheatley was again invited to facilitate the summer retreat, and when Janet said they needed help with their circle process, Meg invited Christina to cofacilitate. In preparation, the group read two Peer-Spirit booklets, *PeerSpirit Council Management in Businesses, Corporations, and Organizations* and *Understanding Shadow and Projection in Circles and Groups.* Meg and Christina worked to help the board refine its sense of purpose and functionality. PeerSpirit agreements were put in place; Christina served as guardian, Meg served as host, and they helped shape the work of the board and the group process that would serve the work. Christina listened to the accumulated frustration around their process. The board members wanted certain conditions of efficiency to be met before they would commit to circle; without clear agreements trust kept eroding and they had accumulated significant shadow as decisions were getting made (or unmade) in committees, in subgroups, or at the hotel bar late at night and not shared with the whole board. It was decided that Christina would return to their next board meeting in Denver in early November and coach the circle process—after which they would formally vote to proceed with circle or abandon it.

Christina remembers walking into a large, windowless conference hall with forty people (half board members and half staff), sitting in a circle of huge circumference with a bare coffee table in the center and a piece of pine knot—an artifact from the mountain—resting on it. Their talking piece was a hand-held microphone. No one referenced the center. No one knew how to intervene if

Exhibit 11.1

FPA Board Agreements
○ We share a commitment to the process and to being "here."
○ We choose to live in a conversational culture employing various modalities of group process. The circle is our home.
○ We assume each other's good intentions and share responsibility for creating an environment of respect.
○ We hold personal material in confidence and keep board decisions confidential as appropriate to the issue.
○ We employ a group guardian to keep an eye on needs, timing, and energy. We agree to pause at the guardian's signal and to call for that signal when we feel the need for a pause.

people went on long tangents, and power struggles were evident around the rim. They had moved the chairs, but they had not shifted the dynamic. They needed to understand and put into language: social container, attachment to center, strong agreements, use of a guardian, clear hosting through agenda items, and agreed ways to make decisions and initiate action. Christina recalls, "We stopped everything and just worked with circle infrastructure, dividing into small groups in the four corners of the room that came back with agreements (see Exhibit 11.1), statements of core beliefs and values, and clarifications of roles for host, guardian, and scribe. As you will note reading these statements, the language is visionary and far-reaching. It provides the outer rim of philosophy inside which the ever-changing board of directors can respond to current need and function.

The group instituted thumb voting as a way to get a sense of cohesiveness in a long conversation or to ascertain readiness to make decisions—and soon members were voting on the work of the subgroups. Christina trained the guardian by opening a chair next to her and inviting various people to hold the chime and practice intervening to pause or correct the course of action as the meeting progressed. The next day, the agenda items went smoothly, and when votes were taken, the board members rolled their chairs forward toward the reenergized center and the staff pushed their chairs back to hold the rim and serve as observers. A solid foundation for circle was in place.

The national board formally adopted circle as its governance, and by the next meeting, the supportive structural language they had developed was standing literally at the back of the circle on laminated foam-core placards at the rim. By the next time PeerSpirit interacted with the board, in May 2005, Marv Tuttle had assumed the executive director position, and the board had voted to downsize membership to eighteen members or less to work more efficiently. Marv speaks easily about the transition:

> "I've lived through a hundred board meetings in the previous association and now with FPA. I've watched our transformation until we can say that circle has truly become our culture on the board. The board members and staff have developed an atmosphere of welcoming contributions, and we feel comfortable with how we have adapted the form. Our national board meetings are usually two and a half days long, and we think of the meeting in half-day segments. We train each other in guardianship by using someone with experience to take the role during intense issues and inviting new people to assume that authority in more routine sessions. Usually, up to five people have the chance to serve as guardian. The chair of the board is the host, and we see the chair as the board's mentor who is experienced in carrying the wisdom of the group and watching over our process. The president-elect serves as the advocate for moving through agenda items—someone who is familiar with topics and issues and who has more freedom to lead content. These three folks and I sit equidistant from each other in the circle so that we can keep an eye on the whole process. We hold the container.
>
> "In the center, we have a mirrored globe that reflects our faces to one another, a journal with thoughts and messages from previous board members so that our story is always with us, and several placards of inspiring quotes from Einstein and others. We have two talking pieces: a feather for checking in and out and deeper councils and a Koosh ball for tossing when we want to pick up the pace and still use a talking piece."

Inevitably in an association environment, leadership changes—both in the board and staff—and the contextual understanding of circle and the story of and importance to the organization needs to be sustained. Transferring the commitment and peer training of circle as new board members join the group has been one of FPA's biggest challenges. Marv explains:

> "People come in knowing we have this circle process, but they've never actually seen it or experienced it, and we have to help them adjust. What fosters integrity in this situation is the understanding

that we are always in circle as a board, even when we leave the hotel—circle is how we treat each other and our relationships and our conversations. There came a time when we were wrestling with our agreements. Folks were not feeling safe in circle. At our 2007 board retreat, it seemed we were wading through unexpressed expectations when we had to make some complex decisions. So Nick (president in 2007 and board chair in 2008) and I went to the Art of Hosting to enhance and broaden the chair's and CEO's skills and attentiveness to circle process. Then we were able to lead the board through a process of recommitment and reaffirmation. For me, this was the most intense experience of falling out of practice and potentially doing harm to our integrity."

Marv regularly speaks to other executive directors and the Colorado association management group about FPA's use of circle process.

"When I tell them we do three-day board meetings in circle with small groups operating in Open Space and that we do World Café with hundreds of members, they don't know what to think. Planners tend to be entrepreneurial, go-getters, quick thinkers, and I try to explain that circle teaches us to hold long, sustained conversations that lead to a clear decision point. We have had to hold very substantial conversations about standards in the financial services industry. For example, it took us five years to come to a decision to press a lawsuit—which we won—with the Securities and Exchange Commission. We were clear going into the suit thanks to the long, clarifying, open-ended conversations we had in circle. Sometimes it makes the hair on the back of my neck stand up when we get to a point of understanding our commitment to an issue or each other. You don't get that in usual meetings."

In 2009, Merv contacted the PeerSpirit office requesting our return for a "circle tune-up" with the new board. Neither of us was available, so we suggested they invite Martin Siesta, a former board member with training in both circle and the Art of Hosting modalities. This marked a celebrated progression in the transmission of skilled circle leadership: the next generation of teachers now exists within the organization itself.

Also in 2009, the FPA staff conducted a "listening tour" among the state chapters. They are seeking ways to foster a culture of conversation throughout the association. Their goal is to permeate the chapters and demonstrate to their membership that collaborative conversations using circle, World Café, or Open Space will foster thoughtful leadership wherever it is used.

Ridge and Valley Charter School

Ridge and Valley Charter School, grades kindergarten through eight, opened September 8, 2004, with ninety students. It is a free public elementary school located in the Appalachian ridge and limestone valley region of northwestern New Jersey. The curriculum for each grade is offered through an integrated program, Earth Literacy, which includes learning about the natural world and how humans can live in a mutually enhancing relationship with the entire community of life.

In 2003, when a group of dedicated parents were struggling with all the details of land acquisition, state regulations, teacher selection, and ideological priorities, PeerSpirit colleague Sarah MacDougall traveled to New Jersey to offer a weekend training retreat. She found a group of wise, educated, and fairly burnt-out parents and community members. Together they worked to attend to the group's depleted energetics and further hone the rotating and shared leadership of circle structure to which they were already dedicated.

Parent, founder, and ongoing trustee Kerry Barnett explained:

"When Sarah first came, we were already five years into the process of launching this school. We had been using circle process for all of our meetings because the open communication circle offers was part of what we intended to offer our children. The school is founded on the premise that humanity's current model of earth exploitation can't continue, and we want to educate our children for the kinds of sustainable adult lives we believe they will be required to face. Our earth stewardship model includes the values of collaboration, respect for each other and other species, and a spirit of lifelong learning."

In these first five years of meetings, the group had had to learn about every aspect of launching a public school—from educational curricula and state educational requirements to real estate law and grant writing. Motivated to find an alternative mode of education for her children that would complement the family's commitment to alternative living at nearby Genesis Farm, Kerry joined the group in 1999 and has been a member of the trustees' circle ever since. The trustees' circle is the equivalent of a traditional school board, except that instead of overseeing a district, it oversees only Ridge and Valley.

Another founding and ongoing trustee, Dave McNulty, is a partner in an e-learning, multimedia, and Web production company in Hope, New Jersey, several miles away. "There are few models for precisely what we are trying to do at the school," he says. "We are determined to build a public institution on a nonhierarchical model. We want to demonstrate that all of us can work together and make decisions, and I have no doubt that we have made better decisions because we have used the circle and PeerSpirit principles."

"We did not know how hard this would be," Kerry explains, "or how many areas we would have to become educated in. However, the biggest education for all of us has come in understanding human relations. As trustees, we have worked explicitly in circle, and it is the reason the school opened at all. We developed sympathy, empathy, love, and trust for one another while working hard to create something we all believed in."

Traci Pannullo, another young parent looking for an alternative to traditional public education for her child, joined the trustees' circle in April 2004, less than six months before the first group of students was slated to begin. She remembers:

"We had just purchased a facility. Everything was happening really fast. Then those acquisition plans fell through, and we had to scramble to find buildings where the first group of students could meet. A local Presbyterian church camp provided a short-term solution while our long-term facility construction was completed. Kindergarten and first grade met in a log structure, and the upper grades each met in a cabin with bunk beds pushed aside and wood stoves for heat. It was all very exciting and incredibly intense, and the hardships created great bonding.

"In those early trustees' circle meetings, I felt something energetically amazing going on between us. I could not articulate it at the time, but there was something very calming and grounding about the ritual elements of the circle: holding the talking piece, pausing to gather one's thoughts, opening with a quote, checking in and checking out—even in the midst of all the chaos of the school's reality."

To illustrate this, Traci loves to share the story of one August night at 2:00 A.M., just before school opened. The trustees' circle was up late doing a final reading of new policies because everything had to be in place in order to legally open the school.

> "Even though everyone was exhausted, there was a sense of determination and commitment. The steadfastness of our teamwork came about as a result of the group's circle work. It was personally transformative for me to experience people working together with such respect and integrity, even in the midst of incredible tension, deadlines, and occasional disagreements. The circle process continually brought us back to the purpose in the center—the pursuit of a common, higher goal."

In February 2005, all of the students, teachers, and administrators moved into their permanent building located on sixteen acres with beautiful views of the Delaware Water Gap. The campus includes classrooms and offices, organic gardens and fields, solar panels, a greenhouse, and a yurt. It is located a short walk away from the Paulinskill River Trail. Student-built birdhouses, debris shelters, herb gardens, miniature villages, trails, campfire circles, compost bins, solar ovens, artwork, picnic tables, and much more soon enhanced the grounds.

One steady personnel presence throughout has been Nanci Dvorsky, a lifelong explorer of alternative education, organic gardening, and sustainability, who was drawn to contribute to the unfolding story of Ridge and Valley Charter School. By summer 2005, Traci Pannullo had resigned from the trustees' circle to become the part-time curriculum coordinator. So now there were two women with history, skill, and circle experience keeping the school stable while other personnel structures were sorted.

The trustees' circle always intended that the school's administrative coordinator, curriculum coordinator, and academic coordinator would work together as a circle. However, the old paradigm of a traditional principal in charge of operations kept emerging. After three years of unsuccessfully working toward a paradigm shift, the trustees' circle once again began to map out a leadership team arrangement that more directly reflected the shared leadership model of the school's charter.

Nanci and Traci, both deeply aligned with the history and heart of the school, were logical choices for the new leadership team. Lisa Masi, founding kindergarten teacher, stepped forward to work with the team and liaison with her fellow teachers (guides) on matters of integrated curriculum and parent relationships. The fourth member of the team is Rowena McNulty (no relation to Dave), who is the differentiated learning coordinator responsible for all special education. With no principal and no superintendent's office, the challenge continues to be a need for clear definition of work responsibilities in the midst of collaborative dialogue.

Nanci recalls:

"We could not have sustained the group work through the early challenges if we had not had that foundational relationship piece that came from reading *Calling the Circle* and then having first Sarah and then Sarah and Ann Linnea come and give us 'tune-ups' on circle practice. Each time we refocus on circle work, it strengthens what we are doing. It helps us on our own steep learning curve, coming out of our hierarchical training and expectation. And we are still circle novices.

"Even in the charter school movement, we are on the fringe. Most other charter schools in New Jersey are urban. They are working to create a safe haven where inner-city kids can begin to get acceptable test scores. We are mostly working with children who have clothes, food, and a warm house who are lost and wandering in a different yet very real way. They live in a culture that is too often a wasteland of consumerism and media-paced communication—and they don't fit. If we can raise children capable of working and living in nontraditional ways, maybe the human crisis we're in won't be endlessly perpetuated."

Dave agrees wholeheartedly.

"Ridge and Valley is a complex mirror of an equally complex society. What sustains us as an organization is that we have children who are happy and eager to attend school. Most parents are really on board about creating and growing a school where children are respected, cherished, and able to develop a joy for living successfully in the larger world. The guides are doing stunning things with their students. And now we have a leadership team that is learning to work together."

Working for their children and on behalf of all children keeps Traci, Kerry, Dave, and Nanci going through trying times. And all four concur that working in circle has created a core dynamic of love, trust, and respect among trustees and administrators. This is the paradigm shift as they see it now: power struggles, shadow elements, and the pressures for the school to meet state requirements are always present and are counterbalanced with the strength of their relationships from years of working through issues in circle process.

People expect to have to battle their point forward in a typical hierarchical setting. Parents come to a school board meeting riled up and ready to fight. At Ridge and Valley, if something is being overlooked, people can slip into an aggressive attitude and <u>abandon the principle of assuming each other's good intentions.</u> Everyone from children to parents to teachers (guides) to leadership team to trustees is working to understand and implement a circular, rotating leadership way of being, and the learning curve is not always smooth.

Sarah and Ann serve as "on call" consultants who work with Ridge and Valley to help people clear accumulated misunderstandings and refresh circle skills. When they make visitations to coach circle practice, they usually address several issues:

- ◉ Reminding everyone that circle-based governance is an attitude and practice of consistency—and looking for any relational places where things have gotten gummed up

- ◉ Helping people refine the process to fit their needs now, recognizing that an agreement that worked three years ago may not fit today or that they may need to strengthen a line of communication—as between the leadership team and parents—so that all parties know how to get concerns expressed and responded to

- ◉ Honoring the groundbreaking nature of what they are doing and helping them keep the larger perspective so that the daily trials are held within the visionary choice they have made

Sarah, a former high school biology teacher who did her doctoral dissertation investigating how circle can transform the field of education, speaks to their roles:

"The school is large enough to act as an organization of incredible complexity and is small enough that almost everyone feels a sense of ownership and stake in the outcome. Children are eager for increasing variety in their educational journeys. Parents are advocating for the particular needs of their children. Teachers want increased curriculum support. Administrators are handling the fiduciary responsibilities along with the daily operations and management. And all this occurs within an environment in which roles are being redefined while responsibilities need to be consistently maintained. Collaborative administration and self-governance is not easy. And the longer and more deeply Ridge and Valley lives this shift, the greater their expectations are for themselves."

Nanci says:

"One of the hardest things about really being a pioneer is that we haven't had another school to look to for help. We are literally making it up as we go. Now we are established enough that we can begin reaching out to other parents and teachers with a dream and say, we made it, here's what worked for us, and we have a sound academic curriculum housed in the delights of nature."

A recent Ridge and Valley graduate was accepted into an elite private high school. She was excited to attend the daylong orientation but came home disappointed in her experience. She reported to her parents that the entire day had been spent in an auditorium listening to speeches, and she had not gotten to know a single other student. She could not understand why they had not done some interactive games and sat everyone in a circle.

In the long run, this will be the great challenge for Ridge and Valley: How will its students translate their early educational experience as they transition into more traditional higher education and the workplace? Will they find in themselves the leadership capacities their parents and guides hope they are grooming them for? Will they find in themselves the courage needed to march to a different drummer? And will they and the community that guides them now be there to call circles of support for building a world modeled and valued in the haven of Ridge and Valley Charter School?

True North Health Care Center

The holistic True North Health Care Center, in Falmouth, Maine, was founded in 2002 as a 501(c)3 nonprofit after a loose association of determined nurses, alternative and complementary practitioners, doctors, Catholic sisters, and technicians met for four years in circle to realize this dream. The center currently consists of a team of dedicated professionals, ranging from physicians to massage therapists, all working in an 8,200-square-foot facility. The facility has ten examination and treatment rooms, a patient resource area with high-speed Internet access, two conference rooms for classes and workshops, and a teaching kitchen where a natural foods chef demonstrates healthy cooking during weekend workshops. People are drawn here either because they are coping with difficult health issues that allopathic medicine or a specific alternative therapy has not resolved or because they are healthy and want to stay that way.

In the formative years before the clinic, Kathryn Landon-Malone, a pediatric nurse practitioner, came across the first edition of *Calling the Circle* and introduced the concepts to the group. "We met twice a month at 7:30 A.M. in the basement of Mercy Hospital in Portland, Maine. Parallel growth processes were going on in many of our lives. There was such tremendous energy in those early meetings; we knew that even if we only checked in, our workdays would be different."

The group dedicated itself to creating a plan for Mercy to launch an inpatient arm of alternative services that the hospital ultimately rejected for monetary reasons. However, this planning circle had become determined to find a way to offer a holistic health care practice to the Portland community. In 2002, using circle as their organizing principle, a broad range of practitioners opened the current center. Medical director Bethany Hays eagerly proclaims, "We use the circle for everything here—our board of directors, our bimonthly meetings with the entire staff, our weekly decision circle. We have found that circle nourishes relationships, and we believe that there is nothing more important than relationships in medicine and health care. Relationships are as necessary as air, water, movement, love, and food. So much of our health care system consists of broken relationships, and circle offers hope to heal this."

Hays brings over thirty years of medical practice to True North, with a specialty in obstetrics and gynecology. She practices functional medicine, which focuses on primary prevention and underlying causes rather than what she calls "symptom fixes." Functional medicine uses the patient story as a key tool in diagnosis and treatment—a ready complement to circle.

True North has been able to apply and adapt PeerSpirit Circle Process based on the original book and their own experience. Although Christina has spoken on narrative medicine at several of True North's conferences, we have not consulted with the group and have celebrated the center's ability to learn on its own. Several current and former staff members offer circle training to other medical practices and are conducting qualitative and quantitative research on the impact of circle in health care settings.

At True North, circle begins with four deep breaths followed by a round of check-in of varying length, depending on time and agenda. Organizers don't appoint a guardian unless they know they're tackling a challenging issue. They use both talking piece and open conversation and seem to organically know when to pick up the talking piece to make sure every voice is being heard. They vote using thumbs up, down, and sideways and decide everything by consensus minus one. Bethany explains:

> "I think it's critical to hear from the people who vote no. We move forward if there is only a single dissent so that one person can't co-opt the work of the circle. (We do, however, ensure that the circle member who is dissenting feels heard before moving on.) We use the circle to accomplish real work, and we need to stand by our decisions, so if we have two no votes, we keep hashing things out."

The center currently has twenty-three practitioners, ranging from specialists in energy medicine to three family practice physicians. A staff of ten supports these practitioners. Over time, the clinic's team commitment to operating entirely in circle grew unwieldy—especially as the scope and scale of True North's work had grown. So in 2007, executive director Tom Dahlborg, who came to the clinic from a more traditional career in health care management, helped design a "circle process survey" to gather information on how circle management might be redesigned for increased relevance. Hays explained, "One survey comment pretty much summed things up: 'Our system is inefficient and cumbersome. There are too many chiefs and not enough accountability. Circle process generally makes more work for staff that are already overloaded.'" So True North, which had based its entire operational organization on circle, began to question the "sacred cow" of circle.

This is a moment of empowerment in a collaborative organization. The founders had designed a structure, lived it, and were experienced enough to redesign it. Tom Dahlborg and Chris Bicknell Marden, director of marketing and development, who both provide support for practitioners—physicians, nurses, technicians, massage therapists, and nutritionists—were members of the long-standing decision circle, where it was decided that the survey results would be tallied and the process reviewed. The decision circle is made up of administrative staff and practitioners who are committed to weekly oversight and confidentiality. Because it handles personnel decisions, it is the only circle not fully transparent. "The decision circle is the place where we have traditionally had the most revealing conversations because a large nucleus of that group has been together a long time and we really trust each other," explained Chris. In powerful councils, the decision circle asked the hard questions: Do we want to keep using circle? In what ways is it effective? In what ways is it ineffective? What do we keep? What do we let go of? Can we make circle and hierarchy work together?

Kathryn noted that many conversations focused on the importance of the relationship and community-building aspects of circle.

> "Circle has taught us how to be better practitioners. As we have developed heart-centered relationships with one another, we are better able to be in 'reverent participatory relationships' with our patients. That is the direct result of circle. Because we work consistently in a circle way, we work differently with our funders, vendors, and patients than most health care systems. We are relationship-oriented. We know how to listen. We can elicit the story of a medical history."

This is not typical language in a health care system. And while highly valued, the practical and business aspects of the clinic needed tending. Chris continued, "We needed a streamlining process behind the scenes. These conversations took us right into our shadow stuff. It was not fun, and we learned some important things."

Both Kathryn Landon-Malone and Bethany Hays cited the importance of the teaching they had received from Christina when she had addressed the True North conference several years earlier. Responding to questions about how to respond to conflict, Christina said, "When you feel the circle wobble, don't abandon the form—lean in and trust it." In the middle of decision circle conversations emphasizing greater time and money efficiency, it would have been easy to blame circle process and make it a scapegoat rather than using circle to find ways to balance the values of relationship with time management, efficiency, and fiscal responsibility.

"I find conflict very challenging," said Chris. "Some of these meetings I walked into with a knot in my stomach and almost always left feeling relieved. I noticed that dealing with conflict in an authentic and heart-centered way allowed us to get to the heart of the matter quickly instead of getting stuck in personality challenges."

As the decision circle met week after week in late 2007, a recurring theme was the need for order and efficiency without sacrificing the relational gifts of circle. The key to unlocking the apparent polarity between circle and hierarchy was the idea that the circle and the triangle (hierarchy) were meant to work together. Hierarchy separated from circle leads to isolated leaders making decisions with limited input. Hierarchy combined with circle establishes a collaborative environment where input concerning impact and consequences is gathered, and leaders feel empowered to act by the whole organization.

Using their commitment to "reverent participatory relationship" and the True North circle process, the decision circle listened carefully to its participants over a period of several months. On November 29, 2007, a document titled "Evolution of Circle at True North" was finalized by the decision circle and then approved by all staff and practitioners. A number of changes to the existing system resulted, including the following:

- Creation of a "connector circle"

- Creation of a leadership triangle consisting of the board, the medical director, and the executive director

- A clear delineation of existing circle responsibilities and meeting frequencies

- Procedures to balance work time in circle with work time to accomplish key tasks

- Encouragement of staff independence

Each of the existing nine circles at True North now has a designated circle connector. Circle connectors are point persons for questions, insights, concerns, and communications. Each of these individuals belongs to a connector circle. A connector at True North may belong to anywhere from two to eight of these circles, which meet anywhere from once a week to three times a year, depending on their function. It may still sound cumbersome to outsiders, but what Dahlborg and the decision circle have done is clarify and structure the kinds of meetings that go on in organizations that usually remain unnamed.

These changes to the existing system can be seen in the True North Circle Connectivity (see Figure 11.1) and the Public Trust Hierarchical Chart (see Figure 11.2). True North's new organizational charts contain some elements of a traditional system, such as a board of directors working directly with a medical and executive director, with each element of that triangle sharing equal power.

"The fact that we designed two separate charts is significant," explained Dahlborg. "They say pretty much the same thing, but in different ways for different people. Those who come from a more circular perspective prefer the True North Circle Connectivity diagram, which rounds out the necessary legal, hierarchical connection between our nonprofit board of directors, medical director

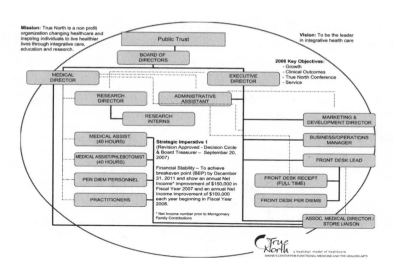

FIGURE 11.1

Hays and practitioners, and myself and support staff. Some members of the True North staff find the Public Trust Hierarchical Chart to be clearer and more precise. We wanted to offer both versions."

During the reevaluation process, the decision circle tallied the number of hours each staff member had been spending in circle meetings and the num-

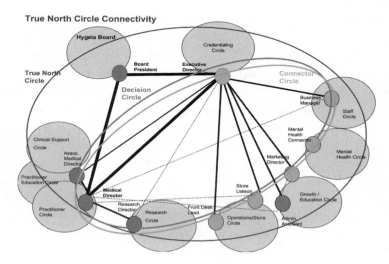

FIGURE 11.2

ber of hours each staff member would now be spending in circle meetings under the evolved model. Under the earlier system, the yearly cost of wages for staff and practitioners to attend circle meetings came to $492,000. Under the evolved model, costs are $360,000, for a savings of $132,000. "These figures represent our best effort to quantify time spent in meetings," explained Tom. "This is a useful accounting for any organization, whether meetings take place in a more hierarchical form or in circle as they do at True North."

True North has worked diligently to examine its inner workings. The openness of its process is a tribute to the organizers' genuine belief in the statement from their Web site: "We feel that circle process is healing our multidisciplinary wounds and that it is the container for the momentum of our strong and fearless group to nurture a professional experience that is beyond our wildest dreams (and keeps getting better). The continuous work of the circle has provided us with the most functional place we have ever worked, where we have fun and take risks because of the trust we have in each other and in spirit."

People at True North acknowledge that looking critically at circle process allowed them to develop an evolved version that better suits "who we are now." For Tom, the combination of good business practices, continuous process improvement, and a heart-centered approach is what makes True North a powerful place.

Reflections

We have watched these colleagues and many others adapt and refine circle to fit a wide variety of settings and applications and still hold the integrity of PeerSpirit's basic infrastructure. We made a decision at the start of our work not to trademark our adaptation of such a universal process and social lineage or to certify facilitators. We have practiced honoring our teachers, sources, and circle's lineage itself and relied on other people's willingness to do the same as they have carried circle process into their own words and work. We have counted on people practicing at the edge of their confidence and learning as they go—as have we. By and large, this has served us all well. We are delighted to offer so many stories of people who have read about PeerSpirit Circle Process and thought, *I can do this.* They tried it, and it worked, and they have figured out how to keep working with circle—with and without our engagement. We consider this a huge indicator of the circle's resilience and capacity to adapt to an ever-changing world.

12

Circle as a Way of Life

Once upon a time, circle was the core of human culture. That time has come round again in a new evolution. The circle way is a take-it-home, take-it-to-work, try-it-anywhere practice. Circle is a life skill with the power to sustain both intimacy and cultural change.

Hurrying through the chaos of the world's busyness, circle offers us opportunities to sit down with each other in the round, to ring the bell and quiet our hearts and minds, and to enter the spaciousness to speak and listen to one another as we find our way forward. This amazing capacity is available to anyone, at any time, with any group of people. Anyone who has read this far now understands how to host the social container; how to place an inviting question into the center, pass a talking piece, pause, and receive people's responses.

We live the circle way one conversation at a time, one group at a time. Through incremental daily changes of mind-set and behavior that make the world around us a friendlier place, we see how the tenets of the circle way can emerge:

- *The circle way is relational.* It occurs wherever people create an intentional social space of compassion and curiosity.

- *The circle way is inclusive and adaptable.* It seeks to restore principles of belonging and to find meaningful ways for everyone to contribute.

183

○ *The circle way is a synthesis of our human journey.* It can occur now because we have the full story of our origins and history, increasingly global literacy, and an interconnected world.

Learning circle is an adventure. We can learn through careful, step-by-step instruction, or we can learn by jumping in and trying it. We can go on to use circle skills in complex situations, or we can enjoy circle as an occasional venture beyond the norm. Circle is like dropping a round, smooth stone into the waters of the social pond. The stories in this final chapter are intended as an invitation and an inspiration to begin incorporating circle and its inherently collaborative way of being into ever-widening circles of application and rings of influence in our lives.

Couples and the Circle Way

It has been our experience that using circle within a partnership greatly enhances communication and supports mutually beneficial outcomes. This example speaks of marriage, but there are many forms of personal and professional partnerships in which similar rituals of communication are needed and could apply.

One of the major causes of miscommunication between partners is introducing a conversation without the time or social container to actually have the conversation. We call this "drive-by commentary," and it can become a way of life for busy, working people. On the way out the door, one partner says to the other, "Honey, we have to talk about finances. See you this evening." Coffee cup is set on the counter, and before the other partner can ask, "Is everything OK?" the first one's gone.

The receiver of this news may respond with fear, defensiveness, or a sense of helplessness or impending doom. When the conversation does occur, it tends to start off with a lot of confusion because so much ambiguity has been generated. And even if the news is good, enough tension has accumulated that each partner tends to have a defensive edge and difficulty hearing the other.

In couples retreat weekends, we give each couple some training in circle structure, an empty basket, and time to create their own agreements, intention, and an informal agenda of what issues they need to talk about. They are invited to fill the basket with meaningful objects for their centerpiece.

Sam and Krista had been married for three decades, raised two children, and were enjoying their two young grandchildren. Both were accomplished professionals at the height of their careers. Drive-by commentary had become habitual—especially during the last years of child rearing, negotiating their work schedule and overseeing the extracurricular lives of two teens. The kids went off to college and then launched into adulthood, and Sam and Krista filled in the spaces with increasingly demanding twelve- to fourteen-hour workdays. Things were OK between them, but they had lost the sense that they were building a life and a life story together.

Krista said, "We wanted something back, a kind of spark, and a sense that we were each other's best friend—and at fifty-five, it's a whole different scene than at twenty-five or thirty-five. We couldn't go back, and we didn't know how to go forward. I wanted to go to therapy, and Sam said, 'Why? Nothing's wrong. If we go to therapy, they'll just find something wrong.' He had a point. So we signed up for a woodsy circle weekend retreat."

Their presenting intention was to practice circle by speaking and listening honestly, making clear decisions, and catching up on what was going on under the surface in each other's lives. They decided to call each other into circle once a week. We suggested a format where each partner would speak uninterrupted for a designated period of time, be responded to by the listener, and then switch roles. After these long check-ins, they could go into conversation council, discuss whatever was needed between them, and check out with a statement of understanding of what they'd learned or committed to. They established several guidelines for themselves (Exhibit 12.1).

No deserting the conversation unless the house is burning down. Their circle ritual is simple. He gets the basket and lays out the center: a small cloth, a few photos, and an heirloom silver spoon for a talking piece. She lights the candle; he rings the bell. They have a brief discussion about what needs to happen next: how long they can be in circle and whether or not their general check-in needs to be followed by specific topics. Sam rings the bell again, and they both

EXHIBIT 12.1

Working Agreements for Couples
○ Make sure we have time to start and finish.
○ Make sure we are both awake and present.
○ Turn off the cell phones.
○ Get comfortable.
○ No interruptions during each other's opening monologues.

sit quietly for a moment. One of them picks up the spoon, and the other sets a little kitchen timer, usually for ten minutes. They each take turns holding the talking piece and expressing everything they can think of about what's going on in their lives. At the end of the ten minutes (which sometimes contains some significant pauses for thinking), the other person spends several minutes reflecting what was heard and asking questions. Then they reverse roles. Once they have each spoken, they place the spoon on the coffee table between them and begin an open conversation about their check-ins and any topics they have cited. They do their best to wind things down in the allotted time—ringing a bell to close the space and returning the circle basket to its place on the dresser.

"I had no idea how hard it would be to say something about myself for ten minutes," Sam reports. "I wasn't tapped into anything underneath my to-do list. Krista would be sitting there. I'd say, 'I'm fine. What else do you want to know?' And she'd smile at me and ask quietly, 'What do you want me to know?' We cut these opening exchanges to five minutes, and then I eventually discovered enough story inside myself to extend the time—and so did she. You get so out of the habit of going into anything in detail because there never seems to be time for anyone to hear the detail. That's the habit we had to change. And we did. We know each other better than ever, and that's pretty great."

The stability that comes from the exchange of sharing story, sharing thoughts and feelings and doubts, is the reward for circle in partnerships. The important components are there: having a beginning and an ending point and an agreed time for meeting, giving each person uninterrupted time to check in as deeply as possible and for the other to listen and then exchange a few minutes of mirroring back what was heard. We have often suggested that people keep a small notebook in their basket and a log of their councils—just a few sentences that leave a map of the conversation or a question to be considered the next time.

As elsewhere, the right question can be a powerful invocation in couples' circles. The son of some friends called us in near tears. "I think my girlfriend is about to break up with me, and I don't want to lose her. We're just not communicating, and I'm doing the best I can. What can I do?"

We thought for a minute, and then a question came to mind. "Create a quiet place with no distractions, and ask her this question," Christina prompted. "'What do you need me to know right now so I can love you better?' See what happens next."

Families and the Circle Way

The challenge of careful listening is magnified in a family setting because there are more people of more ages and more interests. Ann began trying circle with her children when they were teenagers. She set up specific times and protocols for having "conversations of consequence." She soon discovered that when she announced that they would be having a circle, both her teens gave each other that "What did we do now?" look.

Realizing her mistake, Ann stopped using circle at home for a few months. Then she introduced the idea of appreciation circles to Brian and Sally. Once a month, they would all sit after dinner with a candle and a talking piece resting in the middle of the dining room table. When they were ready, one at a time, they would reach for the talking piece and share a story or comment that showed their appreciation for each other member of the family. These experiences were short and often humorous, and they restored the positive impression of circle.

About that same time, Brian came home from yet another soccer game loss in the midst of a miserable season. The sport was a new addition at his high school, and the team was pitted against more experienced teams from bigger schools. "Hey, Mom," he yelled from the kitchen. "I tried that circle stuff with the team, and I think it worked. We lost another game, and the coach asked me to cheer everyone up—to keep us going for the next few weeks. So I put us all in a huddle and asked, 'What's the most important thing we're learning this fall—that's not about winning and losing?' I used the soccer ball for a talking piece, and I didn't know what to use for a centerpiece, so I just stood there myself." Mother and son high-fived each other.

Christina's mother is a vibrant eighty-nine-year-old at the writing of this book. Partly because she has always appeared more youthful than her age, when she turned seventy-five, she requested that her family create a ritual to mark her passage into her elder years. Children, grandchildren, and spouses gathered from Alaska, Washington, and Wisconsin at the Minneapolis home of Connie's older son, Carl.

Together the four siblings, spouses, and six grandchildren created two concentric rings of yarn on the rug of the family den: a red one for the blood line and a green one for those related by marriage. Connie sat in the center. In this appreciation circle, everyone held a carnation and was invited to share a story that honored the family matriarch. Some of the stories were humorous; some were poignant. By the time each story had been told, Connie held a bouquet of flowers. She then shared some reflections on aging and the importance of honoring the voice of elders.

About this same time, Christina regularly hosted "Auntie Camp" for her nieces—four little girls sitting cross-legged on the floor, each one speaking through the voice of a favorite stuffed animal. "Little Tiger says . . . ," "Bearie Bearie says . . ." It was a hilarious check-in full of giggles; even the animals were amused at themselves. What got said during these evenings has disappeared from memory, but the importance of circle in family life has remained. These nieces, now in their twenties, remain willing participants whenever Auntie Christina rings the bell.

Friends and family attend birthdays, weddings, retirements, and anniversaries wanting to honor whoever is being celebrated and to make authentic connection with people they probably don't see very often. The addition of circle creates a container to hold the intentions people bring and their desire to connect more deeply than social banter. Several examples of family ritual have already been presented in these pages.

When Ann's grandson, Jaden, turned four, his parents, Sally and Joe, invited his preschool friends to a local park for bouncing in an inflatable palace, face painting, a Batman piñata, and cake. Afterward, the young family of three, plus three grandparents, an aunt, a friend, and a cousin, all gathered in their apartment. People carried in many gifts from the party and set them in the middle of the living room carpet. Jaden sat down next to his presents and announced, "I want everyone to sit in a circle." We smiled and willingly obeyed. Then the little host announced, "Now I want us to hold hands."

"OK, Mom, he's a convert," laughed Sally. "They do this every morning in preschool, and he sees that people pay better attention if you gather them this way."

Neighbors and the Circle Way

Cynthia Trenshaw likes to tell the story of how she created a circle to address some of the deeper questions about aging that were beginning to nag at her as a sixty-year-old in a new community. After a year or so getting to know a variety of people, Cynthia gathered a small group of new friends and formally created a PeerSpirit circle to address questions of aging. Five years later, the group still meets twice a month. "We are continuously amazed and amused at how we came together, how we have grown, and how deep our individual roots have sunk into the soil of circle. We are now fourteen men and women, aged forty-something to seventy-something—four couples, four singles, and two partnered people who are in the circle without their partners."

Fourteen members has proved to be a good number for ensuring that enough people are always present to sustain the conversation and not so large that it's impossible to remember all the stories. The group operates with a rotating host, guardian, and scribe. Once a year, at a potluck, they think up topical questions of interest and lay out the conversational map for the next twelve months. They hold an annual retreat at a small local conference facility and use the time to share stories and activities that would not fit in their usual two-hour meeting format. They cook together, experiment with arts and crafts projects, enjoy silence and reading, and do whatever else strikes their fancy.

Group members have shared deep conversations about living well and dying well. They have helped each other write advance directives and letters to families explaining their wishes. "We have had to go down some tough roads with one another," explained Cynthia. "We didn't have too much trouble talking about the nitty-gritty stuff of tending to someone who is ill, but when individual members have needed bedside care, we discovered that we are not actually very good at it. We are not trained professionals, and that's OK. We had to learn the boundaries with respect to what we can and cannot do."

In one situation, a husband and wife became seriously ill at the same time. The man had been the steady caregiver in the pair, so when he got ill, the Circle of Caring was called to a new level of commitment, offering help with meals and hospital visitations and organizing professional assistance. "That was a pivotal time for us," explained Cynthia.

"People got stretched pretty thin, and only coming back to circle and talking about these challenges got us through.

"We are supporting each other in what are literally life-and-death topics, and it requires that we do our work around shadow. That's become a term we all know. There have been moments halfway through a long check-in when there was so much tension in the room, I couldn't imagine how we would get through something and leave one another at the end of the evening with a sense of peace. We aren't usually confrontational; rather, we have learned an increasing tolerance for the things in each of us that are not going to change. And we use the center profoundly—that's where our tolerance for each other's personalities resides."

Not surprisingly, the circle has had requests from others who would like to join. Members have handled this by sponsoring several new local groups, and in 2004, Cynthia wrote a booklet on the subject, *Harvest of Years: A PeerSpirit Guide for Proactive Aging Circles.* When a Seattle newspaper story on the group went national, we received hundreds of orders for the booklet, and Cynthia became a telephone circle coach and occasional conference speaker.

Community and the Circle Way

In August 2008, public interest consultant Jim Neale traveled from Halifax, Nova Scotia, to Whidbey Island, Washington, to take the Circle Practicum. A few weeks later, having returned home, he had a great opportunity to try out his new skills. For the past several years, residents of a small agricultural village (established in 1674, population 600) near Halifax had struggled with the question of whether an abandoned rail line which had been converted into a trail that ran through the community should be open to use by motorized vehicles. Many residents were opposed, believing that the community was better served by preserving a serene space suitable for bicycling and safe for the many seniors to walk. Others favored motorized use by all-terrain vehicles whose drivers wanted to access hundreds of kilometers of other trails already open to ATVs, to boost tourism in the region, and to provide a wider range of recreation options.

The issue had created a palpable rift in the community. Discussions began to take place mostly among small special-interest groups. In any "mixed" sessions, residents faced aggressive oppositional views and quickly fell silent. No progress was made over nine months of community meetings. People lapsed into frustration, polarization, exhaustion, and the belief that a good resolution wasn't possible. Jim reported:

> "I was asked to develop a process for the conversations and then facilitate them, ideally producing a consensus (it would never be unanimous) view for trail use and for how to begin a sense of social healing. Having just returned from a PeerSpirit Practicum fully jazzed about

the fruits of circle and eager to give it a try, I was game to experiment. I was also careful to harmonize the approach with the more conservative nature of the community.

"I developed a process that started with consultations with community representatives to envision the kind of community they wanted and to establish the more fundamental and common intention for the community. What emerged was a clear desire for a strong and united community, honoring its long traditions of neighbors helping neighbors."

Jim discovered a shared value for a community that had been harmed by the outbursts of diverse opinion. This is a common consequence in settings where there has not been a group process in place that could deal effectively with differences of opinion. Jim set about trying to rectify the situation by designing a series of three circles, one for each of the three primary special-interest groups:

- Individuals who owned land adjacent to the trail, who would be most affected by the decision

- Hikers

- Motorized vehicle users

He wanted to create an opportunity where people could become comfortable expressing their views without concern about confrontation. After each of the three circles had occurred, he offered a fourth circle for the entire community, where the practiced viewpoints could now be brought forward for the benefit of the whole.

He described the circle process this way:

"In each preparatory circle, we established a center that reflected the shared vision for the community as a town of neighbors helping neighbors. The center point was an antique bowl (representing the long and colorful history of the village) that began empty to represent a 'fresh start.' After checking in, we spent a little time role-playing some of the behaviors people might expect to see in the large circle as they addressed this emotional issue (quiet anger, rage, protectiveness of more frail residents, and so on). The role-plays gave people a chance to put the behaviors they were concerned about out front, ham it up, laugh a little, and become more able to recognize these behaviors and then practice calling for the bell."

This was a creative way to dispel the shadow—to give people an opportunity to play with their own and each other's impulses for control. Then Jim led people into practicing clear statements and neutral language so that they would be confident in their ability to maintain focus and make their point in the midst of whatever energies were swirling in the container of the larger group. He would be the host and guardian and enforce the etiquette of circle process. One of the skills Jim brought into this community process was his ability to coach each of the polarized interest groups and offer each of them a sense that they had his support in making positive contributions to the conversation.

Then came the open circle for all interested community members. Throughout the circle time, Jim invited participants to write their hopes, concerns, and ideas for community healing on small cards and deposit them in the center bowl. He later said, "I did this in part to provide a private and very safe avenue to express views (which proved to be very important to some of the more senior participants), and also, as the bowl filled, the presence of intention grew in strength, scope, and importance—and to my amazement, converged toward a more shared aspiration for the village."

One of the participants, an elderly woman with terminal cancer, lived very close to the trail. The quieter environment needed for her care appeared incompatible with motorized use. "Many of the residents had become involved in this issue to protect her right to live in a health-preserving setting," Jim said.

"As this woman told her story, it became clear that the rift in the community was also a cause of pain for her and that her deepest wish was for reconciliation and healing. She surprised everyone by announcing that for that reason, she was going to support reopening the trail to vehicles.

"She offered a clear and present challenge to the circle that compelled compromise and creativity to find the best possible solution. It was a magnificent breakthrough moment. They reframed what the trail was: not an old rail line but a community commons—shared land. Closing the trail to motorized use would prevent members of the community from using a village commons and was therefore not consistent with the vision they held of a united community. Opening the trail through these conversations of shared hope and sensitivity became the only acceptable conclusion."

This is an example of the alchemy of circle: a conclusion is discovered that no one walked in with, that seems to have grown out of the group process itself. At the end of the evening, Jim reported:

"The session went exceptionally well—like nothing the residents (or I) had experienced before when addressing divisive issues within a small, close, and very conservative community. A strong consensus view emerged that included better understandings, beginnings of real forgiveness, a fresh faith that they could work together to bring about a good end result, and acceptance of the need to move forward even when some people are going to be disappointed by the outcome. Circle provided an extremely powerful alternative to conversations of self-interest and reinforced basic community values."

The townspeople felt resolved, but Jim was still nervous. The actual owner of the rail bed, and the entity that had commissioned Jim to lead this process, was the provincial Department of Natural Resources (DNR). Upon reporting the results, Jim was concerned that the minister, a political representative, might choose to decide in favor of more powerful minority interests and override the consensus wishes of the community. In that case, dynamics would not simply revert to the previous state; they'd be worse. "Having raised the expectations of citizens, if the DNR made a political choice, it would deepen distrust of government and the malaise of residents. This would be a concern in any organizationally based circle work I can imagine doing, where group progress could be overturned by a higher authority." While this is a worthy caution, in this case, the consensus recommendation was accepted, the trail reopened, and healing began.

Circle is a portable craft. To almost every meeting she attends, Christina carries *tingsha* bells, a talking piece, and an ability to synthesize thematic conversational threads. Ann brings her listening ear, a kitchen timer, and an ability to ask the question that opens the door to personal storytelling.

People know when they're not being respectful of one another. Almost everyone has enough skill to help bring a situation back to productiveness if a tiny opening appears. Circle as community intervention can be a whole process, carefully thought out as Jim modeled, or some aspect of circle can be introduced into a moment where it's needed. We just need patience to watch for the moment when an intervention will most likely work and the courage to assume a bit of leadership.

At a gathering to address the future of a local landmark, Christina was standing against the back wall in a large crowd. At one point, there were many community members talking over one another. To gain the attention of the moderators, she loudly rang the *tingsha* bells she carried in her jacket pocket. People were so surprised at the high resonating sound that everyone stopped talking for a few seconds. The pause gave her a chance to say, "I rang the bell because I can't hear what anyone is saying when everyone is talking at once. Could we go back to raising hands and waiting for the moderator to call on us?" People complied, and order was restored. The moderator looked relieved.

Twenty minutes later, the energy in the room had again increased, and people were interrupting one another to get their opinion or question expressed. Someone from the audience called out, "Where is that lady with the bells?" Obligingly, Christina rang them again.

From the back of the room, without any role in the proceedings other than that of an interested citizen, she could not call this town meeting to order—but she could call it to pause, and in that pause, the possibility for order rests in the hands of the majority. There is the opportunity for civility to prevail, for leadership to swirl out of the crowd and to insist that the underlying values of community and neighborliness be carried through the conversational thread. Jim Neale and the citizens of his Nova Scotia town practiced civility; the Kufunda villagers in Zimbabwe practiced it; the church that surrounded Pastor Larry practiced it. Just as the wisdom we need is in the room, the core values we need are in the room and can remind us who we are.

Circle works in the world we have. It works in the concentric rings around our lives at work, at home, and in our communities. And it is the deepest prayer of this book that hundreds, thousands, and tens of thousands of self-empowered circle practitioners will call on circle to work in the world of the future.

The Future and the Circle Way

When you leave this book, you will have acquired the tools to make a better world—certainly to make your own personal world better. Better in what ways? We don't know; you know. Sit down and talk your dreams into being so that your actions are clear and grounded in strong principles. The promise that we made—that we can mold and change the world of human interaction to fit our needs—is true.

The ecophilosopher Joanna Macy refers to the time we are living in as the "Great Turning." She says in a video on her Web site, "The Great Turning is a name for the essential adventure of our time: the shift from the industrial growth society to a life-sustaining civilization." The concept is echoed by Thomas Berry, who refers to it as the "Great Work." It is taught in college courses. E. F. Schumacher references it in his "Small Is Beautiful" movement. The alternative economist David Korten has written a book titled *The Great Turning: From Empire to Earth Community*. We are all living in an experience larger than our ability to perceive, swallowed into the light and shadow of our turning times.

In the early 1990s, we became aware that circle process was coming through a number of voices and lineage streams. In the early 2000s, we became aware that a culture of conversation was going global through a number of circle-based methodologies and variations. Now we are aware that a community of visionary social scientists is calling forth the next stage of social evolution. Macy says this is the third great revolution. "The 'life-sustaining society' that is emerging," Macy says, "needs structures that are deeply rooted in common human values and resilient enough to take us into the future."

We would like to nominate the circle as a structure for helping us safely make this turn. Everything and anything we do with circle today, tomorrow, and in reaction to reading this book is practice for holding on to our civility in the chaos of enormous change.

The image of the Great Turn empowers everyone: everyone can turn. We can make daily turns in our lives that head us toward the life-sustaining society, and then we can take leadership in our spheres of influence to help others take turns toward such a society.

Put a dozen people in the circle and ask the question "What is coming?" and we get a dozen answers. Technological marvels? Social collapse? The fifth great extinction or the next great leap for humankind? Put a hundred people into circles, and we get a hundred answers.

We don't know, and we have choices to make and things to do despite our not knowing.

Circle gives us space to sit down in our not knowing, to hear each other out, and to hold on to the story while taking the next step forward. Circle gives us a container for receiving difference without doing violence to one another. The skills of hosting, of guardianship, of participation and leadership from the rim are among the most needed skills of the age. Circle holds us in the great work we have to do.

The circle is a seed of human civilization. It has existed since the dawn of our time here. Tremendous changes have swirled around this tenacious gift to humanity. Wars have raged. Armies have conquered. People have nearly died out and then multiplied wildly. And all the while, our understanding of circle has continued to grow, strengthen, and adapt. Circle has waited time and again for someone to put a common intention in the middle, to pass the talking piece, and to create a listening space that calls forth people's good hearts and willingness to cooperate. We know how to do this. The youngest among us have always known. The oldest among us have remembered.

The way forward is seeded in the way we stop, what we will consider, and then what we do as a result. As we lean into this ancient lineage, our work in circle is to create the world we want within the world we have. Circle and its components are the seeds. Circle is the pattern.

We have changed the chairs. Now we can change the world.

Circle in the Heart of Stone

Christina Baldwin

There is a river cottage that has been in a friend's family for generations, a summer home for the city folks built by the country cousins.

There is a ritual for getting here—a circuitous meandering off the interstate through several small towns, taking sharp-angled turns at the edges of cornfields, down one county road and then another, no street signs, a route they all know in their blood, and I by acquaintanceship and a lucky sense of direction.

There is a ritual for getting here—the driveway unmarked, a quarter mile of sandy parallel tire tracks between Grandpa Zimmer's cornfield and the stand of scrub oak he cut for firewood before central heating came to the white frame house that sits on the rise at river's edge.

There is a ritual for getting here—because in the middle of this drive there hides the remains of a granite boulder and everyone who comes, be they family or friend, must ease their car over this slab rock without gutting the mechanics and bleeding oil or gasoline on the sand. The rock is part of the ritual. You learn to turn at the white flag and go slow over that rock, or you'll be getting the tow truck to take you back to town.

The boulder is navigable now, though I've watched my friend drop to her knees in an auto showroom and gauge the distance from floor to chassis, seeing this heirloom rock in her mind and not buying a new car that couldn't make it to the cottage.

The boulder is navigable now because, summer after summer, when it was the size of a bathtub, as long and as high, Grandpa Zimmer spent his evenings straddling rock and working away at the surface with a diamond-headed auger, drilling small, round circles into the surface of the stone. And autumn after autumn, when the freeze came, Grandpa Zimmer filled those holes with buckets of river water. And winter after winter, the ice did its work and blew up more of his boulder. Bit by bit. Water set on stone.

Water crystals expanding against granite seem no match for each other, yet the soft, burbling river sets to its winter task: persistent, changing form to meet the need. The need here, in the bowel of the rock, is to bore within, to be the circle in the center of the stone.

It is autumn on our planet. We stand in the middle of great change and cannot see what transformation is coming any more than the river can see itself cooling at the end of summer.

The boulder is the patriarchal way; the auger is the energy of circle boring into granite; and you and I are the water at work. You and I are the water, willing to set ourselves to the next task.

You and I are the water, H_2O, the molecular heart of the planet. Eighty percent of everything on earth is water. You and I are the water. We are the majority of everything. We can be steam, be river, be rain and rainbow. We can be ice, talking to the granite one molecule at a time, convincing the rock to let go, to let itself be slivered: to be slivered small enough to be carried by water, to become sand, to rest on the banks of a river.

Come sit with me on this boulder. We will take turns boring the auger into stone. It is not such hard work when more than one is working. We will tell each other stories. We will help each other with the tasks of our lives. We will wear this stone away without violence. There has been enough violence.

We will talk to the granite.

We will not give up.

We will be like drops of water falling on a stone.

GLOSSARY

Agreements   Guidelines or rules for respectful engagement that provide an interpersonal safety net for participating in conversations. Agreements remain constant as leadership rotates—they are the circle's self-governance.

Archetype   A collectively inherited idea, pattern, thought, or image universally present; a prototype or model.

Center   The middle of the circle, where a visual representation of the group's intention resides. The center serves as a stabilizing reference point in circle process and is the hub of the wheel of group energetics.

Check-in   An opportunity for everyone to introduce himself or herself and respond to an opening question. Usually the first conversation that occurs in a circle meeting.

Check-out   Just as a circle meeting is carefully begun, so it is carefully concluded by inviting a brief statement from each individual about what the person learned, heard, appreciated, or is committed to doing. Usually the closing conversation in a circle meeting.

Circle   A group process that calls on an infrastructure of collaborative leadership functions where people establish a social safety and take time to make authentic, thoughtful contributions toward fulfilling their intention for gathering. As a universal archetype, the circle symbolizes wholeness, inclusion, openness, and boundary.

Collaborative conversation   Any of the conversations that happen in circle, World Café, Open Space, or other formats that encourage the wisdom of each voice to be heard and respected.

Collective shadow (collective unconscious)   Unconscious behavior, projection, and transference that occur on the societal or macro level. The consequence of seeing the world divided into "us" and "them." See also Individual shadow.

Consensus   The willingness of a group to move forward on a decision or action. This process occurs when all participants have come to agreement before a decision goes forward or action is taken. It does not require the same degree of enthusiasm from all participants, but it does require that each person approve the group's action.

Conversation council   A form of dialogue practiced in circle process when participants desire a more informal structure or a quickened pace of contribution and response. Conversation flows freely through open dialogue that is guided by the host and guardian and a group that continues to observe the infrastructure of circle process they have set in place. See also Talking piece council and Silence as council.

Energetics   The study of nonverbal interactions that occur between people, individually and collectively, and the attention given to various circle practices that stabilize people's nonverbal experience during circle meetings.

Guardian   A circle member responsible for keeping the circle centered and focused on its intent. The guardian holds a bell and rings it to signal a pause. After ten to fifteen seconds of silence, the bell is run again, and the guardian states the reason for the pause. Anyone may ask the guardian to ring the bell at any time. The guardian role usually rotates among group members from one session to the next.

Hierarchy   A system of organization that follows well-defined patterns of priority that allows the carrying out of clearly delineated tasks with little or no debate.

Host   The person who prepares the space where a circle conversation will be held, often helps define the scope of that conversation, and then participates in it from a position of peer leadership.

Individual shadow   A concept originated by the Swiss psychiatrists Carl Gustav Jung and Marie-Louise van Franz referring to aspects of ourselves we have been unable to know. Shadow theory states that people have both an accepted self and a hidden or forbidden self of which they are unaware. Shadow work is a way to talk about the confusing issues that arise whenever people get together. See also Collective shadow, Interior shadow, Projected shadow, and Transference shadow.

Intention   The understanding of why people are present, what they expect to happen, and what they commit to doing and experiencing together.

Interior shadow   Personal behaviors we don't perceive in the same way that others tend to perceive them, such as speaking in a loud voice that we consider jovial but others interpret as aggressive.

Interpersonal space   The space in which verbal and nonverbal interactions between two or more people occur.

Invitation   A verbal or written statement explaining why a group is coming together, who will be or needs to be present, and what contributions are expected of the recipient.

Neutral language   The ability to talk about what's happening without instigating shame or blame. Neutral language is often self-referencing ("This is what I am experiencing at this moment . . .") or invitational ("I suggest that we . . .") rather than commanding, accusatory, or directive.

Personal hoop   A First Nations term to describe a personal energy field, the assumed psychosocial space surrounding each person. The term implies a sense of boundary that is maintained by the individual and respected by others.

Personal preparation   Whatever individuals do to shift from the fast pace of modern culture to the slower pace of circle. It may consist of simple centering activities, such as quiet breathing, listening to music, or a walk in nature.

Practices   The three skills of circle participation: attentive listening, intentional speaking, and attending to the well-being of the group.

Principles   Three fundamental tenets of circle process: rotating leadership, shared responsibility, and reliance on the wholeness of the group.

Projected shadow   Qualities we ascribe to other people that we don't know how to deal with inside ourselves. These can be positive or negative—for example, assuming that someone is more or less capable and then behaving as if that assumption were true without evaluating the person objectively.

Rim   The outside edge of the circle, where each person sits as a circle participant.

Scribe   The circle member who volunteers to record group process by gathering insights and essence statements and noting decisions. Recording can be done using a journal, a laptop computer, a flip chart, or any other convenient means.

Silence council   Employing silence in the usually verbal processes of circle. Silence may be offered in a few seconds after the ringing of the bell by the guardian or for a few minutes at the opening or closing of a circle. Silent council may also be offered during times of conflict as a way for the group to stay calmly together while seeking a way forward.

Singing bowl   A metal or crystal bowl that resonates when struck with a wooden stick or other implement chosen to produce pleasing chimelike sound by the guardian.

Social container   The interactive space in a circle conversation in which all exchanges, be they challenging or easy, are received and considered with respect by everyone participating in the dialogue.

Spiritual practice   Any ritualized gesture that helps us tune in or stay attuned to an intuitive sense of guidance in the course of a day. It can coincide with religious observances or be performed on its own.

Start-point   A small event at the beginning of circle process that signals a shift from social space to circle space—often a reading, a song, or a moment of silence.

Story   Narrative; a way of talking or writing about human experience that combines chronology, character, scene, and insight.

Synergy   The phenomenon whereby combined interaction among people produces a total effect greater than the sum of the individual parts; an experience of harmony established between intention and action.

Talking piece   Any object designated to grant the person holding it the right to speak without interruption. Objects are selected that reflect the setting and personality of the group and the purpose of the circle process.

Talking piece council   A formal pattern for conducting a meeting that involves passing permission to speak from person to person through the use of a talking piece. The purpose is to hear each voice, garner insights, and seek collective wisdom. Talking piece council slows down dialogue and interaction. See also Conversation council and Silence council.

Thumbs vote   A system of signals for checking for consensus: thumb up = "I'm in favor"; thumb sideways = "I still have a question"; thumb down = "I don't think this is the right way to go." Clarifying conversations occur when a sideways or downward thumb is shown.

Tingsha   A set of brass cymbals, originally from Tibetan Buddhist practice, often used by the guardian, valued for their pleasant tone and reverberating quality.

Transference shadow   Projecting onto a person in the present unfinished business from a person in the past. For example, reacting to a current colleague on the basis of unresolved issues in your relationship with a parent when you were younger.

Transpersonal space   Interactions that belong to the collective and not just individuals. In circle, this space is usually referenced as being located in the center. Transpersonal space creates a sense of "third presence" and implies that a zone of neutrality is available to each individual in the conversation.

Triangle   The typical arrangement of hierarchical leadership, with decision makers at the top and followers at the bottom. As a universal archetype, the triangle symbolizes triad relationships (mother/father/child, body/mind/spirit), chain of command, or hierarchies of consciousness, status, or complexity.

NOTES

Foreword

1. Humberto Maturana (with G. Verden-Zöller), "Biology of Love," in *Focus Heilpädagogik*, ed. G. Opp and F. Peterander. Munich and Basel: Reinhardt, 1996.

Chapter 1

1. This is a favorite invocation that we use in many settings. This version appears in Christina Baldwin's *Storycatcher*, pp. 55–56.
2. Pinker, *Language Instinct*, p. 353.

Chapter 2

1. This document is available on our Web site, http://www.peerspirit.com, in a growing number of languages.

Chapter 4

1. This story is told in its entirety as a PeerSpirit Circle Tale, archived in July 2007 on our site, http://www.peerspirit.com. See also the Web site of Matthias zur Bonsen, http://www.all-in-one-spirit.de/.

Chapter 7

1. Bohm, *On Dialogue*, pp. 16–17.

Chapter 9

1. Zweig and Abrams, *Meeting the Shadow*, p. 3.
2. Ibid.

Chapter 10

1. Baldwin, *Storycatcher*, pp. 3–4.
2. A rondeval is a traditional hut with walls made from rocks collected in the fields. It is held together with dung and covered with a thatch roof.
3. Miombo woodlands form a broad belt across south-central Africa from Angola in the west to Tanzania in the east. The woodland contains grasses and shrubs and various tree species that shed their leaves for short periods during the dry season to preserve moisture.
4. "Ndira, a lifelong campaigner for political change, had been arrested more than 30 times but has kept up his opposition to the government that has led Zimbabweans to the lowest life expectancy in the world. His remains—a crushed skull, a bullet wound through the chest and blood-stained shorts—are a depressing metaphor for Zimbabwe in the aftermath of a stolen election." Daniel Howden and Raymond Whitaker, reporting in *The Independent*, June 2, 2008.

5. The Research and Advocacy Unit is a nongovernmental organization working on providing specialist assistance in research and advocacy in the field of human rights, democracy, and governance in Zimbabwe.

6. Mahatma Gandhi, *The Essential Writings of Mahatma Gandhi,* ed. Raghavan Iyer. New Delhi: Manzar Khan/Oxford University Press, 1996, p. 242.

Chapter 11

1. See Brown and Isaacs, *World Café,* pp. 96–98.

BIBLIOGRAPHY AND RESOURCES

Books by the Authors

Baldwin, Christina. *Calling the Circle: The First and Future Culture.* New York: Bantam Doubleday Dell, 1998.

———. *Lifelines: How Personal Writing Can Save Your Life.* Louisville, Colo.: Sounds True, 2005.

———. *Life's Companion: Journal Writing as a Spiritual Quest,* 2nd ed. New York: Bantam Doubleday Dell, 2007.

———. *The Seven Whispers: Spiritual Practice for Times Like These.* Novato, Calif.: New World Library, 2002.

———. *Storycatcher: Making Sense of Our Lives Through the Power and Practice of Story.* Novato, Calif.: New World Library, 2005.

Linnea, Ann. *Deep Water Passage: A Spiritual Journey at Midlife.* New York: Pocket Books, 1993.

———. *Keepers of the Trees: The Re-Greening of North America.* New York: Skyhorse, 2010.

Linnea, Ann, Marina Lachecki, Joseph Passineau, and Paul Treuer. *Teaching Kids to Love the Earth.* Minneapolis: University of Minnesota Press, 1991.

Publications Available Through PeerSpirit, Inc.

Baldwin, Christina, and Ann Linnea. *A Guide to PeerSpirit Circling.*

———. *PeerSpirit Council Management in Businesses, Corporations, and Organizations.*

Conklin, Cheryl, and Ann Linnea. *Understanding Energetics in Circles and Groups.*

Gilliam, Craig, and Christina Baldwin. *PeerSpirit Circling in Congregational Life.*

Jordan, Meredith, and Christina Baldwin. *Understanding Shadow and Projection in Circles and Groups.*

Thompson, Pamela A., and Christina Baldwin. *PeerSpirit Circling for Nursing Leadership: A Model for Conversation and Shared Leadership in the Workplace.*

Trenshaw, Cynthia. *A Harvest of Years: A PeerSpirit Guide for Proactive Aging Circles.*

Other Works Consulted

Arrien, Angeles. *The Fourfold Way: Walking the Paths of the Warrior, Teacher, Healer, and Visionary.* San Francisco: HarperSanFrancisco, 1993.

Bohm, David. *On Dialogue,* ed. Lee Nichol. London: Routledge, 1996.

Bolen, Jean S. *The Millionth Circle: How to Change Ourselves and the World—The Essential Guide to Women's Circles.* York Beach, Maine: Conari Press, 1999.

Brown, Juanita, with David Isaacs and the World Café Community. *The World Café: Shaping our Futures Through Conversations that Matter.* San Francisco: Berrett-Koehler, 2005.

Cahill, Sedonia, and Joshua Halpern. *The Ceremonial Circle: Practice Ritual and Renewal for Personal and Community Healing.* New York: HarperCollins, 1992.

Cooperrider, David, and Diana Whitney. *Appreciative Inquiry: A Positive Revolution in Change*: San Francisco: Berrett-Koehler, 2005.

———. *Appreciative Inquiry Handbook.* San Francisco: Berrett-Koehler, 2003.

Dressler, Larry. *Standing in the Fire: Leading High-Heat Meetings with Calm, Clarity, and Courage.* San Francisco: Berrett-Koehler, 2010.

Guilfoyle, Jeanne. *The Wheaton Franciscan Heritage.* Chicago: Arcadia, 2009.

Harrison, Roger. *Consultant's Journey: A Dance of Work and Spirit.* San Francisco: Jossey-Bass, 1995.

Holman, Peggy, Tom Devane, and Steven Cady. *The Change Handbook: The Definitive Resource on Today's Best Methods for Engaging Whole Systems.* San Francisco: Berrett-Koehler, 2007.

Jung, Carl G. *The Symbolic Life.* Princeton, N.J.: Princeton University Press, 1976.

Koloroutis, Mary, ed. *Relationship-Based Care: A Model for Transforming Practice.* Minneapolis, Minn.: Creative Health Care Management, 2004.

Korten, David C. *The Great Turning: From Empire to Earth Community.* San Francisco: Berrett-Koehler, 2006.

MacDougall, Sarah N. *Calling on Spirit: An Interpretive Ethnography of PeerSpirit Circles as Transformative Process.* Santa Barbara, Calif.: Fielding Graduate University, 2005.

Maslow, Albert H. "A Theory of Human Motivation." *Psychological Review* 50 (1943): 370–96.

Owen, Harrison. *Open Space Technology: A User's Guide,* 3rd ed. San Francisco: Berrett-Koehler, 2008.

———. *Wave Rider: Leadership for High Performance in a Self-Organizing World.* San Francisco: Berrett-Koehler, 2009.

Palmer, Parker J. *The Courage to Teach: Exploring the Inner Landscape of a Teacher's Life.* San Francisco: Jossey-Bass, 1998.

———. *A Hidden Wholeness: The Journey Toward an Undivided Life.* San Francisco: Jossey-Bass, 2004.

Peddigrew, Brenda. *Original Fire: The Hidden Heart of Religious Women.* Charleston, S.C.: BookSurge, 2008.

Pinker, Stephen. *The Language Instinct: How the Mind Creates Language.* New York: Morrow, 1994.

Pranis, Kay, Barry Stuart, and Mark Wedge. *Peacemaking Circles: From Crime to Community.* St. Paul, Minn.: Living Justice Press, 2003.

Rosenberg, Marshall B. *Nonviolent Communication: A Language of Compassion.* Encinitas, Calif.: PuddleDancer, 1999.

Seed, John, Joanna Macy, and Pat Fleming. *Thinking like a Mountain: Toward a Council of All Beings.* Philadelphia: New Society, 1998.

Spring, Cindy, Charles Garfield, and Sedonia Cahill. *Wisdom Circles: A Guide to Self-Discovery and Community Building in Small Groups.* New York: Hyperion, 1998.

Van der Post, Laurens. *Jung and the Story of Our Time.* New York: Vintage Books, 1976.

Wheatley, Margaret J. *Finding Our Way: Leadership for an Uncertain Time.* San Francisco: Berrett-Koehler, 2005.

————. *Leadership and the New Science: Discovering Order in a Chaotic World, 3rd ed.* San Francisco: Berrett-Koehler, 2006.

————. *Turning to One Another: Simple Conversations to Restore Hope to the Future.* San Francisco: Berrett-Koehler, 2002.

WindEagle and RainbowHawk. *Heart Seeds: Messages from the Ancestors.* Minneapolis, Minn.: Beaver's Pond Press, 2003.

Zimmerman, Jack, and Virginia Coyle. *The Way of Council,* 2nd ed. Putney, Vt.: Bramble Books, 2009.

Zweig, Connie, and Jeremiah Abrams. *Meeting the Shadow: The Hidden Power of the Dark Side of Human Nature.* Los Angeles: Tarcher, 1991.

Useful Web Sites

The Appreciative Inquiry Commons: http://www.appreciativeinquiry.case.edu

The Art of Hosting Conversations That Matter: http://www.artofhosting.org/

Berkana Institute: http://www.berkana.org/

Center for Courage and Renewal: http://www.couragerenewal.org/

Great Turning (Joanna Macy): http://www.joannamacy.net/index.html

Kufunda Village: http://www.kufunda.org/

Open Space Technology: http://www.openspaceworld.org/

PeerSpirit, Inc.: http://www.peerspirit.com

Positive Futures Network (Yes! Magazine): http://www.yesmagazine.org/

E. F. Schumacher Society: http://www.smallisbeautiful.org/

Storycatcher Network: http://www.storycatcher.net

World Café: http://www.theworldcafe.com

ACKNOWLEDGMENTS

When we were preparing to submit the proposal for this book, we sat down with our dear colleague and office manager, Debbie Dix, asked her to read it and tell us what she thought. We three, who are the entire staff of PeerSpirit, Inc., know that writing, launching, and supporting a book takes an ongoing effort and commitment from all of us. We are profoundly grateful for this team, for the circle in the office as well as in the work, and for Debbie's skilled and steadfast contributions to PeerSpirit and to us.

Thank you to Meg Wheatley for collegiality that has deepened into friendship and for carrying our pages to Berrett-Koehler and advocating for this project. We are delighted to be working with this company, to have met Steve Piersanti and Jeevan Sivasubramaniam and our editor, Johanna Vondeling.

This writing occurred during a period of strenuous work that informed and enriched the stories and content of the book and strained our abilities to contribute to our local community and to relax with family and friends. We thank you for understanding and valuing what we do, especially when it so often conflicts with what we might be doing together! We are especially grateful to have four vibrant living parents, Leo Baldwin, Connie McGregor, and Frank and Astrid Brown, who continue to be proud of us, as we are of them. We stand gladly in the generations, including Ann's grown children, Brian Schimpf and Sally Schimpf, and grandson, Jaden Villarreal.

As for our friends, you know who you are—and we bow in gratitude for all exchanges of the heart, large and small.

We offer thanks to the Calling the Circle Foundation and are particularly grateful to Martin Siesta and the legacy of his mentoring aunts, Theda, Rita, and Marie, for their support during our writing time.

To all who appear in this book—by name and by pseudonym—please know that your stories are offered as teaching tales toward the common good.

The following colleagues are named in the book through contributing stories and personal references: Angeles Arrien, Kerry Barnett, Matthias zur Bonsen, Juanita Brown, Terry Chase, Chris Corrigan, Gigi Coyle, Guy Cumbie, Thomas Dahlborg, Stephen Diwauripo, Nanci Dvorsky, Susan Edstrom,

Roq Gareau, Angelina Gibson, Bethany Hays, Ruben Castilla Herrera, Jutta Herzog, David Isaacs, Elizabeth Jetton, David Korten, Fran Korten, David Kyle, Kathryn Landon-Malone, Sarah MacDougall, Joanna Macy, Chris Bicknell-Marden, Bonnie Marsh, Janet McCallen, David McNulty, Rowena McNulty, Cathy Michaels, Judy Mladineo, Sikhethiwe Mlotsha, Toke Paludan Møller, Jerry Nagel, Jim Neale, Monica Nissen, Marsha Paludan, Traci Pannullo, Colleen Person, Kay Pranis, RainbowHawk, Bev Reeler, Steve Ryman, Mary K. Sandford, Martin Siesta, Pamela Austin Thompson, Cynthia Trenshaw, Marvin Tuttle, Margaret J. Wheatley; the Wheaton Franciscans—especially the leadership team with whom we worked: Sisters Alice Drewek, Pat Norton, Gabriele Uhlein, and Marge Zulaski; WindEagle, and Jack Zimmerman.

In addition we also wish to acknowledge circles of colleagues who have contributed to our understanding and development of this work over the years: Ruth Anderson and the School for Servant Leadership and the circle colleagues in Greensboro, North Carolina; Barbara Belknap; Phil Cass and the Art of Hosting community in Columbus, Ohio; Jackie Claunch, Cheryl Conklin, Marie Dumais, Beth Elmore, Sharon Faulds, Susan Fekety, Caitlin Frost, Kim Gilbreath, W. Craig Gilliam, Jeanne Guy, Roger Harrison, Bev Haskins, Kim Howlett, Firehawk Hulin, Meredith Jordan, Jim Kellar, Kristen Lombard; Mary Martin, Sandy MacIver, Cathy McKenzie, and Royal Roads University; Linda Moore, Mary O'Connor, Harriet Peterson, Pele Rouge, Sibyl Dana Reynolds, Sharon Schindler Rising, Pamela Sampel, Linda Secord, Mark Secord, Virginia Harvey Shapiro, Sandy Smith, Jane Swanson, Clare Taylor, Kit Wilson and the Grandmothers Council.

More recently, our international networks have come to include people who came into our lives through From the Four Directions and the Art of Hosting: Kathy Jourdain, Marianne Knuth and the members of Kufunda village (Harare, Zimbabwe), Tim Merry, Cristina Molinar, Zoe Nicholson, Teresa Posakony, Kerry Sandison, Maria Scordialos, Bob Stilger, Sarah Whiteley, Tenneson Woolf; and friends from the Wilderness Guides lineage, Sheila Belanger, Anne Hayden, Meredith Little, Lynnaea Lumbard, Rick Paine, and Anne Stine.

There are hundreds of alumni of our circle trainings and thousands from consulting and seminars—we see your faces and hear you ring the bell that calls the circle in. May it serve.

C. B. & A. L.

ABOUT THE AUTHORS

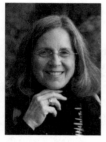

CHRISTINA BALDWIN is an author, teacher, consultant and co-originator of PeerSpirit Circle Process with more than thirty years' experience as a seminar presenter. She has written eight books and contributed three classics to the international renaissance in personal writing and story. *Life's Companion: Journal Writing as a Spiritual Practice,* was revised and reissued in 2007 after 100,000 original sales and *Storycatcher: Making Sense of Our Lives Through the Power and Practice of Story,* is a seminal work on the necessity of story to communicate in all areas of professional and personal life. As a primary thought leader in understanding personal story, she began, with Ann Linnea, to study personal growth and group dynamics, and wrote *Calling the Circle: The First and Future Culture* to explain how collaborative conversation could release needed wisdom and lead to well-informed action and activism. Since 2000, she has also written *The Seven Whispers: Spiritual Practice for Times like These* and recorded an entire curriculum, *"Lifelines, How Personal Writing Can Save Your Life."* She earned a Bachelor of Arts degree in English with honors at Macalester College, and a Master of Science degree in educational psychology at Columbia Pacific University. She currently lives on Whidbey Island, near Seattle, from which she travels extensively to lecture, teach, and call people and organizations into conversations of heart, meaning, and activism.

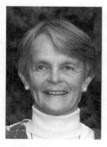

ANN LINNEA is a writer, educator, facilitator, mentor and guide with decades of experience serving the art of dialogue in a fascinating range of settings. Whether guiding people on a wilderness quest or presenting a workshop to business leaders, she embodies the stewardship of wild things that has characterized her life and work. She began her writing career in Utah, composing hiking and skiing guides during her years as a U.S. Forest Service naturalist in the 1970s. In 1991, Ann co-wrote the award-winning *Teaching Kids to Love the Earth.* In 1992, she designed her own mid-life rite of passage and became the first woman to circumnavigate Lake Superior by sea kayak (an 1,800-mile journey). *Deep Water Passage: A Spiritual Journey at Midlife*, describes this journey, portraying her extraordinary physical courage and even more extraordinary spiritual trial and transformation. Besides *The Circle Way*, her most recent work is *Keepers of the Trees: A Guide to Re-Greening North America*. Ann graduated from Iowa State University with honors and distinction in botany and holds a master of education degree from the University of Idaho. When replenishing herself at home on Whidbey Island, she enjoys gardening, hiking, kayaking, and motor-scootering. She has two grown children and one adorable grandson.

Ann and Christina founded their educational company, PeerSpirit, Inc., in 1994. Since then, they have offered training in PeerSpirit Circle Process throughout the United States and Canada, Europe, and southern Africa and they are soon to bring their work to Australia and New Zealand. The full-range of their contribution is documented on their website, http://www.peerspirit.com, where many downloadable resources are available in several languages.

INDEX

About Berrett-Koehler Publishers

Berrett-Koehler is an independent publisher dedicated to an ambitious mission: Creating a World That Works for All.

We believe that to truly create a better world, action is needed at all levels—individual, organizational, and societal. At the individual level, our publications help people align their lives with their values and with their aspirations for a better world. At the organizational level, our publications promote progressive leadership and management practices, socially responsible approaches to business, and humane and effective organizations. At the societal level, our publications advance social and economic justice, shared prosperity, sustainability, and new solutions to national and global issues.

A major theme of our publications is "Opening Up New Space." They challenge conventional thinking, introduce new ideas, and foster positive change. Their common quest is changing the underlying beliefs, mindsets, institutions, and structures that keep generating the same cycles of problems, no matter who our leaders are or what improvement programs we adopt.

We strive to practice what we preach—to operate our publishing company in line with the ideas in our books. At the core of our approach is *stewardship*, which we define as a deep sense of responsibility to administer the company for the benefit of all of our "stakeholder" groups: authors, customers, employees, investors, service providers, and the communities and environment around us.

We are grateful to the thousands of readers, authors, and other friends of the company who consider themselves to be part of the "BK Community." We hope that you, too, will join us in our mission.

Be Connected

Visit Our Website

Go to www.bkconnection.com to read exclusive previews and excerpts of new books, find detailed information on all Berrett-Koehler titles and authors, browse subject-area libraries of books, and get special discounts.

Subscribe to Our Free E-Newsletter

Be the first to hear about new publications, special discount offers, exclusive articles, news about bestsellers, and more! Get on the list for our free e-newsletter by going to www.bkconnection.com.

Get Quantity Discounts

Berrett-Koehler books are available at quantity discounts for orders of ten or more copies. Please call us toll-free at (800) 929-2929 or email us at bkp.orders@aidcvt.com.

Host a Reading Group

For tips on how to form and carry on a book reading group in your workplace or community, see our website at www.bkconnection.com.

Join the BK Community

Thousands of readers of our books have become part of the "BK Community" by participating in events featuring our authors, reviewing draft manuscripts of forthcoming books, spreading the word about their favorite books, and supporting our publishing program in other ways. If you would like to join the BK Community, please contact us at bkcommunity@bkpub.com.